T0289398

Sleep Deficiency and Health

Editor

MELISSA P. KNAUERT

CLINICS IN CHEST MEDICINE

www.chestmed.theclinics.com

June 2022 • Volume 43 • Number 2

ELSEVIER

1600 John F. Kennedy Boulevard • Suite 1800 • Philadelphia, Pennsylvania, 19103-2899

http://www.theclinics.com

CLINICS IN CHEST MEDICINE Volume 43, Number 2
June 2022 ISSN 0272-5231, ISBN-13: 978-0-323-89724-2

Editor: Joanna Collett
Developmental Editor: Karen Justine Solomon

Clinics in Chest Medicine (ISSN 0272-5231) is published quarterly by Elsevier Inc., 360 Park Avenue South, New York, NY 10010-1710. Months of issue are March, June, September, and December. Periodicals postage paid at New York, NY and additional mailing offices. Subscription prices are $408.00 per year (domestic individuals), $1049.00 per year (domestic institutions), $100.00 per year (domestic students/residents), $436.00 per year (Canadian individuals), $1091.00 per year (Canadian institutions), $499.00 per year (international individuals), $1091.00 per year (international institutions), $100.00 per year (Canadian Students), and $230.00 per year (International Students). International air speed delivery is included in all Clinics subscription prices. All prices are subject to change without notice. **POSTMASTER:** Send address changes to Clinics in Chest Medicine, Elsevier Health Sciences Division, Subscription Customer Service, 3251 Riverport Lane, Maryland Heights, MO 63043. **Customer Service: Telephone: 1-800-654-2452** (U.S. and Canada); **1-314-447-8871** (outside U.S. and Canada). **Fax: 1-314-447-8029. E-mail: journalscustomerservice-usa@elsevier.com (for print support); journalsonlinesupport-usa@elsevier.com (for online support).**

Reprints. For copies of 100 or more of articles in this publication, please contact the Commercial Reprints Department, Elsevier Inc., 360 Park Avenue South, New York, NY 10010-1710. Tel.: 212-633-3874; Fax: 212-633-3820; E-mail: reprints@elsevier.com.

Clinics in Chest Medicine is covered in *MEDLINE/PubMed (Index Medicus), Current Contents/Clinical Medicine, EMBASE/Excerpta Medica, Science Citation Index,* and *ISI/BIOMED.*

Contributors

EDITOR

MELISSA P. KNAUERT, MD, PhD
Assistant Professor of Medicine, Department of Internal Medicine, Section of Pulmonary, Critical Care, and Sleep Medicine, Yale School of Medicine, New Haven, Connecticut, USA

AUTHORS

OLUROTIMI ADEKOLU, MD
Attending Physician, Pulmonary, Critical Care and Sleep, Starling Physicians, Bloomfield, Connecticut, USA

OLUFUNKE AFOLABI-BROWN, MBBS
Division of Pulmonary and Sleep Medicine, Children's Hospital of Philadelphia, Philadelphia, Pennsylvania, USA

CARMELA ALCÁNTARA, PhD
School of Social Work, Columbia University, New York, New York, USA

MOLLY E. ATWOOD, PhD
Department of Psychiatry and Behavioral Sciences, Johns Hopkins School of Medicine, Baltimore, Maryland, USA

NAJIB AYAS, MD, MPH
Department of Medicine, University of British Columbia, Leon Judah Blackmore Centre for Sleep Disorders, University of British Columbia Hospital, Vancouver, British Columbia, Canada

BRETT BAUMANN, MD
Department of Medicine, University of British Columbia, Vancouver, British Columbia, Canada

SAMANTHA CONLEY, PhD
Nurse Scientist, Nursing Research Division, Department of Nursing, Mayo Clinic, Rochester, Minnesota, USA

ARLIN DELGADO, MD
Department of Obstetrics and Gynecology, Morsani College of Medicine, University of South Florida, Tampa, Florida, USA

AMIR GOHARI, BSc
Department of Medicine, University of British Columbia, Vancouver, British Columbia, Canada

JOSEPH T. HEBL, BA
Oregon Health & Sciences University, School of Medicine, Portland, Oregon, USA

CAMILLA M. HOYOS, MPH, PhD
Centre for Sleep and Chronobiology, Woolcock Institute of Medical Research, The University of Sydney, Faculty of Science, School of Psychology and Brain and Mind Centre, Sydney, Australia

YOURI HWANG, MSN, FNP-C
PhD Candidate, Yale School of Nursing, West Haven, Connecticut, USA

CHANDRA L. JACKSON, PhD, MS
Epidemiology Branch, Department of Health and Human Services, National Institute of Environmental Health Sciences and National Institute on Minority Health and Health Disparities, Research Triangle Park, North California, USA; Intramural Program, Department of Health and Human Services,

National Institute on Minority Health and Health Disparities, Bethesda, Maryland, USA

RACHEL JEN, MD
Department of Medicine, University of British Columbia, Vancouver, British Columbia, Canada

DAYNA A. JOHNSON, PhD, MPH, MSW, MS
Department of Epidemiology, Rollins School of Public Health, Emory University, Atlanta, Georgia, USA

ROO KILLICK, MBBS, FRACP, PhD
Centre for Sleep and Chronobiology, Woolcock Institute of Medical Research, The University of Sydney, Sydney, Australia

MELISSA P. KNAUERT, MD, PhD
Assistant Professor of Medicine, Department of Internal Medicine, Section of Pulmonary, Critical Care, and Sleep Medicine, Yale School of Medicine, New Haven, Connecticut, USA

JENNIFER LANGSTENGEL, MD
Fellow, Pulmonary Critical Care and Sleep Medicine, Yale University, New Haven, Connecticut, USA

SARAH LOGAN, PhD, RN
Research Assistant, Yale School of Nursing, West Haven, Connecticut, USA

JUDETTE M. LOUIS, MD, MPH
Department of Obstetrics and Gynecology, Morsani College of Medicine, University of South Florida, Tampa, Florida, USA

WISSAM MANSOUR, MD
Assistant Professor of Medicine, Duke University School of Medicine, Department of Internal Medicine, Division of Pulmonary, Allergy and Critical Care Medicine, Durham, North Carolina, USA

ANDREW W. McHILL, PhD
Sleep, Chronobiology, and Health Laboratory, School of Nursing, Oregon Institute of Occupational Health Sciences, Oregon Health & Science University, Portland, Oregon, USA

BRIENNE MINER, MD, MHS
Assistant Professor of Medicine, Section of Geriatrics, Yale School of Medicine, New Haven, Connecticut, USA

MELISA E. MOORE, PhD
Division of Pulmonary and Sleep Medicine, Department of Children and Adolescent Psychiatry and Behavioral Sciences, Children's Hospital of Philadelphia, Philadelphia, Pennsylvania, USA

CHIDINMA OHANELE, MPHc
Department of Epidemiology, Rollins School of Public Health, Emory University, Atlanta, Georgia, USA

MONICA ROOSA ORDWAY, PhD, APRN, PPCNP-BC
Associate Professor, Yale School of Nursing, West Haven, Connecticut, USA

ROBERT L. OWENS, MD
Associate Professor of Medicine, Division of Pulmonary, Critical Care and Sleep Medicine, University of California, San Diego, La Jolla, California, USA

JANE ALEXANDRA PAPPAS, MM
Medical Student, San Juan Bautista School of Medicine, Caguas, Puerto Rico

NANCY S. REDEKER, PhD, RN
Professor of Nursing and Medicine, UCONN School of Nursing, Beatrice Renfield Term Professor of Nursing Emeritus, Yale University, University of Connecticut School of Nursing, Storrs, Connecticut, USA

LACHLAN STRANKS, MBBS
Centre for Sleep and Chronobiology, Woolcock Institute of Medical Research, The University of Sydney, Sydney, Australia; The University of Adelaide, Faculty of Health and Medical Sciences, Adelaide, Australia

BERNIE Y. SUNWOO, MBBS
Associate Professor of Clinical Medicine, Division of Pulmonary, Critical Care and Sleep Medicine, University of California, San Diego, San Diego, California, USA

ELOISE HANNAH SUTTON, MS
Post-graduate Fellow, Yale School of Nursing, West Haven, Connecticut, USA

IGNACIO E. TAPIA, MD
Division of Pulmonary and Sleep Medicine, Children's Hospital of Philadelphia, Philadelphia, Pennsylvania, USA

JOSIE VELASCO, BS
Sleep, Chronobiology, and Health Laboratory, School of Nursing, Oregon Institute of Occupational Health Sciences, Oregon Health & Science University, Portland, Oregon, USA

H. KLAR YAGGI, MD, MPH
Professor of Internal Medicine (Pulmonary, Critical Care and Sleep Medicine), Vice Chief of Research, Pulmonary, Critical Care and Sleep Medicine, Associate Director, Yale Pulmonary/Critical Care Fellowship Program, Pulmonary, Critical Care and Sleep Medicine, Director, Yale Centers for Sleep Medicine, Pulmonary, Critical Care and Sleep Medicine, West Haven, Connecticut, USA

ANDREY ZINCHUK, MD, MHS
Assistant Professor, Section of Pulmonary, Critical Care and Sleep Medicine, Department of Internal Medicine, Yale School of Medicine, New Haven, Connecticut, USA

Contents

CLINICS IN CHEST MEDICINE

FORTHCOMING ISSUES

September 2022
Critical Care
Gregory A. Schmidt and Jacqueline Kruser, *Editors*

December 2022
Advances in Cystic Fibrosis
Clemente J Britto and Jennifer L. Taylor-Cousar, *Editors*

March 2023
LungTransplantation
Luis Angel and Stephanie M. Levine, *Editors*

RECENT ISSUES

March 2022
Bronchiectasis
James D. Chalmers, *Editor*

December 2021
Pleural Disease
David Feller-Kopman and Fabien Maldonado, *Editors*

September 2021
Gender and Respiratory Disease
Margaret A. Pisani, *Editor*

Preface
Sleep Deficiency and Health

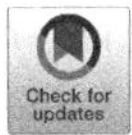

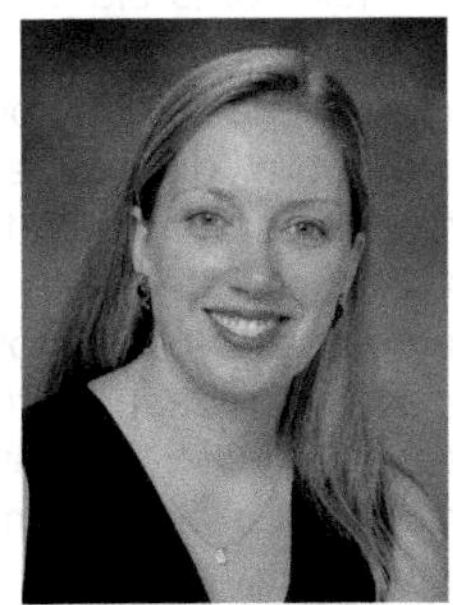

Melissa P. Knauert, MD, PhD
Editor

Sleep deficiency, including short sleep duration, poor sleep quality, mistimed sleep, and diminished daytime function, is a significant public health threat. Though there is increasing recognition of the importance of sleep to human health, a significant proportion of studied populations around the world has sleep duration or quality that is less than recommended; other domains of sleep deficiency are less well studied but also appear to have a high prevalence. In this issue of *Clinics in Chest Medicine*, experts from an array of biomedical disciplines discuss the many facets of sleep deficiency in diverse populations and across the human lifespan.

Our collection starts with the work of Gohari and colleagues, who provide an epidemiologic overview of sleep deficiency. Occupation, social demands, psychiatric disorders, medical disorders, and sleep disorders are key contributing factors to sleep deficiency. Furthermore, the authors highlight the tremendous morbidity related to sleep deficiency that negatively impacts cognition, alertness, mood, behavior, cardiometabolic health, renal function, immune system function, and respiratory physiology. We follow this introduction with Johnson and colleagues' discussion of disparities affecting minoritized racial/ethnic groups with a focus on the increased burden of obstructive sleep apnea (OSA) seen in these groups. Minoritized groups have a higher prevalence of OSA, more severe OSA, and lower treatment adherence. However, there is evidence that culturally tailored evidence-based interventions for OSA improve awareness, diagnosis, and treatment of OSA among minoritized racial/ethnic groups. It is critically important that we continue to expand evidence in this domain. Next, Redeker and colleagues provide a symptoms perspective on sleep deficiency. Using exemplars from chronic heart failure, inflammatory bowel disease, and breast cancer, the authors explore the interplay of key symptoms of excessive daytime symptoms and fatigue with chronic illness. Multiple aspects of sleep deficiency contribute to excessive daytime sleepiness and fatigue. These sleep-related symptoms are associated with poor quality of life and function and difficulty with cognition and self-management.

Our collection then turns to sleep deficiency in specific age groups. This important issue can affect young children, teens, working adults, and the elderly in varied ways. Ordway and colleagues discuss how stress and sleep interact in our youngest sleepers. Sleep in early childhood is influenced by social and ecological variables that are unique to this age group. Behavioral sleep interventions hold great promise in improving children's sleep and overall health. Afolabi-Brown and colleagues then dive into adolescent sleep problems. Reasons for sleep deficiency in adolescence include physiologic changes with delays in circadian phase, medical sleep disorders, and social, cultural, and environmental factors. Early school start times negatively impact sleep in adolescents and are associated with poorer outcomes in overall health, well-being, and performance; delay in school start times reverses many of these ill effects.

From there, we learn about sleep in adulthood, including sleep deficiency related to work schedules, pregnancy, and aging. First, Hebl and colleagues discuss the impact of prolonged work

Clin Chest Med 43 (2022) xiii–xiv
https://doi.org/10.1016/j.ccm.2022.02.014

and social schedules, exemplified by shift work, late-night weekends, and early morning work/ school start times (ie, social jetlag) on sleep. The authors discuss how common practices like shift work and social jetlag contribute to sleep disruption, circadian misalignment, and adverse health outcomes. Next, Delgado and colleagues describe the overlap of pregnancy and sleep deficiency. Sleep deficiency in pregnancy is associated with an increased risk of adverse maternal outcomes, including gestational diabetes, hypertensive disorders, and depression. The authors highlight the importance of evaluating socioeconomic factors and social determinants of health to best address sleep health disparities in this at-risk population. Finally, Pappas and Miner discuss the changes in sleep and circadian rhythms in older adults. Causes of sleep deficiency in older age are multifactorial, including medical and psychiatric diseases, medication and substance use, social isolation, loneliness, loss of physical function, caregiving, and bereavement. In addition, sleep deficiency has been associated in older adults with increased mortality, cognitive impairment, depression, and impaired physical function.

In the latter part of the collection, we look at acute and chronically ill populations. Mansour and Knauert discuss the risk factors and unique vulnerability of acutely ill hospitalized patients. Contributing factors include preexisting medical conditions, illness severity, the hospital environment, and treatment-related effects. Hospitalized patients are particularly vulnerable to the adverse health effects of sleep deficiency that can impact multiple organ systems. Key next steps in hospital sleep promotion include improving sleep measurement techniques and harmonizing study protocols and outcomes to strengthen existing evidence for inpatient sleep promotion interventions.

As our focus then shifts to chronic illness and sleep deficiency, Langstengel and Yaggi discuss the epidemic of opioid use disorder and its intersection with sleep deficiency. Strikingly, sleep deficiency is present in 75% of patients with opioid use disorder. This review highlights the bidirectional mechanisms between opioid use disorder and sleep deficiency and the potential to target sleep deficiency with therapeutic interventions to promote long-term recovery among patients. Next, Atwood discusses the interplay of psychiatric disorders and sleep deficiency. There is a significant relationship between sleep deficiency and unipolar and bipolar depression, anxiety disorders, and posttraumatic stress disorder. Furthermore, there is evidence for sleep as a causal factor in the development of psychiatric disorders and a factor related to the outcome and recurrence of psychopathology. Future work will continue to explore sleep deficiency as an important treatment target for comorbid sleep and psychiatric disorders.

Next, Killick and colleagues discuss the important interplay of cardiometabolic disease and sleep. Epidemiologic studies have demonstrated that short sleep duration is associated with an increased risk of cardiometabolic health outcomes, including cardiovascular disease mortality, coronary heart disease, type 2 diabetes mellitus, hypertension, and metabolic syndrome. This review describes the primary evidence for these associations, proposed mechanisms, and potential sleep deficiency countermeasures. Sunwoo and Owens then discuss chronic lung disease and sleep deficiency. Poor sleep is a common complaint among those with chronic lung disease, and multiple factors contribute to sleep deficiency in this group. Notably, primary sleep disorders, such as OSA and restless leg syndrome, can coexist and need specific treatment. Treatment of OSA in those with chronic lung disease is associated with improved morbidity and mortality. Finally, Adekolu and Zinchuk finish our collection with a discussion of OSA and sleep deficiency. Sleep deficiency in patients with OSA includes the presence of comorbid conditions, such as insomnia, circadian misalignment disorders, and periodic limb movements of sleep. The cooccurrence of these conditions with OSA likely plays a role in pathogenesis, clinical presentation, and management of OSA. Considering these conditions and their treatment in evaluating sleep deficiency in OSA may help improve patient outcomes.

This collection provides a window into this widespread health threat conveyed by sleep deficiency that affects patients across their lifespan. Our authors highlight gaps in research and the need to learn more about the causes, consequences, and treatments of sleep deficiency.

Melissa P. Knauert, MD, PhD
Department of Internal Medicine
Section of Pulmonary, Critical Care, and Sleep Medicine
Yale University School of Medicine
300 Cedar Street
P.O. Box 208057
New Haven, CT 06520-8057, USA

E-mail address:
melissa.knauert@yale.edu

Sleep Deficiency
Epidemiology and Effects

Amir Gohari, BSc[a], Brett Baumann, MD[a], Rachel Jen, MD[a,b], Najib Ayas, MD, MPH[a,b,*]

KEYWORDS

• Cardiovascular health • Diabetes • Arthritis • Sleep disorders • Sleep deficiency
• Gastroesophageal reflux disease • Shift work • Epidemiology

KEY POINTS

- Sleep deficiency, due to reduced duration, abnormal timing, or quality of sleep, is prevalent in modern society, with as many as a third of developed countries' populations being affected by sleep deficiency.
- Contributing factors to sleep deficiency include occupation, social demands, psychiatric disorders, physical disorders, sleep disorders, ethnicity, age, marital status, sex, and hospitalization.
- Sleep deficiency influences cognition, alertness, mood, diabetes, cardiovascular health, renal function, immune system, and respiratory physiology.

INTRODUCTION

Sleep is an important determinant of physical and mental health. Sleep deficiency, defined as insufficient quantity or quality of sleep for optimal function, is common in modern society.[1] Sleep deficiency can result from inadequate total sleep duration, shift in timing of sleep, or interruptions to regular sleep. Since the 1960s, studies have shown that those who regularly sleep less than the recommended duration or experience interruptions to nighttime sleep have greater risks of long-term adverse health outcomes. Sleep debt, often accumulated because of work demands, lifestyle, societal responsibilities, and medical/psychiatric disorders, can cause psychological dysfunction, decreased cognitive performance, and adverse cardiometabolic effects.[2] This review aims to summarize the epidemiology and effects of sleep deficiency.

PREVALENCE

It is clear that sleep deficiency is prevalent,[2] although the exact extent is unclear, given that most studies rely on surveys and self-reported measures to estimate the prevalence of sleep deficiency.[3] In the United States, only 65% of adults report sleeping the recommended 7 hours or more per 24 hours, leaving one-third of the population at risk of sleep deficiency.[4,5] It should be noted that sleep deficiency is more common in some populations based on ethnicity, occupation, and medical, psychiatric, and social factors, as discussed in the "Contributing Factors" section of this review.

The prevalence of sleep deficiency due to short sleep is increasing. In a review of 8 studies ranging from 1975 to 2006 in the United States, the odds of sleeping less than 6 hours per 24 hours increased by a factor of 1.19 (95% confidence interval [CI]: 1.00, 1.42; $P = 0.05$) over the study period among full-time employed American adults.[6] In another review of 9 studies from Finland ranging from 1972 to 2005, researchers observed a decrease of about 18 minutes in sleep duration over the 33-year period, but no significant increase in adults reporting less than 6 hours of sleep per 24 hours.[7] Using 3 representative cohorts of 38-

[a] Department of Medicine, University of British Columbia, 317 - 2194 Health Sciences Mall, Vancouver, BC V6T 1Z3, Canada; [b] Judah Blackmore Centre for Sleep Disorders, Univeristy of British Columbia Hospital, Ground Floor, Room G34A Purdy Pavilion, 2221 Wesbrook Mall, Vancouver, BC V6T 2B5, Canada
* Corresponding author: 7th Floor, Diamond Centre, 2775 Laurel Street, Vancouver, British Columbia V5Z 1M9, Canada
E-mail address: NAyas@providencehealth.bc.ca

Clin Chest Med 43 (2022) 189–198
https://doi.org/10.1016/j.ccm.2022.02.001

and 50-year-old women in 1968 to 1969, 1980 to 1981, and 2004 to 2005, a similar study in Sweden showed that sleep duration decreased by about 15 minutes during the 36 years of observation among 38-year-old women, but no change in sleep duration was observed among 50-year-old women.[8] The proportion of women complaining of sleeping problems almost doubled, from 17.7% in 1968 to 31.7% in 2004 for 38-year-old women, and from 21.6% to 41.8% for 50-year-old women.

Information on the prevalence of sleep deficiency due to poor sleep quality is limited. Sleep interruptions are a frequent cause of decreased sleep quality.[9] Some reasons for sleep interruptions include sleep disorders, nocturia, thirst, psychological burdens, and environmental factors. These factors are common, with approximately 20% of Americans suffering from sleep disorders[2] and 50% of older Americans experiencing ≥2 nocturia episodes per night.[10] In a study of 2144 participants aged 43 to 71 years in Spain, the prevalence of poor sleep quality, defined as a score of greater than 5 on the Pittsburgh Sleep Quality Index (PSQI), was estimated at 40% with 10% of participants reporting sleep interruptions.[11] In another study of 222 hypertensive patients in Italy, the prevalence of poor sleep quality (PSQI>5) was 40%, with 70% of patients reporting sleep interruptions.[12] In an analysis of 9 studies with 9103 participants in Ethiopia, the average prevalence of poor sleep quality was estimated at 50% using PSQI, with sleep interruptions not discussed.[13] These studies of multiple different populations showcase the prevalence of nonoptimal sleep quality as a contributor to sleep deficiency.

CONTRIBUTING FACTORS TO SLEEP DEFICIENCY

Occupational Factors

Sleep deficiency can be driven by occupational factors, including long work hours and shift work. In a study of full-time British civil servants, working more than 55 hours a week was related to shortened sleeping hours (odds ratio [OR] = 1.98; 95% CI: 1.05, 3.76), difficulty falling asleep (OR = 3.68; 95% CI: 1.58, 8.58), and waking without feeling refreshed (OR = 1.98; 95% CI: 1.04, 3.77), when compared with working 35 to 55 hours a week.[14] In another study of 429 participants, using the PSQI, those working more than 48 hours a week had lower quality of sleep than those working less than 48 hours.[15] These studies suggest that working longer hours influence both sleep duration and sleep quality.

Shift work is another major contributor to sleep deficiency and one area that we can most directly note the negative effects of poor sleep timing. In the United States, 15% to 30% of the adult population are shift workers, often needing to work during the normal sleep period.[16–18] Shift work can challenge regular sleep schedules and is associated with sleep deficiency and daytime sleepiness.[19,20] Shift workers often need to sleep during the day; however, daytime sleep is often shorter and of lower quality than nighttime sleep.[16,21] Several studies have associated working night shifts with sleep durations of 5 to 6 hours per day, with day sleep being 1 to 4 hours shorter than night sleep.[22] In addition, night shifts have been reported to reduce total sleep duration more than evening shifts. Sleep patterns during shift work are consistent with the sleep patterns observed during restricted sleep schedules. Many workers, including those in health care and 24/7 services, work long shifts, night shifts, or irregular shifts, posing challenges to regular undisrupted night sleep.[2] Work shifts that are long or irregular can displace or interrupt regular sleeping patterns, respectively, contributing to sleep deficiency.[16] With the economic considerations of modern society, sleep deficiency among workers can have negative socioeconomic effects.[16,19]

It is estimated that 70% of college students in the United States get less than the recommended 8 hours of sleep per night and 50% report daytime sleepiness.[23] While taking on academic and nonacademic responsibilities, students with busy schedules sleep less, contributing to sleep deficiency in this group. Contributors to sleep deficiency among college students include bedtime technology use, alcohol, caffeine, stimulants, and sleep disorders. Students rely on technology to complete many of their academic tasks; near bedtime, technology use can create arousals, decrease sleep, and affect circadian rhythms. To combat sleepiness, students drink caffeine and energy drinks, potentially decreasing sleep. Coffee is very popular among college students, and approximately 50% of American college students drink greater than one energy drink per month, with 70% doing so due to sleep deficiency.[24,25] About 14% use stimulants, altering sleep architecture and further contributing to sleep deficiency in college students.[23] Approximately 4 of 5 college students drink alcohol, with excess alcohol consumption associated with decreased sleep duration and sleep quality through relaxation of upper airway dilator muscles and inducing snoring and sleep apnea.[26,27] Sleep disorders, including obstructive sleep apnea (OSA), insomnia, and restless legs syndrome (RLS), are also common among college students and can contribute to sleep loss. In a survey of 1845 students, 27% were found to be at a risk of a sleep disorder.[28]

Social Factors

Internet and television (TV) are common in our modern society. Among adolescents, 97% report having electronic media devices in their bedroom, and those with more devices were found to sleep less and experience more daytime sleepiness.[29] With 55% of American adolescents accessing the internet after 9 PM and 82% watching TV at night, internet and TV play important roles in contributing to sleep deficiency among adolescents.[29] In California, a study of adolescents demonstrated that adolescents having technology use rules at home spent on average 35 more minutes in bed.[30]

Homelessness is a socioeconomic factor associated with sleep deficiency.[31] In the United States, there are 554,000 homeless individuals on any given night.[31,32] Homeless individuals sleep less and are more tired during the day compared with the general population.[31] In a survey of 32 homeless Americans, 75% of them reported getting less than 7 hours of sleep per night, with 92.7% of these individuals being interested in receiving intervention to obtain better sleep. In a study of 103 homeless individuals in the United States, around 50% of the participants experienced sleep interruptions[33]; substance use as a sleeping aid, environmental impacts including food insecurity, and mental health have been proposed as contributing factors to sleep deficiency among homeless.[22,30] Other social factors, such as smoking and tobacco use, have also been associated with insufficient sleep.[4]

Psychiatric Disorders

Psychiatric disorders can contribute to sleep deficiency. Psychiatric disorders, including depression, bipolar disease, and attention-deficit hyperactivity disorder (ADHD), are common among those with sleeping difficulties.[2,34] The prevalence of sleep disorder symptoms in psychiatric outpatients has been estimated at around 40%.[35] The relationship between sleeping disorders and psychiatric disorders is bidirectional and complex; improvements in either disorder can benefit the other disorder group.[36]

Depression is a common psychiatric disorder among those with sleeping difficulties. In a study of 772 participants, those with insomnia were 9.8 times more likely to have depressive disorders than those without insomnia.[37] Patients with depression can have difficulties falling and staying asleep at night, reducing their sleep duration and sleep quality. In bipolar disorder, the depressive episodes can have the same contributing effect on sleep deficiency and the manic episodes can reduce the sense of needing sleep.[38] Therefore, those with bipolar disorder report frequent nighttime awakenings, reduced sleep quality, and a reduction of sleep duration.[39] During the depressive episodes, insomnia, difficulty waking up, and excessive daytime sleepiness are common. ADHD is another psychiatric disorder that contributes to sleep deficiency. ADHD patients with inattentive symptoms go to bed around 1.5 hours later than individuals without ADHD symptoms and experience increased daytime sleepiness.[40] In addition to these effects, ADHD patients with hyperactive-impulsive and inattentive symptoms also experience lower sleep quality as suggested by higher PSQI values.

Medical Disorders

Physical disorders, such as arthritis and gastroesophageal reflux disorder (GERD), can also reduce sleep duration and quality.[41] Patients with arthritis experience inflammation and discomfort that can hinder sleep.[42] Approximately 50% to 70% of adults with rheumatoid arthritis report sleep complaints, including difficulty initiating sleep, nonoptimal sleep quality, nonrestorative sleep, waking up during the night, and excessive daytime sleepiness. In a 2003 poll from the United States, insomnia was the most common sleep issue (56%) reported by adults with arthritis aged 55 years and older, with 15% sleeping less than 6 hours per night, contributing to sleep debt. GERD can also induce sleep deficiency. It is thought that GERD can result in upper airway inflammation, increasing the risk of OSA, and induce nighttime arousals through initiation of swallowing for esophageal clearance.[43,44] In a study of 83 individuals with GERD and 75 controls, OSA and reduced sleep quality were more common among GERD patients (65% and 60%) than controls (48% and 39%).[43]

Sleep Disorders

Sleep disorders are common causes of sleep deficiency. It is estimated that 50 to 70 million Americans suffer from sleep disorders, contributing to the prevalence of sleep deficiency.[2] OSA, the most common sleep-related breathing disorder, affects almost one billion adults worldwide and is characterized by repetitive upper airway collapse leading to episodic arousals, asphyxia, and nocturnal hypoxemia.[45–47] OSA is associated with disruption of sleep and often presents as excessive daytime sleepiness.[45] It is thought that arousals during regular nighttime sleep, inflammation, and oxygen desaturation due to upper airway collapsibility affect sleep quality and architecture.[48] Patients with OSA suffer from sympathetic activation, arousals from sleep, heart rate acceleration, vasoconstriction, and high blood pressure,[49] potentially accentuating the negative effects of sleep deficiency on patients' health.

Insomnia, defined as having difficulty falling or staying asleep,[50] is another contributing factor to sleep deficiency. The prevalence of insomnia is variable based on the definition and study population used, but is generally approximated at 30%, with women and elders being more affected by insomnia. Insomnia and OSA are often co-occurring and referred to as comorbid insomnia and sleep apnea (COMISA).[51–53] In a study of 2044 Australian adults, insomnia occurred more frequently among participants with OSA (22.3%) compared with participants without OSA (14.3%, $P = 0.01$), and OSA occurred more often among participants with insomnia (10.2%) compared with those without insomnia (6.2%; $P = 0.01$).[51] COMISA results in additive impairments to patients' sleep, daytime functioning, and cardiometabolic well-being.[54] In a study of 685 individuals, hypertension and diabetes were more common in COMISA patients (54.3% and 13.3%) than those with sleep-disordered breathing (41.9% and 10.1%) or insomnia (10.1% and 1.8%) alone.[52] Sleep interruptions associated with OSA, and shorter sleep associated with insomnia can account for the additive effects in COMISA.[54]

Restless legs syndrome (RLS), characterized by uncomfortable leg symptoms and abnormal leg movements during sleep, is another common sleep disorder that can cause sleep disturbance and deficiency.[55] The symptoms of RLS include feeling of discomfort during evening and night, which is relieved by leg movements during sleep, causing many patients difficulty falling asleep.[2] The discomfort associated with RLS can also cause patients to wake up during sleep, causing sleep interruptions. RLS affects between 5% to 15% of the population with its prevalence increasing with age.[55]

Other Contributing Factors

Other factors that contribute to sleep deficiency include ethnicity, age, marital status, sex, and hospitalization. In the United States, sleep deficiency is more common in African Americans, Native Hawaiians/Pacific Islanders, and multiracial individuals.[5] Sleeping less than 7 hours per 24 hours period is most common among adults less than 65 years of age, those unable to work, and those divorced, widowed, or separated.[5] Females report a higher prevalence of sleep interruptions (15%) compared with males (5%).[11] In patients who are hospitalized, frequent disruptions to sleep due to care provision and loud environment are also common.[41,56]

EFFECTS OF SLEEP DEFICIENCY

Daytime Sleepiness and Cognitive Effects

Decreased duration of sleep results in daytime sleepiness and an increased sleep drive.[57] In sleep restriction experiments, regularly sleeping 6 hours or less per night can result in cognitive performance deficits equivalent to 24 hours of total sleep deprivation; 24 hours of total sleep deprivation causes cognitive impairment similar to a blood alcohol concentration of 100 mg/dL.[57–59] Attention deficiency and sleepiness due to sleep deprivation are correlated with brief mental lapses that increase the risk of motor vehicle crashes with approximately 9% of crashes attributable to reduced sleep.[1] In a study of 3201 participants, sleeping 6 hours, compared with 7 or 8 hours, per night was associated with a 33% increased crash risk.[1] Working memory, visuomotor performance, and ability to perform tasks that require higher cognitive function have also been shown to decrease with sleep deprivation.[58] In studies comparing workers, those who work longer hours exhibit more performance deficiency than those who work shorter hours. When compared to those who work regular hours, shift workers exhibit more performance deficiency and daytime sleepiness.[20]

Sleep quality can also affect cognitive performance.[60] In a study of 60 participants, the relationship between sleep quality and cognitive performance was evaluated.[61] Objective sleep quality was assessed using polysomnographic recordings with sleep latency, frequency of nocturnal awakenings, sleep efficiency, and sleep duration as clinical sleep variables; subjective sleep quality was assessed using sleep diaries. In those with no reported insomnia, objective and subjective good night of sleep was related to increased cognitive performance. In individuals with insomnia who were drug-free, an objective good night of sleep was associated with better cognitive performance, and in individuals with insomnia using benzodiazepines, the impression of having slept well was related to better cognitive performance. In another study of 157 older adults, those with poor sleep quality (PSQI >5) were more likely to have deficits in concentration.[62]

Sleep deficiency has been associated with dementia.[63] Using data from 7959 participants of the Whitehall II study, Sabia and colleagues report higher dementia risk associated with sleeping 6 hours or less at age 50 and 60 years (HR = 1.22 and 1.37; 95% CI: 1.01, 1.48 and 1.10, 1.72, respectively), compared with 7 hours of sleep. Persistent short sleep compared with persistent normal sleep at age 50, 60, and 70 years was associated with a 30% rise in dementia risk independently of sociodemographic, behavioral, cardiometabolic, and mental health factors. In another study of 2812 American adults greater than 65 years of age, sleep duration of ≤5 hours and sleep latency of greater than 30 minutes were associated with incident dementia (HR = 2.04 and 1.45; 95% CI: 1.26, 3.33 and 1.03, 2.03, respectively).[64]

Effects on Mood

Sleep restriction can affect mood and mental health. Sleep deficiency increases irritability, moodiness, drowsiness, suicide risk, and decreases frustration tolerance.[4] When sleep is restricted, adolescents tend to complain most commonly of tiredness upon awakening (46%), whereas university students mention excessive drowsiness (50%), and working adults report tension (49%).[65] Sleep deficiency is also related to depression. In a survey of 277 female college students in the United States, self-reported poor sleep was associated with depression (OR = 2.8; 95% CI: 1.3, 5.8).[66]

Weight Gain

Sleep deficiency is a risk factor for obesity.[67] One mechanism through which sleep may affect obesity risk is the balance between ghrelin, a hunger-promoting hormone, and leptin, a satiety-promoting hormone. With experimentally induced sleep restriction, ghrelin increases and leptin decreases, contributing to feelings of hunger.[68] In this regard, some studies show a 14% increase in caloric intake, particularly for carbohydrate-rich nutrients, in sleep-deficient individuals sleeping 4.5 hours per night compared with those sleeping 8.5 hours per night. These studies suggest that increased food intake due to sleep deficiency associated with hunger can be a mechanism for increased obesity risk among these patients. In a study of 68,183 women followed up for 16 years, women sleeping 5 hours or less per night gained 1.14 kg (95% CI: 0.49, 1.79) more than women sleeping 7 hours per night.[69] Weight gain of 15 kg and higher over 16 years was 32% more likely in women sleeping 5 hours or less per night compared with women sleeping 7 to 8 hours per night.

In a study of 56,500 adults, those reporting a sleep duration of less than 7 hours had a 6% higher probability of obesity compared with those sleeping 7 to 8 hours.[68,70] In a more recent prospective study of over 160,000 adults age 20 to 80 years, sleep duration of less than 6 hours per day was independently associated with an increased risk for central obesity by 12%, low high-density lipoprotein by 7%, hypertriglyceridemia by 9%, and metabolic syndrome by 9%.[71] Obesity is related to increased cardiovascular risk, further contributing to the cost of sleep deficiency.[72] In an analysis of 18 studies with 604,509 adults, 5 hours of sleep per night was associated with a pooled obesity OR of 1.55 (95% CI: 1.43,1.68; $P < 0.0001$) with a sleep duration dose effect such that for each additional hour of sleep per night, body mass index (BMI) decreased by 0.35 kg/m^2.[68,73] Sleep disorders, including OSA, have also been associated with obesity.[74]

Diabetes

Diabetes risk is increased with sleep deficiency. With sleep deficiency, cortisol levels rise leading to increased blood glucose,[70] predisposing to or worsening diabetes. Other mechanisms for increased risk of diabetes in short sleep include weight gain, insulin resistance, and increased inflammation.[75] Suppression of slow-wave sleep and rapid eye movement sleep has also been associated with insulin resistance.[76] In a prospective study of over 160,000 adults age 20 to 80 years, sleep duration of less than 6 hours per day was independently associated with an increased risk for elevated fasting glucose by 6%.[71] In the Sleep Heart Health Study, in comparison to sleeping 7 to 8 hours per night, sleeping 5 hours or less was associated with 2.5 times, and sleeping 6 hours was associated with 1.7 times increase in likelihood of having diabetes. Both sleep-deficient groups were more likely to display impaired glucose tolerance compared with those sleeping the regular 7 to 8 hours per night.[77] As diabetes and obesity are related, effects of sleep deficiency on diabetes risk can also be confounded by BMI or through weight gain.[78]

Cardiovascular Effects and Hypertension

Sleep deficiency is associated with increased cardiovascular disease (CVD) risk. Sleep deficiency is believed to influence CVD through diurnal patterns of blood pressure and heart rate, insulin sensitivity, the activity of the autonomic nervous system, inflammation, and salt and fluid homeostasis.[79] Sleep disorders, such as OSA, can accentuate some of these effects on cardiovascular health. Intermittent hypoxemia and fluctuations in intrathoracic pressure are common in OSA and can negatively impact cardiovascular health through endothelial damage, decreased myocardial contractility, and induction of oxidative stress and inflammation.[79,80] Sleep also may indirectly influence CVD risk via its effects on behaviors such as physical activity,[79] with those sleeping less reporting decreased physical activities[81] contributing to CVD. Through both the physiologic responses and associated behaviors mentioned, suboptimal sleep can lead to obesity and diabetes and have pronounced influences on CVD risk factors including inflammation, sympathetic activation, and hypertension[82]; in this section, we will highlight these mentioned factors in more detail.

Inflammation is a contributor to CVD risk in sleep deficiency. In an experiment with 19 adults, participants sleep restricted to 4 hours in bed per night had an elevated C-reactive protein (CRP) of 145% of baseline levels, whereas participants who spent 8 hours in bed per night had no significant increase in their CRP levels.[83] Elevated CRP levels, suggesting increased inflammation, in sleep-deficient patients can negatively influence their cardiovascular health in the long term. Hypertension and sympathetic activation are closely related in the context of sleep deficiency and are both risk factors for CVD in sleep-deficient patients. In an experiment with 10 adults, interruptions induced by auditory stimuli were associated with elevation of blood pressure at night.[84] In sleep disorders such as OSA, interruptions to sleep are common, and include arousals due to apneas.[85] Increased sympathetic tone resulting in peripheral vasoconstriction and increased arterial pressure is a mediator in cardiovascular risk associated with disordered sleep, including OSA.[86] Patients with severe OSA tend to present with blunted nocturnal dips of blood pressure (nondipping profile) and an elevated blood pressure during the day, suggesting increased basal sympathetic tone.[85,86]

Compared with inflammation and increased sympathetic tone, hypertension is more widely investigated as a mediator of CVD risk in sleep-deficient patients. In a study of over 4500 adults from the National Health and Nutrition Examination Survey in the United States, hypertension was associated with sleeping 5 hours per night compared with sleeping 7 to 8 hours per night after adjusting for confounders (OR = 1.32; 95% CI: 1.02, 1.71).[87] Another study has estimated that every hour decrease of sleep is associated with a 37% higher odds of incident hypertension.[88] In a prospective study of over 160,000 adults age 20 to 80 years, sleep duration of less than 6 hours per day was independently associated with an increased risk for hypertension by 8%.[71] In a study of 36 hypertensive patients, experimental sleep deprivation was associated with higher mean 24-h systolic blood pressure, with this difference most pronounced at night ($P < .01$).[89] Increased blood pressure during night is a strong predictor of CVD.[90] Coronary artery calcification, a predictor for coronary heart disease (CHD), is also negatively associated with sleep duration, with every extra hour of sleep per night being associated with a 33% lower odds of coronary artery calcification.[91] In the Nurses' Health Study, the risk ration for incident CHD over 10 years was 1.45 (95% CI: 1.1, 1.92) for women reporting 5 hours of sleep compared with 8 hours of sleep per night.[92]

Other Effects

Other effects of sleep deficiency include impaired renal function, immunosuppression, and changes in respiratory physiology. In a prospective cohort study of 4238 participants from the Nurses' Health Study, in comparison to those sleeping 7 to 8 hours per night, the adjusted odds ratio for impaired renal function were 1.79 (95% CI: 1.06, 3.03) for those sleeping 5 hours or less per night and 1.31 (95% CI: 1.01, 1.71) for those sleeping 6 hours per night.[93] There was also a decline in the estimated glomerular filtration rate of 1.2 mL/min/1.73 m^2/y and 0.9 mL/min/1.73 m^2/y for individuals sleeping 5 hours or less per night and 6 hours per night, respectively. Immunosuppression is another effect of sleep deficiency. Those who are sleep deficient are more immunosuppressed and more prone to common colds.[94] Sleep deprivation has been reported to dampen the immune response following vaccinations, rendering vaccines less helpful.[95] Sleep deprivation has also been shown to decrease ventilatory responses to hypercapnia and hypoxia.[96] Therefore, sleep deficiency can give rise to impaired renal function, immunosuppression, and changes in respiratory physiology.

SUMMARY

Sleep deficiency is common in modern society and has become a topic of interest among researchers. In this article, we reviewed the common contributing factors associated with sleep deficiency, including occupational factors, social factors, and medical/psychiatric disorders. The effects of sleep deficiency include daytime sleepiness, impaired cognitive function, mood disorders, obesity, diabetes, CVD, hypertension, inflammation, and other disorders. It is important for medical professionals and health care teams to educate their patients about sleep deficiency.

DISCLOSURE

Dr. Jen was funded by an Investigator Award from the Vancouver Coastal Health Research Institute.

REFERENCES

1. Gottlieb DJ, Ellenbogen JM, Bianchi MT, et al. Sleep deficiency and motor vehicle crash risk in the general population: a prospective cohort study. BMC Med 2018;16(1):44.
2. Institute of Medicine (US) Committee on Sleep Medicine and Research. In: Colten HR, Altevogt BM, editors. Sleep disorders and sleep deprivation: an unmet public health problem. Washington, DC: National Academies Press (US); 2006.
3. Basner M, Dinges DF. Sleep duration in the United States 2003-2016: first signs of success in the fight against sleep deficiency? Sleep 2018;41(4):1. New York, N.Y.
4. Chattu VK, Manzar MD, Kumary S, et al. The Global problem of insufficient sleep and its serious public health implications. Healthcare (Basel) 2018;7(1):1.
5. Liu Y, Wheaton AG, Chapman DP, et al. Prevalence of healthy sleep duration among adults — United States, 2014. MMWR Morb Mortal Wkly Rep 2016; 65(6):137–41.
6. Knutson KL, van Cauter E, Rathouz PJ, et al. Trends in the prevalence of short sleepers in the USA: 1975—2006. Sleep 2010;33(1):37–45. New York, N.Y.
7. Kronholm E, Partonen T, Laatikainen T, et al. Trends in self-reported sleep duration and insomnia-related symptoms in Finland from 1972 to 2005: a comparative review and re-analysis of Finnish population samples. J Sleep Res 2008;17(1):54–62.
8. Rowshan Ravan A, Bengtsson C, Lissner L, et al. Thirty-six-year secular trends in sleep duration and sleep satisfaction, and associations with mental stress and socioeconomic factors - results of the Population Study of Women in Gothenburg, Sweden: thirty-six-year secular trends in women's sleep. J Sleep Res 2010;19(3):496–503.
9. Bing MH, Moller LA, Jennum P, et al. Prevalence and bother of nocturia, and causes of sleep interruption in a Danish population of men and women aged 60–80 years. BJU Int 2006;98(3):599–604.
10. Soysal P, Cao C, Xu T, et al. Trends and prevalence of nocturia among US adults, 2005-2016. Int Urol Nephrol 2020;52(5):805–13.
11. Madrid-Valero JJ, Martínez-Selva JM, Ribeiro do Couto B, et al. Age and gender effects on the prevalence of poor sleep quality in the adult population. Gac Sanit 2017;31(1):18–22.
12. Bruno RM, Palagini L, Gemignani A, et al. Poor sleep quality and resistant hypertension. Sleep Med 2013; 14(11):1157–63.
13. Manzar MD, Bekele BB, Noohu MM, et al. Prevalence of poor sleep quality in the Ethiopian population: a systematic review and meta-analysis. Sleep Breath 2020;24(2):709–16.
14. Virtanen M, Ferrie JE, Gimeno D, et al. Long working hours and sleep disturbances: the whitehall ii prospective cohort study. Sleep 2009;32(6):737–45. New York, N.Y.
15. Afonso P, Fonseca M, Pires JF. Impact of working hours on sleep and mental health. Occup Med (London) 2017;67(5):377–82.
16. Boivin DB, Boudreau P. Impacts of shift work on sleep and circadian rhythms. Pathol Biol (Paris) 2014;62(5):292–301.
17. Wang D, Ruan W, Chen Z, et al. Shift work and risk of cardiovascular disease morbidity and mortality: a dose–response meta-analysis of cohort studies. Eur J Prev Cardiol 2018;25(12):1293–302.
18. Lawson CC, Whelan EA, Eileen N, et al. Rotating shift work and menstrual cycle characteristics. Epidemiology 2011;22(3):305–12.
19. Al Lawati NM, Patel SR, Ayas NT. Epidemiology, risk factors, and consequences of obstructive sleep apnea and short sleep duration. Prog Cardiovasc Dis 2009;51(4):285–93.
20. Yazdi Z, Sadeghniiat-Haghighi K, Loukzadeh Z, et al. Prevalence of sleep disorders and their impacts on occupational performance: a comparison between shift workers and nonshift workers. Sleep Disord 2014;2014:870320–5.
21. Czeisler CA, Buxton OM. Human circadian timing system and sleep-wake regulation. In: Kryger M, Roth T, Dement WC, editors. Principles and practice of sleep medicine. Sixth ed. Elsevier; 2017. p. 362–76.
22. Åkerstedt T, Wright KP. Sleep loss and fatigue in shift work and shift work disorder. Sleep Med Clin 2009; 4(2):257–71.
23. Hershner SD, Chervin RD. Causes and consequences of sleepiness among college students. Nat Sci Sleep 2014;6:73–84.
24. O'Brien MC, McCoy TP, Rhodes SD, et al. Caffeinated cocktails: energy drink consumption, high-risk drinking, and alcohol-related consequences among college students. Acad Emerg Med 2008;15(5): 453–60.
25. White A, Hingson R. The burden of alcohol use: excessive alcohol consumption and related consequences among college students. Alcohol Res 2013;35(2):201–18.
26. Park S, Oh M, Lee B, et al. The effects of alcohol on quality of sleep. Korean J Fam Med 2015;36(6): 294–9.

27. Cui R, Iso H. Alcohol and sleep-disordered breathing. In: Watson RR, editor. Modulation of sleep by obesity, diabetes, age, and diet. Elsevier Inc; 2015. p. 349–52.
28. Gaultney JF. The prevalence of sleep disorders in college students: impact on academic performance. J Am Coll Health 2010;59(2):91–7.
29. Cain N, Gradisar M. Electronic media use and sleep in school-aged children and adolescents: a review. Sleep Med 2010;11(8):735–42.
30. Bowers JM, Moyer A. Adolescent sleep and technology-use rules: results from the California Health Interview Survey. Sleep Health 2020;6(1): 19–22.
31. Gonzalez A, Tyminski Q. Sleep deprivation in an American homeless population. Sleep Health 2020; 6(4):489–94.
32. Taylor A, Murillo R, Businelle MS, et al. Physical activity and sleep problems in homeless adults. PLoS One 2019;14(7):e0218870.
33. Redline B, Semborski S, Madden DR, et al. Examining sleep disturbance among sheltered and unsheltered transition age youth experiencing homelessness. Med Care 2021;59(Suppl 2): S182–6.
34. Wajszilber D, Santiseban JA, Gruber R. Sleep disorders in patients with ADHD: impact and management challenges. Nat Sci Sleep 2018;10:453–80.
35. Hombali A, Seow E, Yuan Q, et al. Prevalence and correlates of sleep disorder symptoms in psychiatric disorders. Psychiatry Res 2019;279:116–22.
36. Krystal AD. Psychiatric disorders and sleep. Neurol Clin 2012;30(4):1389–413.
37. Taylor DJ, Lichstein KL, Durrence HH, et al. Epidemiology of insomnia, depression, and anxiety. Sleep 2005;28(11):1457–64. New York, N.Y.
38. Winokur A. The relationship between sleep disturbances and psychiatric disorders: introduction and overview. Psychiatr Clin North Am 2015;38(4): 603–14.
39. Moreira CA, Afonso P. The sleep changes in bipolar disorder. Eur Psychiatry 2015;30:1124.
40. Gamble KL, May RS, Besing RC, et al. Delayed sleep timing and symptoms in adults with attention-deficit hyperactivity disorder: a controlled actigraphy study. Chronobiol Int 2013;30(4): 598–606.
41. Stewart NH, Arora VM. Sleep in hospitalized older adults. Sleep Med Clin 2018;13(1):127–35.
42. Abad VC, Sarinas PSA, Guilleminault C. Sleep and rheumatologic disorders. Sleep Med Rev 2008; 12(3):211–28.
43. Fujiwara Y, Arakawa T, Fass R. Gastroesophageal reflux disease and sleep disturbances. J Gastroenterol 2012;47(7):760–9.
44. Vela MF, Kramer JR, Richardson PA, et al. Poor sleep quality and obstructive sleep apnea in patients with GERD and Barrett's esophagus. Neurogastroenterol Motil 2014;26(3):346–52.
45. Peppard PE, Young T, Barnet JH, et al. Increased prevalence of sleep-disordered breathing in adults. Am J Epidemiol 2013;177(9):1006–14.
46. Benjafield AV, Ayas NT, Eastwood PR, et al. Estimation of the global prevalence and burden of obstructive sleep apnoea: a literature-based analysis. Lancet Respir Med 2019;7(8):687–98.
47. Zhang Y, Ren R, Yang L, et al. Arousal during sleep is associated with hypertension in obstructive sleep apnea. Sleep 2019;42(Supplement_1):A234. New York, N.Y.
48. Ralls F, Cutchen L. A contemporary review of obstructive sleep apnea. Curr Opin Pulm Med 2019;25(6):578–93.
49. Venkataraman S, Vungarala S, Covassin N, et al. Sleep apnea, hypertension and the sympathetic nervous system in the adult population. J Clin Med 2020;9(2):591.
50. Roth T. Insomnia: definition, prevalence, etiology, and consequences. J Clin Sleep Med 2007;3(5 suppl):S7–10.
51. Sweetman A, Melaku YA, Lack L, et al. Prevalence and associations of co-morbid insomnia and sleep apnoea in an Australian population-based sample. Sleep Med 2021;82:9–17.
52. Cruz MME, Salles C, Gozal D. A reappraisal on the associations between sleep-disordered breathing, insomnia and cardiometabolic risk. Am J Resp Crit Care Med 2021;203(12):1583–4.
53. Sweetman A, Lack L, Bastien C. Co-Morbid insomnia and sleep apnea (comisa): prevalence, consequences, methodological considerations, and recent randomized controlled trials. Brain Sci 2019;9(12):371.
54. Sweetman AM, Lack LC, Catcheside PG, et al. Developing a successful treatment for co-morbid insomnia and sleep apnoea. Sleep Med Rev 2017; 33:28–38.
55. Ohayon MM, O'Hara R, Vitiello MV. Epidemiology of restless legs syndrome: a synthesis of the literature. Sleep Med Rev 2012;16(4):283–95.
56. Buxton OM, Ellenbogen JM, Wang W, et al. Sleep disruption due to hospital noises: a prospective evaluation. Ann Intern Med 2012;157(3):170–9.
57. van Dongen HP, Maislin G, Mullington JM, et al. The cumulative cost of additional wakefulness: dose-response effects on neurobehavioral functions and sleep physiology from Chronic sleep restriction and total sleep deprivation. Sleep 2003;26(2):117–26. New York, N.Y.
58. Alhola P, Polo-Kantola P. Sleep deprivation: impact on cognitive performance. Neuropsychiatr Dis Treat 2007;3(5):553–67.
59. Dawson D, Reid K. Fatigue, alcohol and performance impairment. Nature 1997;388(6639):235. London.

60. Scullin MK, Bliwise DL. Sleep, cognition, and normal aging: integrating a half century of multidisciplinary research. Perspect Psychol Sci 2015;10(1):97–137.
61. Bastien CH, Fortier-Brochu É, Rioux I, et al. Cognitive performance and sleep quality in the elderly suffering from chronic insomnia: relationship between objective and subjective measures. J Psychosom Res 2003;54(1):39–49.
62. Nebes RD, Buysse DJ, Halligan EM, et al. Self-reported sleep quality predicts poor cognitive performance in healthy older adults. J Gerontol B Psychol Sci Soc Sci 2009;64B(2):180–7.
63. Sabia S, Fayosse A, Dumurgier J, et al. Association of sleep duration in middle and old age with incidence of dementia. Nat Commun 2021;12(1): 2289.
64. Robbins R, Quan SF, Weaver MD, et al. Examining sleep deficiency and disturbance and their risk for incident dementia and all-cause mortality in older adults across 5 years in the United States. Aging 2021;13(3):3254–68. Albany, NY.
65. Oginska H, Pokorski J. Fatigue and mood correlates of sleep length in three age-social groups: school children, students, and employees. Chronobiol Int 2006;23(6):1317–28.
66. Wilson KT, Bohnert AE, Ambrose A, et al. Social, behavioral, and sleep characteristics associated with depression symptoms among undergraduate students at a women's college: a cross-sectional depression survey, 2012. BMC Women's Health 2014;14(1):8.
67. Ogilvie RP, Patel SR. The epidemiology of sleep and obesity. Sleep Health 2017;3(5):383–8.
68. Beccuti G, Pannain S. Sleep and obesity. Curr Opin Clin Nutr Metab Care 2011;14(4):402–12.
69. Patel SR, Malhotra A, White DP, et al. Association between reduced sleep and weight gain in women. Am J Epidemiol 2006;164(10):947–54.
70. Buxton OM, Marcelli E. Short and long sleep are positively associated with obesity, diabetes, hypertension, and cardiovascular disease among adults in the United States. Soc Sci Med 2010;71(5): 1027–36.
71. Deng H, Tam T, Zee BC, et al. Short sleep duration increases metabolic impact in healthy adults: a population-based cohort study. Sleep 2017;40(10). New York, N.Y.
72. Alpert MA, Omran J, Bostick BP. Effects of obesity on cardiovascular hemodynamics, cardiac morphology, and ventricular function. Curr Obes Rep 2016;5(4):424–34.
73. Cappuccio FP, Taggart FM, Kandala N, et al. Meta-analysis of short sleep duration and obesity in children and adults. Sleep 2008;31(5):619–26. New York, N.Y.
74. Romero-Corral A, Caples SM, Lopez-Jimenez F, et al. Interactions between obesity and obstructive sleep apnea: implications for treatment. Chest 2010;137(3):711–9.
75. Grandner MA, Seixas A, Shetty S, et al. Sleep duration and diabetes risk: population trends and potential mechanisms. Curr Diab Rep 2016;16(11):1–14.
76. Dutil C, Chaput J. Inadequate sleep as a contributor to type 2 diabetes in children and adolescents. Nutr Diabetes 2017;7(5):e266.
77. Gottlieb DJ, Punjabi NM, Newman AB, et al. Association of sleep time with diabetes mellitus and impaired glucose tolerance. Arch Inten Med 2005; 165(8):863–7.
78. Ayas NT, White DP, Al-Delaimy WK, et al. A prospective study of self-reported sleep duration and incident diabetes in women. Diabetes Care 2003;26(2):380–4.
79. Jackson CL, Redline S, Emmons KM. Sleep as a potential fundamental contributor to disparities in cardiovascular health. Annu Rev Public Health 2015; 36(1):417–40.
80. Bradley TD, Floras JS. Obstructive sleep apnoea and its cardiovascular consequences. Lancet 2009;373(9657):82–93.
81. Zimberg IZ, Dâmaso A, Del Re M, et al. Short sleep duration and obesity: mechanisms and future perspectives. Cell Biochem Funct 2012;30(6):524–9.
82. Fioranelli M, Bottaccioli AG, Bottaccioli F, et al. Stress and inflammation in coronary artery disease: a review psychoneuroendocrineimmunology-based. Front Immunol 2018;9:2031.
83. van Leeuwen, Wessel MA, Lehto M, et al. Sleep restriction increases the risk of developing cardiovascular diseases by augmenting proinflammatory responses through IL-17 and CRP. PLoS One 2009;4(2):e4589.
84. Carrington MJ, Trinder J. Blood pressure and heart rate during continuous experimental sleep fragmentation in healthy adults. Sleep 2008;31(12):1701–12. New York, N.Y.
85. Bilo G, Pengo MF, Lombardi C, et al. Blood pressure variability and obstructive sleep apnea. A question of phenotype? Hypertens Res 2019;42(1):27–8.
86. Hermida RC, Crespo JJ, Domínguez-Sardiña M, et al. Bedtime hypertension treatment improves cardiovascular risk reduction: the Hygia Chronotherapy Trial. Eur Heart J 2020;41(48):4565–76.
87. Gangwisch JE, Heymsfield SB, Boden-Albala B, et al. Short sleep duration as a risk factor for hypertension: analyses of the first National Health and Nutrition Examination Survey. Hypertension 2006; 47(5):833–9.
88. Knutson KL, Van Cauter E, Rathouz PJ, et al. Association between sleep and blood pressure in midlife:

the CARDIA sleep study. Arch Intern Med 2009;169(11):1055–61.
89. Lusardi P, Zoppi A, Preti P, et al. Effects of insufficient sleep on blood pressure in hypertensive patients: a 24-h study. Am J Hypertens 1999;12(1):63–8.
90. Calhoun DA, Harding SM. Sleep and hypertension. Chest 2010;138(2):434–43.
91. King CR, Knutson KL, Rathouz PJ, et al. Short sleep duration and incident coronary artery calcification. JAMA 2008;300(24):2859–66.
92. Ayas NT, White DP, Manson JE, et al. A prospective study of sleep duration and coronary heart disease in women. Arch Intern Med 2003;163(2):205–9.
93. McMullan CJ, Curhan GC, Forman JP. Association of short sleep duration and rapid decline in renal function. Kidney Int 2016;89(6):1324–30.
94. Cohen S, Doyle WJ, Alper CM, et al. Sleep habits and susceptibility to the common cold. Arch Intern Med 2009;169(1):62–7.
95. Bollinger T, Bollinger A, Skrum L, et al. Sleep-dependent activity of T cells and regulatory T cells. Clin Exp Immunol 2009;155(2):231–8.
96. White DP, Douglas NJ, Pickett CK, et al. Sleep deprivation and the control of ventilation. Am Rev Respir Dis 1983;128(6):984.

The Need for Social and Environmental Determinants of Health Research to Understand and Intervene on Racial/Ethnic Disparities in Obstructive Sleep Apnea

Dayna A. Johnson, PhD, MPH, MSW, MS[a,*], Chidinma Ohanele, MPHc[a], Carmela Alcántara, PhD[b], Chandra L. Jackson, PhD, MS[c,d]

KEYWORDS

• Obstructive sleep apnea • Health disparities • Sleep disparities • Health equity interventions • Race • Sleep-disordered breathing

KEY POINTS

- Obstructive sleep apnea (OSA) is disproportionately prevalent and severe among racial/ethnic minority children and adults.
- Asian, especially Chinese and Japanese, Black, and Hispanic/Latinx adults and children have a particularly high prevalence of undiagnosed and untreated OSA.
- There is limited research among American Indian children and adults.
- The most commonly studied social determinant of health, neighborhood environment, partially explains racial/ethnic disparities in OSA for adults and children.
- Culturally tailored evidence-based interventions that leverage social determinants of health frameworks have been shown to reduce the burden of OSA among racial/ethnic minorities.

INTRODUCTION

Sleep disorders and sleep health inequities are a public health burden. Obstructive sleep apnea (OSA), a sleep-disordered breathing (SDB) disorder, is highly prevalent[1,2] and has been implicated as an emerging risk factor for hypertension, type 2 diabetes, CVD, and mortality.[3–7] CVD-related outcomes and early mortality are

Funding: This work was, in part, supported by National Heart, Lung, and Blood Institute, (NHLBI) K01HL138211and HL125748. This work was funded, in part, by the Intramural Program at the NIH, National Institute of Environmental Health Sciences (Z1A ES103325-01).

[a] Department of Epidemiology, Rollins School of Public Health, Emory University, 1518 Clifton Road NE, CNR Room 3025, Atlanta, GA 30322, USA; [b] School of Social Work, Columbia University, 1255 Amsterdam Avenue, Room 917, New York, NY 10027, USA; [c] Epidemiology Branch, Social and Environmental Determinants of Health Equity, National Institute of Environmental Health Sciences, National Institutes of Health, 111 T.W. Alexander Drive, Room A327, Research Triangle Park, 27709 Post: P.O. Box 12233, Mail Drop A3-05, NC 27709, USA; [d] Intramural Program, Department of Health and Human Services, National Institute on Minority Health and Health Disparities, Bethesda, MD, USA

* Corresponding author. Department of Epidemiology, Rollins School of Public Health, Emory University, 1518 Clifton Road NE, Room 3025, Atlanta, GA 30322.

E-mail address: dayna.johnson@emory.edu

Clin Chest Med 43 (2022) 199–216
https://doi.org/10.1016/j.ccm.2022.02.002
0272-5231/22/

disproportionately prevalent among minoritized racial/ethnic groups.[8,9] Emerging evidence suggests that sleep disorders and adverse sleep health contribute to cardiovascular and overall health disparities.[10–13] Thus, addressing the burden of sleep disorders, particularly OSA, will likely aid in the reduction of sleep and health disparities. As a result of the urgent need to address racial/ethnic disparities in OSA, herein, the authors (1) review and summarize the literature disclosing the current state of scientific knowledge on racial/ethnic disparities in OSA, (2) discuss the social determinants investigated, (3) review treatments with demonstrated effectiveness, (4) discuss promising evidence-based interventions, and (5) conclude with future research directions in hopes of informing the development and rigorous testing of interventions designed to attenuate or eliminate disparities.

LITERATURE REVIEW STRATEGY

Focused on racial/ethnic disparities in SDB (especially OSA), we define "race" as a social construct with biological consequences that result from social, economic, and environmental determinants that are differentially experienced across racial/ethnic groups as a result of historical racist and discriminatory practices, laws, and policies based on race/ethnicity.[14] As defined by the National Institute on Minority Health and Health Disparities, a health disparity is "a health difference, on the basis of one or more health outcomes that adversely affects disadvantaged populations."[15] Further, disparities are defined as inequities between racial groups that are preventable and unfair/unjust[16] and are related to any differences that are not due to clinical need or preferences for health care services.[17] Relatedly, social determinants are considered the broad range of economic, social, neighborhood, and environmental factors as well as policies that influence access to opportunities and resources that can in turn directly or indirectly shape health.[18]

To review the literature on OSA disparities, the authors searched PubMed, Medline (Ovid), EMBASE, Google Scholar, and The Cochrane Library May-June 2021. The following search terms were used to identify English-language articles published in peer-reviewed journals without study design restrictions: 'OSA'/exp, 'sleep apnea syndromes'/exp, 'sleep disordered breathing'/exp, disparit*, health disparit*, 'social determinants of health', continental population groups, 'population group'/exp, ethnic groups, (race* or racial* or minorit* or cultur*):ti,ab, ethnic*:ti,ab, black*:ti,ab, ((african or asian or mexican) adj american*):ti,ab, (Hispanic* or latin* or spanish).ti,ab, (white* or Caucasian* or European*):-ti,ab, Asian*:ti,ab, Native*:ti,ab, Aborig*:ti,ab, Indian*:ti,ab, Pacific:ti,ab, Subcontinent:ti,ab, Chicano:ti,ab, Amish:ti,ab, arab*:ti,ab, Inuit*:ti,ab, jew*:ti,ab, Indigenous:ti,ab, colo?r*ti:ab, 'socioeconomics'/exp, 'socioeconomic factors'/exp, working poor, poverty, vulnerable populations, (socioeconomic* or poverty or poor or ses or social class* or employ* or unemploy* or income or education* or underserve* or vulnerable*):ti,ab, and (sex* or bisex* or homosex* or heterosex* or lesbian* or transgender* or lgbt). The search was limited to studies conducted in the United States (US); however, when deemed appropriate and useful, examples were drawn from research outside the US. Although no restrictions were placed on the date of publication, most of the articles were published starting in the early 2000s. Based on the aforementioned criteria, this search yielded 82 published articles, and later the authors summarize the literature on OSA or SDB among minoritized racial/ethnic groups including African American, Asian, Hispanic/Latinx, and American Indian (or Native American) children as well as adults.

RACIAL/ETHNIC DISPARITIES IN SLEEP-DISORDERED BREATHING INCLUDING OBSTRUCTIVE SLEEP APNEA

OSA is prevalent among minoritized racial/ethnic children and adults (**Table 1**) with the prevalence ranging from 5% to 86%.[19,20] Compared with non-Hispanic White adults, African American or Black adults have a higher prevalence of sleep apnea syndrome (apnea-hypopnea index [AHI] $\geq$5 plus sleepiness), daytime sleepiness, snoring, and more severe sleep apnea.[19,21–24] Among a clinical sample, African American men had a higher AHI, an objective measure of OSA, than White men of the same age while accounting for body mass index (BMI).[25] Similar findings are shown among elderly samples.[22] In addition to the high prevalence of OSA, there was also a high burden of undiagnosed OSA. Data from a US-based cohort study found that only 16.2% of African Americans who had polysomnography-defined moderate or severe sleep apnea reported a physician diagnosis[19]; this is supported by research among the largest longitudinal cardiovascular cohort study, the Jackson Heart Study. Johnson and colleagues reported that among 852 African Americans in Jackson, MS, 24% had moderate or severe sleep apnea with 95% being undiagnosed.[26] These results underscore the need for screening in this population.

A similar OSA burden for adults is also observed among African American pediatric populations. A

Table 1
Studies reporting on racial/ethnic disparities in obstructive sleep apnea (N = 24)

Study	Sample	Diagnostic Assessment	Obstructive Sleep Apnea Definition	Main Findings
Geovanini et al,[4] 2018	390 African American 13 Chinese 430 Hispanic 511 White adults (mean age = 68 y) Male (47%) Female (53%)	In-lab PSG	No OSA (AHI<5), mild (AHI = 5–14), moderate (AHI = 15–29), and severe (AHI ≥ 30)	30% African American, 4% Chinese, 35% Hispanic, and 31% White adults had moderate OSA 27% African American, 0.5% Chinese, 42% Hispanic, and 30.5% White adults had severe OSA
Johnson et al,[5] 2018	664 Black (mean age = 64.9 y) Male (30.9%) Female (69.1%) Jackson, MS residents	In-home sleep apnea test (type 3 sleep apnea device)	Moderate or severe OSA defined as REI ≥15	26% prevalence of moderate-to-severe sleep apnea
Chen et al,[19] 2015	612 Black (mean age = 68.8 y) Male (44.4%) Female (55.6%) 262 Chinese (mean age = 67.7 y) Male (49.6%) Female (50.4%) 528 Hispanic (mean age = 68.6 y) Male (47%) Female (53%) 828 White adults (mean age = 68.8 y) Male (46.1%) Female (53.9%)	In-lab PSG & self-reported doctor diagnosed sleep apnea, Sleep Questionnaire Survey	AHI>5 and categorized as mild (AHI = 5–14), moderate (AHI = 15–29), and severe (AHI ≥ 30)	17.9% White, 17.5% Black, 20.5% Hispanic, and 21.6% Chinese participants had moderate SDB 12.4% White, 14.9% Black, 17.7% Hispanic, and 17.8% Chinese had severe SDB 9.0% of participants reported doctor diagnosed sleep apnea
Jean-Louis et al,[20] 2008	421 Black adults Adherent (mean age = 51 y) Male (43%) Female (57%) Nonadherent (mean age = 52 y)	In-lab PSG	AHI ≥5	91% of patients received a sleep apnea diagnosis and treatment

(*continued on next page*)

Table 1
(continued)

Study	Sample	Diagnostic Assessment	Obstructive Sleep Apnea Definition	Main Findings
	Male (38%) Female (62%)			
Redline et al,[21] 1997	253 African American Control Family (mean age = 32.6 y) Male (38%) Female (62%) Index Family (mean age = 34.8 y) Male (53%) Female (47%) 622 White Control Family (mean age = 31.7 y) Male (47%) Female (53%) Index Family (mean age = 32.6 y) Male (49%) Female (51%)	In-home sleep monitor	RDI> 5, 10, and 15 for subjects < 25 y, 26–55 y, and > 55 y, respectively	SDB was twice as prevalent among African Americans than in Whites
Ancoli-Israel et al,[22] 1995	54 African American adults (mean age = 70.8 y) Male (43%) Female (57%) 352 White adults (mean age = 72.8 y) Male (47%) Female (53%)	In-home sleep monitor	RDI>5	17% of African Americans and 8% of Whites had severe SDB
Scharf et al,[23] 2004	128 African American (mean age = 44.9 y) Male (50%) Female (50%) 102 White adults (mean age = 49.2 y)	In-lab PSG	RDI>5	53.9% of African Americans and 48% of White adults had more severe sleep apnea

	Male (57.8%) Female (42.1%)			
O'Connor et al,[24] 2003	643 American Indian Male (43%) Female (57%) 90 Asian-Pacific Islander Male (51%) Female (49%) 648 Black Male (41%) Female (59%) 296 Hispanic Male (42%) Female (58%) 11,517 non-Hispanic white adults Male (46%) Female (54%)	The Sleep Habits Questionnaire & In-lab PSG	Frequent snoring defined as snoring 3–5 nights a week or more Breathing pauses defined as cessation of breathing during sleep SDB defined as AHI≥15	Persistent snoring was more common among Black (21%), Hispanic (29%) women, and Hispanic (52%) men, compared with non-Hispanic White adults (39% male 19% female) Breathing pauses was more common among American Indians (23% male, 10% female)
Pranathiageswaran et al,[25] 2013	340 African American Male (45%) Female (55%) 132 White adults Male (70%) Female (30%)	In-lab PSG	AHI>5	The median AHI was 32.7 for African American patients and 22.4 for White patients
Johnson et al,[26] 2018	852 African American (mean age = 63.1 y) Male (34%) Female (66%) Jackson, MS residents	In-home sleep apnea test (type 3 sleep apnea device)	AHI ≥15	23.6% prevalence of moderate-to-severe OSA
Goldstein et al,[27] 2011	155 Black/African American 41 Hispanic 133 White 17 other children Male (48.5%) Female (51.5%)	Questionnaire-PSQ, Sleep-Related Breathing Disorders Scale	SDB defined as mean PSQ score> 0.33	SDB was found in 11.6% of Black children, 9.8% of Hispanic children, and 6.8% of white children
Rosen et al,[28] 2001	Term children 166 Black 268 White 22 other (mean age = 9.6 y)	In-home monitor	SDB defined as (1) AHI≥5 event/h (2) Obstructive apneas ≥1 event/h, regardless of	SDB was found in 4.8%, 8.1%, and 8.7% of Black children, and 1.0%, 1.4%, and 2.2% of White children, detailed

(*continued on next page*)

Table 1
(continued)

Study	Sample	Diagnostic Assessment	Obstructive Sleep Apnea Definition	Main Findings
	Male (51%) Female (49%) Preterm children 144 Black 233 White 17 Other (mean age = 9.3 y) Male (51%) Female (49%)		desaturation (3) Combination of criteria (1) & (2)	by the apnea hypopnea index, the obstructive apnea index, and the combined definition, respectively
Stepanski et al,[29] 1999	68% African American 19% Latino 12% White 1% Arabic children (mean age = 5.9 y) Male (52%) Female (48%)	Clinical, PSG, and audiovisual data	SDB defined as (1) frequent (≥5/h) episodes of upper airway obstruction (2) Oxygen desaturation (<90%), sleep fragmentation, or cardiac arrhythmia in association with episodes of upper airway obstruction	65% of African American, 62% Latino, and 68% of White children were diagnosed with SDB
Seixas et al,[31] 2016	1035 Black/African American adults (mean age = 62 y) Male (31%) Female (69%)	Questionnaire: Apnea Risk Evaluation System	OSA defined as Apnea Risk Evaluation score ≥6	77% prevalence of moderate-to-high risk of OSA
Thomas et al,[32] 2020	206 African American adults (mean age = 55.6 y) Male (33%) Female (67%)	In-home sleep apnea test (type 3 sleep apnea device)	REI4% ≥15 events/h	26.2% had moderate-to-severe sleep apnea
Yano et al,[33] 2020	789 Black adults (mean age = 63 y) Male (26%) Female (74%))	In-home sleep apnea test (type 3 sleep apnea device)	SDB defined as (1) continuous variables (REI4P, REI3P, Sat<90, MinSaO_2) in the primary analysis (2) a categorical variable in secondary analyses, where REI<5, REI ≥5 and < 15, REI ≥15 and < 30, and REI ≥30 is	14.7% prevalence of moderate OSA and 8.9% of severe OSA

			unaffected OSA, mild OSA, moderate OSA, severe OSA, respectively	
Leong et al,[34] 2013	40 South Asian adults (mean age = 43.8 y) Male (40%) Female (60%) 268 White European adults (mean age = 46.6 y) Male (27.6%) Female (72.4%)	In-home monitor	OSA defined as AHI ≥ 5 events/h	85% of South Asian and 66% of White adults had OSA
Ong et al,[35] 1998	105 Asian adults (mean age = 41.5 y) Male (87.6%) Female (12.4%) 99 White adults (mean age = 41.2 y) Male (87.9%) Female (12.1%)	The Sleep Questionnaire and Assessment of Wakefulness & In-lab PSG	Severe OSA defined as (1) RDI≥50 (2) SaO_2≤69%	25% of Asians and 11.1% of White patients had severe OSA (RDI≥50) 20.6% of Asians and 4.2% of White patients had severe OSA (SaO_2≤69%)
Genta et al,[36] 2008	54 Japanese adults (mean age = 53.3 y) 466 White adults (mean age = 50.6 y)	In-lab PSG	OSA defined as AHI ≥5 events/h	The proportion of individuals with OSA was 89% for Japanese descendants and 88% White patients
Lee et al,[37] 2010	76 Chinese adults (mean age = 49.5 y) Male (82.9%) Female (18.1%) 74 White adults (mean age = 48.5 y) Male (79.7%) Female (21.3%)	In-lab PSG	OSA defined as AHI ≥5 events/h	The severity of OSA was (35.3 ± 26.1 events/h) for Chinese patients and (25.2 ± 16.3 events/h) for White patients
Shafazand et al,[38] 2012	99 Cuban 63 Puerto Rican 4 Mexican 9 Caribbean 35 Central American 49 South American 23 Other adults (mean	STOP Bang Questionnaire & In-lab video PSG	SDB defined as AHI ≥5 events/h	63% of participants had moderate-to-severe SDB (AHI ≥ 15)

(*continued on next page*)

Table 1
(continued)

Study	Sample	Diagnostic Assessment	Obstructive Sleep Apnea Definition	Main Findings
	age = 54 y) Male (62%) Female (38%)			
Yamagishi et al,[39] 2010	211 Hispanic adults (mean age = 61.6 y) Male (48%) Females (52%) 978 Japanese adults (mean age = 63 y) Male (46%) Female (54%) 246 White adults (mean age = 62 y) Male (44%) Female (56%)	In-lab (single-channel airflow monitor)	SDB defined as RDI ≥15 events/h	36.5% of Hispanic, 33.3% White, and 18.4% Japanese participants had SDB
Redline et al,[40] 2014	Dominican 448 male (mean age = 38.9 y) 840 female (mean age = 39.6 y) Central American 588 male (mean age = 38.2 y) 905 female (mean age = 41.4 y) Cuban 897 male (mean age = 45.7 y) 1011 female (mean age = 47.1 y) Mexican 2297 male (mean age = 38.0 y) 3807 female (mean age = 39.4 y) Puerto Rican 943 male (mean age = 42.0 y) 1348 female (mean age = 44.9 y)	In-home sleep apnea monitor—Apnea Risk Evaluation System	SDB severity defined as minimal (AHI ≥5), moderate (AHI ≥15), and severe (AHI ≥30)	9.8% of participants had moderate or severe SDB

	South American 390 male (mean age = 40.2 y) 550 female (mean age = 44.5 y) Mixed or other adults 184 male (mean age = 34.4 y) 232 female (mean age = 35.3 y)			
Alshehri et al,[41] 2020	3779 Hispanic/Latino adults (mean age = 55.32 y) Male (42.1%) Female (57.9%)	In-home sleep monitor—Apnea Risk Evaluation System	Continuous AHI with 3% of desaturation	Mean AHI: 8.46 ± 13.4

Note: The articles are listed in the order presented in the article.

Abbreviations: RDI, Respiratory Disturbance Index; REI, Respiratory Event Index.

study of young children found that snoring, a symptom of OSA, but not sleep-disordered breathing, was more common among Black children compared with their White counterparts.[27] However, other studies have reported an SDB disparity. In a study of 8- to 11-year-old children, African American children were more likely to have SDB compared with White children.[28] The investigators of the prior study reported preterm status as a significant risk factor for increased SDB risk in African American children. Future studies should explore preterm status as a contributor to SDB. Interestingly, a study of African American, Hispanic/Latinx, White, and Arabic children and adolescents referred for sleep center evaluation found a similar severity of SDB by race/ethnicity but yet, found more frequent and more severe oxygen desaturation by pulse oximetry in African American children.[29] The study findings suggested African American children may be at increased risk for cardiovascular consequences of SDB.

The high prevalence of OSA is particularly problematic among African Americans, given the higher burden of CVD risk factors that emerge earlier in life.[3] For instance, a recent study found childhood OSA persisted to adolescence and that it was associated with hypertension in adolescence.[30] Studies within African Americans have shown that OSA is associated with resistant hypertension,[5] uncontrolled blood pressure,[31] nighttime blood pressure,[32]and higher blood glucose levels.[33] Furthermore, in diverse samples, researchers have found that the association between sleep apnea and CVD is stronger among African Americans.[4] OSA is likely a target to reduce CVD among African Americans.

Similar to African Americans, Asian populations have a particularly high prevalence of OSA. Although sleep data among Asian Pacific Islander–identified ethnic groups are scant, data outside the US suggest Asian ethnicity is associated with OSA. For instance, a study in England found South Asian adults had a higher prevalence and greater severity of OSA than White European study participants.[34] In fact, among a clinical adult sample of Asian and White patients in the US, Asian patients had more severe polysomnography-measured OSA but no observed differences in severity of questionnaire-based symptoms.[35] Asian adults may underreport symptoms, which should be further explored. Furthermore, data from the Multi-Ethnic Study of Atherosclerosis demonstrated that Chinese Americans had higher odds of objectively measured SDB, with differences most evident after adjusting for BMI.[19] In the prior study, Chinese individuals had the lowest prevalence of doctor-diagnosed OSA,[19] which may be attributable to social factors or structural barriers that adversely affect access to care, leading to underdiagnoses while underscoring the need for screening. Similar findings exist among Japanese descendants. In a study of White and Japanese men in São Paulo Brazil, the investigators reported that the risk of OSA associated with obesity is likely largely underrecognized among Japanese descendants.[36] This finding suggests there may be a delay or underdiagnosis of OSA among obese Japanese descendants. Although acknowledging that some of the OSA burden among Asian populations may be attributable to variations in craniofacial anatomy,[37] strategies are needed to screen and treat Asian subgroups with unrecognized, underdiagnosed OSA potentially due to social determinants of health.

Hispanic/Latinx populations are also disproportionately burdened by OSA. In a study among a clinical cohort of US Hispanic/Latinx adults in South Florida, 63% of the participants who underwent polysomnography had moderate-to-severe OSA.[38] In a cross-cultural study of Hispanics/Latinx, White Americans, and Japanese adults in Japan, Hispanic/Latinx adults had a higher prevalence of SDB than White and Japanese participants.[39] However, BMI explained the differences. When examining OSA among pediatric samples, a study of young children found that snoring was more common among Hispanic/Latinx than non-Hispanic/Latinx White children.[27] Similarly, in an adult population, snoring was also more common in Hispanic/Latina women, even after adjustment for BMI.[24] Targeting snoring among this population may reduce OSA burden.

Given the heterogeneity of the Hispanic/Latinx population, conducting within-group analyses is critically important. In the Hispanic Community Health Study/Study of Latinos, SDB was assessed among Hispanic/Latino individuals of diverse backgrounds. Redline and colleagues found that 25.8% of the study population met minimal criteria for SDB (AHI $\geq$5).[40] Although not statistically significant, the age-adjusted prevalence of moderate or severe SDB was highest among Puerto Rican women and lowest among South American women.[40] Among men, the prevalence of SDB was highest among Cuban and "mixed/other" men and least prevalent among Puerto Rican and South American men.[40] Consistent with data among African Americans, SDB is associated with an increased prevalence of diabetes and hypertension among Hispanic/Latinx populations,[40,41] and the associations vary by Hispanic/Latino group, thus underscoring the importance of conducting within-group studies and OSA as a target to reduce the CVD burden among Hispanic/Latinx populations.

Overall, American Indian (or Native American) populations are underrepresented in sleep research. In one study with a racially/ethnically diverse sample, which included 5% American Indian adults, breathing pauses were more common among American Indians in comparison to non-Hispanic White adults.[24] The prior result suggests that there may be a disproportionate burden of OSA among American Indian populations, but more research is needed.

SOCIAL DETERMINANTS OF OBSTRUCTIVE SLEEP APNEA

The social determinants of OSA disparities are poorly understood. Limited literature shows that neighborhood environment is a contributor to OSA and OSA disparities.[42–46] Although determinants are likely multifactorial, the most commonly studied social determinant of health is of the neighborhood environment, and most of the literature on neighborhood environment and OSA has been conducted among pediatric populations. These studies have shown that living in a socioeconomically disadvantaged neighborhood increases the risk of OSA.[44,46] For instance, among a sample of children in Canada, Brouillette and colleagues reported that the highest probability of OSA prevalence was observed among children referred from the most disadvantaged census tracts.[46] A study among children in Canada found that children with OSA were more likely to reside in disadvantaged neighborhoods.[46] Neighborhood disadvantage likely contributes to OSA risk disparities, as neighborhood environments are shaped by racial residential segregation from health-promoting resources, socioeconomic status (SES), and immigration status.[47] As a result of historical discriminatory housing practices and environmental racism, minoritized racial/ethnic groups are more likely to live in lower SES neighborhoods and are exposed to more environmental hazards.[48] For example, ambient air pollution is associated with disturbed sleep and OSA.[49–56] Air pollution can negatively affect the nervous system, and can cause oxidative stress or inflammatory damage, which contributes to disturbed sleep.[57] In addition to air pollution, socially disadvantaged neighborhoods tend to have less access to high-quality medical care, sleep physicians, and behavioral sleep medicine providers.[58] Taken together, this evidence supports that neighborhood environment is associated with OSA.

A growing literature has shown that neighborhood environment partially explains racial/ethnic disparities in OSA. In 2 studies among adolescents, the investigators found that 50% to 55% of the racial/ethnic disparities in OSA was attributable to neighborhood environment.[44,45] More specifically, neighborhood poverty explained the racial disparity in pediatric OSA syndrome.[45] Neighborhood poverty may act as a proxy for adverse environmental exposures that increase OSA risk. In a separate study, residence in a disadvantaged neighborhood and African American race predicted OSA in middle childhood.[59] Similar data among adults are lacking. OSA is often undiagnosed in minoritized populations, thus disturbed sleep, measured as wakefulness after sleep onset (WASO), may serve as proxy or symptom. In a sample of adults, neighborhood disadvantage explained 24% of the racial disparity in WASO.[60] Although neighborhood disadvantage, often a measure of SES, is associated with OSA, most studies have reported a null finding between individual-level SES and OSA.[61,62] The health disparities literature has shown that racial/ethnic minorities are more likely to live in environments below their individual SES level,[63,64] which may explain the prior result.

In addition to neighborhood environment, individual-level factors such as exposure to secondhand smoke can increase the risk of OSA. In a study of African American, White, and additional races (not specified in the article), children with exposure to secondhand smoke had more severe OSA, and this was more common among non-Hispanic White children.[65] Aside from secondhand smoke, asthma and obesity are known individual-level risk factors of OSA. Among a diverse sample of urban adolescents, moderate persistent asthma was associated with higher odds of symptoms.[66] However, a study among Black, Hispanic/Latinx, and White adolescents found that asthma reduced the likelihood of severe OSA by approximately 14% among obese patients and 8% among nonobese patients; and obesity was associated with severe OSA.[67] More research is needed to further understand the association between asthma and OSA and variation by obesity status and setting (urban vs rural).

Adult and pediatric studies have reported the racial/ethnic differences in OSA may be explained by differences in BMI.[24,39,67] Obesity is a known individual-level risk factor for OSA, and racial/ethnic minorities are more likely to be obese,[68] which is partially due to social and structural determinants of health. Racial/ethnic minorities are more likely to live in disadvantaged neighborhoods that often are food deserts (eg, an area that lacks fresh good-quality food). These areas are often limited in access to healthy foods, particularly fruits and vegetables, which can increase risk of obesity. Also, neighborhood crowding is more prevalent, which is associated with BMI and OSA.[42] Racial/ethnic minorities are also exposed to more structural racism and to psychosocial stressors including interpersonal racism and discrimination, which are associated with obesity.[69]

Psychosocial factors may also be individual-level determinants of OSA among racial/ethnic minorities. In a sample of African Americans with metabolic syndrome, Ceide and colleagues reported that anxiety and depression were associated with greater odds of OSA[62]; this is consistent with an OSA screening tool developed by Johnson and colleagues that included depression in the model to predict OSA among African Americans.[70] Psychosocial factors may be salient individual-level risk factors for OSA among racial/ethnic minorities.

RACIAL/ETHNIC DISPARITIES IN TREATMENT OF OBSTRUCTIVE SLEEP APNEA

The role of social determinants of health is important to consider in the treatment of OSA. Access to care and health insurance are contributing factors to disparities in treatment. Among a study of White, Black, and additional races (not specified in the article) who attended either a voluntary hospital (VH) or a minority serving institution (MSI), 42% of the MSI patients with OSA failed to follow-up for treatment, compared with 7% of the VH group.[71] The investigators report a similar prevalence of OSA in the VH and MSI patient groups. In exploring the reasons for this difference, the MSI group had either public health insurance (Medicaid) or no health insurance, which limits the access to treatment outside of the institution. This result highlights access to care as a potential structural barrier to treatment of OSA.

Data regarding racial/ethnic differences in continuous positive airway pressure (CPAP) adherence are mixed although most of the studies suggest lower acceptance by racial/ethnic minorities. A study among African American and White patients showed similar CPAP acceptance rates, defined as the mean number of self-reported hours per week of CPAP use.[23] The optimal levels of CPAP were the same by race, which suggests that the tendency for airway closure was similar; therefore, in theory the treatment should not be more difficult in one race compared with the other. However, data from a multicenter clinical trial showed that CPAP acceptance was lower in Black compared with non-Black participants, and the participants from the lowest SES zip codes were of Black race (59%).[72] The prior study also demonstrated that CPAP acceptance was lower among those in the lowest quartile SES zip codes. Similar data exist among older adults with neurologic disorders, which have shown that adherence to OSA treatment is less likely among Black and Hispanic/Latino older adults compared with their White counterparts.[73] A study conducted in an urban public hospital found that race was associated with CPAP nonadherence. In fact, African Americans were 5 times as likely to be nonadherent than White adults.[74] However, the sample size for White patients was small (6%). There is a need to understand the barriers to CPAP adherence among racial/ethnic minority groups and if individualized combination therapies (eg, CPAP and mandibular repositioning devices) based on needs could improve adherence and treatment effectiveness.

HEALTH EQUITY INTERVENTIONS TARGETING OBSTRUCTIVE SLEEP APNEA

Intervention approaches that leverage social determinants of health frameworks have been developed to address racial/ethnic disparities in OSA. One strategy to reduce sleep disparities is to improve OSA diagnosis and treatment among the populations most at risk. For example, Jean-Louis and colleagues conducted a randomized controlled trial using a culturally tailored web-based application to improve OSA self-efficacy among community-dwelling Black adults.[75,76] Participants were provided access to the Tailored Approach to Sleep Health Education (TASHE) intervention for 2 months and were assessed at 3 intervals. Participants exposed to the TASHE content described improved OSA self-efficacy at 2 months compared with individuals who received the sleep health education.[76] Similarly, a study by Jean-Louis and colleagues assessed the effectiveness of a telephone-delivered intervention to improve OSA evaluation and treatment among Blacks with metabolic syndrome.[77] To improve these outcomes, participants received culturally and linguistically tailored health messages from a health educator to assess their challenges and willingness to change behavior. The intervention was effective in increasing sleep consultations and evaluations.[77] These prior studies are an example that tailored approaches are beneficial intervention strategies for increasing OSA assessment. In addition, peer-based approaches are also beneficial. In a population of African Americans, a peer-based sleep health education and social support approach was used to increase OSA assessment and treatment.[78] As part of the intervention, participants received 10 counseling sessions with a sleep health educator to encourage screening, diagnosis, and treatment adherence.[78] Preliminary findings showed that fewer African Americans in the control condition scheduled an OSA assessment appointment compared with those in the intervention.[78]

Similar data among pediatric populations are lacking. However, among a pediatric study of 136 children, the importance of social determinants of health was underscored. There were longer intervals from baseline evaluation to polysomnography (PSG) among children with public insurance. Thus, the investigators concluded that PSG may be a deterrent for children with public health insurance or low SES.[79] This study provides a great example for the need to understand social determinants contributing to OSA disparities, particularly surrounding delay in care with PSG and surgery for children with sleep-disordered breathing. In addition, as obesity is a strong risk factor for OSA, weight loss interventions also promoting family cohesion and emotional involvement have been shown to enhance weight loss among African Americans and may prove important for addressing pediatric OSA.[80]

FUTURE RESEARCH DIRECTIONS

In this review, the authors identified both contextual-level factors (including social determinants such as neighborhood environment) and individual-level clinical and psychosocial factors as potential contributors to racial/ethnic disparities in OSA risk, prevalence, and treatment over the life course. They also reviewed promising data from efficacy trials of social determinants of health-informed interventions that targeted OSA screening and treatment in African American adults through the delivery of culturally and linguistically tailored sleep health education about OSA. Although these represent important scientific advances in addressing racial/ethnic disparities in OSA prevalence and treatment, the authors identify 3 future research directions that represent key scientific opportunities in contemporary sleep medicine.

First, prevalence of OSA is high and seems to vary by race/ethnicity; therefore, the authors urge clinicians and researchers to consider the testing and implementation (if effective) of tailored risk factor assessments across race/ethnicity groups in order to move more individuals to treatment. For example, Johnson and colleagues developed a screening tool for African Americans with better predictive properties than more commonly used screening tools.[70] Similarly, a sex-specific screening tool designed for Hispanic/Latinx populations was also more predictive.[81] Both of these tools are available online.[70,81] Importantly, none of these tailored screening tools target pediatric OSA, which warrants future research.

Second, it is critical for the sleep medicine field to expand its focus from investigation of precision medicine that focuses on genetic factors in SDB to "precision public health."[82] Although scientific evidence has demonstrated the heritability of multiple aspects of OSA[83] including differences in craniofacial structural features leading to differential susceptibility,[37] nongenetic factors (eg, food deserts or swamps in low-income communities) can contribute to differential group vulnerability through social disadvantage, leading to, for instance, increased obesity risk. The precision public health approach will expand the field's opportunity to intervene by supporting the identification of multilevel influences (not mainly genetic with limited intervention levers) on sleep-disordered breathing across the life course. These efforts can inform the development of, for example, multifactorial community-level interventions that reflect multifactorial and modifiable determinants.[84] Moreover, because health insurance provisions alone will not address disparities caused by broader societal forces, there is a clear need for research comprehensively investigating the broad structural and individual-level social as well as environmental determinants of sleep health beyond the neighborhood. For instance, future research could determine the influence of underresourced, obesogenic residential as well as occupational environments on OSA risk overall and in terms of racial/ethnic disparities in OSA. Noting the importance of using proactive population-level efforts to change adverse social and physical environments that will likely reduce (vs merely document) OSA risk, additional investigations could include (but are not limited to) the effects of structural racism that can lead to differential exposure to household income and wealth; air pollution; occupational hazards; insecurity in terms of housing, job, and food; access to sleep specialists in underserved areas; and health (including sleep) literacy influenced by differences in educational attainment. Adverse social and physical exposures could, for instance, increase obesity risk, a strong OSA risk factor. Relatedly, these efforts must be coupled with theory-informed research (eg, intersectionality) that examines how multiple social identities (eg, race, ethnicity, gender, sexual orientation) that reflect differential access to power, privilege, and marginalization intersect with these structural and individual-level exposures to shape OSA risk.[85] In addition, it is critical to conduct more within racial/ethnic group studies to in order to identify the drivers of OSA within the population. Furthermore, socially vulnerable groups such as individuals who are minoritized and women need to be thoughtfully included in recent efforts to identify OSA phenotypes through clustering algorithms that can contribute to more personalized care or treatment.[86] In terms of symptom subtypes, it is important to know which phenotypes are associated with CVD across diverse populations as current data.[87–89] This recommendation also applies to research focused on identifying potentially superior measures (eg, hypoxic burden) to AHI.[90–92]

Third, there is an urgent need to move beyond the mere documentation of racial/ethnic disparities in OSA prevalence and treatment to the rigorous development, testing, and (if effective) wide implementation and dissemination of health equity–focused multilevel interventions for OSA across the life course. For example, Bonuck and colleagues, designed a multilevel intervention for parent-child dyads in Head Start programs that involved individual-level sleep education, a sleep media campaign, a local sleep medicine specialist in the community, and knowledge-translation strategies to change policy.[93] The prior study is currently in progress; to-date results have not been published. More studies that consider the nesting of individuals within environments with a variety of adverse and health-promoting exposures that are also culturally and linguistically tailored and that leverage the engagement of individuals along with their networks of social support are needed. Similarly, collaborative interventions that involve physicians, clinical settings, school, and community (including for example community health workers) may be the most advantageous for reducing burden of OSA among racial/ethnic minority pediatric and adult populations,[27] although this research is in its infancy. Equally important will be the systematic evaluation of interventions and their implications for health equity in order to guard against potential unintended consequences such as the widening versus narrowing of health disparities.[94] Further, interventions that target improvement of patient-provider communication as well as bolster patient satisfaction, self-efficacy, or build trust across racial/ethnic groups may represent promising and new avenues of research. To that end, a recent individual-level randomized controlled trial found that CPAP plus motivational enhancement, a behavioral intervention that targets ambivalence and self-efficacy, compared with CPAP alone increased CPAP adherence of 99 minutes in adults with moderate-to-severe OSA and cardiovascular morbidity.[95] Notably, greater than 85% of participants in this trial were non-Hispanic White, underscoring significant gaps in the testing of these evidence-based treatments that promote adherence in health disparity populations at risk of OSA and at greater risk of being undertreated for OSA. Similar data are needed among pediatric populations. There is a clear need to devote resources to conduct research and intervene earlier in the life course. Future intervention research should seek to further diversify the sample composition of sleep medicine clinical trials in order to increase the generalizability of study findings[95,96] and apply rigorous theory-informed implementation science frameworks and methods,[97,98] as well as community-based participatory research principles and precision public health[84] to identify implementation strategies and community-generated solutions to address racial/ethnic disparities in OSA prevalence and treatment.

CLINICS CARE POINTS

- Apply a health equity lens to patient care.
- Consider how OSA treatment and treatment adherence is affected by both structural and individual-level factors, and aim to address these factors.
- Include OSA patients as stakeholders in clinical decision making.
- Develop cultural tailored and competent materials in OSA-related interventions.

DISCLOSURE

The authors have no conflicts of interest to report.

REFERENCES

1. Lee W, Nagubadi S, Kryger MH, et al. Epidemiology of obstructive sleep apnea: a population-based perspective. Expert Rev Respir Med 2008;2:349–64.
2. Peppard PE, Young T, Barnet JH, et al. Increased prevalence of sleep-disordered breathing in adults. Am J Epidemiol 2013;177:1006–14.
3. Olafiranye O, Akinboboye O, Mitchell JE, et al. Obstructive sleep apnea and cardiovascular disease in blacks: a call to action from the Association of Black Cardiologists. Am Heart J 2013;165: 468–76.
4. Geovanini GR, Wang R, Weng J, et al. Association between obstructive sleep apnea and cardiovascular risk factors: variation by age, sex, and race. the

multi-ethnic study of atherosclerosis. Ann Am Thorac Soc 2018;15:970–7.

5. Johnson DA, Thomas SJ, Abdalla M, et al. Association between sleep apnea and blood pressure control among blacks: jackson heart sleep Study. Circulation 2018;139(10):1275–84.
6. Jehan S, Farag M, Zizi F, et al. Obstructive sleep apnea and stroke. Sleep Med Disord 2018;2:120–5.
7. Kendzerska T, Gershon AS, Hawker G, et al. Obstructive sleep apnea and incident diabetes. A historical cohort study. Am J Respir Crit Care Med 2014;190:218–25.
8. Graham G. Disparities in cardiovascular disease risk in the United States. Curr Cardiol Rev 2015;11: 238–45.
9. Carnethon MR, Pu J, Howard G, et al. American Heart Association Council on E, Prevention, Council on Cardiovascular Disease in the Y, Council on C, Stroke N, Council on Clinical C, Council on Functional G, Translational B and Stroke C. Cardiovascular Health in African Americans: A Scientific Statement From the American Heart Association. Circulation 2017;136:e393–423.
10. Jackson CL, Redline S, Emmons KM. Sleep as a potential fundamental contributor to disparities in cardiovascular health. Annu Rev Public Health 2015; 36:417–40.
11. Curtis DS, Fuller-Rowell TE, El-Sheikh M, et al. Habitual sleep as a contributor to racial differences in cardiometabolic risk. Proc Natl Acad Sci U S A 2017;114:8889–94.
12. Knutson KL, Van Cauter E, Rathouz PJ, et al. Association between sleep and blood pressure in midlife: the CARDIA sleep study. Arch Intern Med 2009;169: 1055–61.
13. Bowman MA, Buysse DJ, Foust JE, et al. Disturbed sleep as a mechanism of race differences in nocturnal blood pressure non-dipping. Curr Hypertens Rep 2019;21:51.
14. Smedley A, Smedley BD. Race as biology is fiction, racism as a social problem is real: anthropological and historical perspectives on the social construction of race. Am Psychol 2005;60:16–26.
15. Alvidrez J, Castille D, Laude-Sharp M, et al. The National Institute on minority health and health disparities research framework. Am J Public Health 2019; 109:S16–20.
16. McGuire TG, Alegria M, Cook BL, et al. Implementing the Institute of Medicine definition of disparities: an application to mental health care. Health Serv Res 2006;41:1979–2005.
17. Le Cook B, McGuire TG, Zuvekas SH. Measuring trends in racial/ethnic health care disparities. Med Care Res Rev 2009;66:23–48.
18. Braveman P, Egerter S, Williams DR. The social determinants of health: coming of age. Annu Rev Public Health 2011;32:381–98.
19. Chen X, Wang R, Zee P, et al. Racial/ethnic differences in sleep disturbances: the multi-ethnic study of atherosclerosis (MESA). Sleep 2015;38:877–88.
20. Jean-Louis G, von Gizycki H, Zizi F, et al. Evaluation of sleep apnea in a sample of black patients. J Clin Sleep Med 2008;4:421–5.
21. Redline S, Tishler PV, Hans MG, et al. Racial differences in sleep-disordered breathing in African-Americans and Caucasians. Am J Respir Crit Care Med 1997;155:186–92.
22. Ancoli-Israel S, Klauber MR, Stepnowsky C, et al. Sleep-disordered breathing in African-American elderly. Am J Respir Crit Care Med 1995;152: 1946–9.
23. Scharf SM, Seiden L, DeMore J, et al. Racial differences in clinical presentation of patients with sleep-disordered breathing. Sleep Breath 2004;8: 173–83.
24. O'Connor GT, Lind BK, Lee ET, et al, Sleep Heart Health Study I. Variation in symptoms of sleep-disordered breathing with race and ethnicity: the Sleep Heart Health Study. Sleep 2003;26:74–9.
25. Pranathiageswaran S, Badr MS, Severson R, et al. The influence of race on the severity of sleep disordered breathing. J Clin Sleep Med : JCSM 2013;9:303–9.
26. Johnson DA, Guo N, Rueschman M, Wang R, Wilson J and Redline S. Prevalence and Correlates of Obstructive Sleep Apnea among African Americans, the Jackson Heart Study. 2018.
27. Goldstein NA, Abramowitz T, Weedon J, et al. Racial/ethnic differences in the prevalence of snoring and sleep disordered breathing in young children. J Clin Sleep Med 2011;7:163–71.
28. Rosen RC, Zozula R, Jahn EG, et al. Low rates of recognition of sleep disorders in primary care: comparison of a community-based versus clinical academic setting. Sleep Med 2001;2:47–55.
29. Stepanski E, Zayyad A, Nigro C, et al. Sleep-disordered breathing in a predominantly African-American pediatric population. J Sleep Res 1999; 8:65–70.
30. Fernandez-Mendoza J, He F, Calhoun SL, et al. Association of pediatric obstructive sleep apnea with elevated blood pressure and orthostatic hypertension in adolescence. JAMA Cardiol 2021;6(10): 1144–51.
31. Seixas A, Ravenell J, Williams NJ, et al. Uncontrolled blood pressure and risk of sleep apnea among blacks: findings from the Metabolic Syndrome Outcome (MetSO) study. J Hum Hypertens 2016; 30.149–52.
32. Thomas SJ, Johnson DA, Guo N, et al. Association of obstructive sleep apnea with nighttime blood pressure in African Americans: the Jackson Heart Study. Am J Hypertens 2020;33(10):949–57.
33. Yano Y, Gao Y, Johnson DA, et al. Sleep characteristics and measures of glucose metabolism in blacks:

the Jackson Heart Study. J Am Heart Assoc 2020; e013209.
34. Leong WB, Arora T, Jenkinson D, et al. The prevalence and severity of obstructive sleep apnea in severe obesity: the impact of ethnicity. J Clin Sleep Med 2013;9:853–8.
35. Ong KC, Clerk AA. Comparison of the severity of sleep-disordered breathing in Asian and Caucasian patients seen at a sleep disorders center. Respir Med 1998;92:843–8.
36. Genta PR, Marcondes BF, Danzi NJ, et al. Ethnicity as a risk factor for obstructive sleep apnea: comparison of Japanese descendants and white males in Sao Paulo, Brazil. Braz J Med Biol Res 2008;41: 728–33.
37. Lee RW, Vasudavan S, Hui DS, et al. Differences in craniofacial structures and obesity in Caucasian and Chinese patients with obstructive sleep apnea. Sleep 2010;33:1075–80.
38. Shafazand S, Wallace DM, Vargas SS, et al. Sleep disordered breathing, insomnia symptoms, and sleep quality in a clinical cohort of U.S. Hispanics in south Florida. J Clin Sleep Med : JCSM : official Publ Am Acad Sleep Med 2012;8:507–14.
39. Yamagishi K, Ohira T, Nakano H, et al. Cross-cultural comparison of the sleep-disordered breathing prevalence among Americans and Japanese. Eur Respir J 2010;36:379–84.
40. Redline S, Sotres-Alvarez D, Loredo J, et al. Sleep-disordered breathing in Hispanic/Latino individuals of diverse backgrounds. The Hispanic Community Health study/study of Latinos. Am J Respir Crit Care Med 2014;189:335–44.
41. Alshehri MM, Alqahtani AS, Alenazi AM, et al. Associations between ankle-brachial index, diabetes, and sleep apnea in the Hispanic community health study/study of Latinos (HCHS/SOL) database. BMC Cardiovasc Disord 2020;20:118.
42. Johnson DA, Drake C, Joseph CL, et al. Influence of neighbourhood-level crowding on sleep-disordered breathing severity: mediation by body size. J Sleep Res 2015;24:559–65.
43. Billings ME, Gold D, Szpiro A, et al. The Association of Ambient Air Pollution with sleep apnea: the multi-ethnic study of atherosclerosis. Ann Am Thorac Soc 2018;16(3):363–70.
44. Spilsbury JC, Storfer-Isser A, Kirchner HL, et al. Neighborhood disadvantage as a risk factor for pediatric obstructive sleep apnea. J Pediatr 2006;149: 342–7.
45. Wang R, Dong Y, Weng J, et al. Associations among neighborhood, race, and sleep apnea severity in children. A Six-City Analysis. Ann Am Thorac Soc 2017;14:76–84.
46. Brouillette RT, Horwood L, Constantin E, et al. Childhood sleep apnea and neighborhood disadvantage. J Pediatr 2011;158:789–795 e1.
47. Johnson DA, Al-Ajlouni YA, Duncan DT. Connecting neighborhoods and sleep health. Social Epidemiol Sleep 2019;409.
48. Gee GC, Payne-Sturges DC. Environmental health disparities: a framework integrating psychosocial and environmental concepts. Environ Health Perspect 2004;112:1645–53.
49. Zanobetti A, Redline S, Schwartz J, et al. Associations of PM10 with sleep and sleep-disordered breathing in adults from seven U.S. urban areas. Am J Respir Crit Care Med 2010;182:819–25.
50. DeMeo DL, Zanobetti A, Litonjua AA, et al. Ambient air pollution and oxygen saturation. Am J Respir Crit Care Med 2004;170:383–7.
51. Shen YL, Liu WT, Lee KY, et al. Association of PM2.5 with sleep-disordered breathing from a population-based study in Northern Taiwan urban areas. Environ Pollut 2017;233:109–13.
52. Gerbase MW, Dratva J, Germond M, et al. Sleep fragmentation and sleep-disordered breathing in individuals living close to main roads: results from a population-based study. Sleep Med 2014;15:322–8.
53. Gislason T, Bertelsen RJ, Real FG, et al. Self-reported exposure to traffic pollution in relation to daytime sleepiness and habitual snoring: a questionnaire study in seven North-European cities. Sleep Med 2016;24:93–9.
54. Mehra R, Redline S. Sleep apnea: a proinflammatory disorder that coaggregates with obesity. J Allergy Clin Immunol 2008;121:1096–102.
55. Lopez-Jimenez F, Sert Kuniyoshi FH, Gami A, et al. Obstructive sleep apnea: implications for cardiac and vascular disease. Chest 2008;133:793–804.
56. MacNell NS, Jackson CL, Heaney CD. Relation of repeated exposures to air emissions from swine industrial livestock operations to sleep duration and awakenings in nearby residential communities. Sleep Health 2021;7(5):528–34.
57. Wu W, Jin Y, Carlsten C. Inflammatory health effects of indoor and outdoor particulate matter. J Allergy Clin Immunol 2018;141:833–44.
58. Thomas A, Grandner M, Nowakowski S, et al. Where are the Behavioral Sleep Medicine providers and where are they needed? A geographic assessment. Behav Sleep Med 2016;14:687–98.
59. Spilsbury JC, Storfer-Isser A, Rosen CL, et al. Remission and incidence of obstructive sleep apnea from middle childhood to late adolescence. Sleep 2015;38:23–9.
60. Fuller-Rowell TE, Curtis DS, El-Sheikh M, et al. Racial discrimination mediates race differences in sleep problems: a longitudinal analysis. Cultur Divers Ethnic Minor Psychol 2017;23:165–73.
61. Xie DX, Wang RY, Penn EB, et al. Understanding sociodemographic factors related to health outcomes in pediatric obstructive sleep apnea. Int J Pediatr Otorhinolaryngol 2018;111:138–41.

62. Ceide ME, Williams NJ, Seixas A, et al. Obstructive sleep apnea risk and psychological health among non-Hispanic blacks in the Metabolic Syndrome Outcome (MetSO) cohort study. Ann Med 2015;47:687–93.
63. Reardon SF, Fox L, Townsend J. Neighborhood income composition by household race and income, 1990–2009. Ann Am Acad Pol Soc Sci 2015;660:78–97.
64. Sharkey P. Spatial segmentation and the black middle class. AJS 2014;119:903–54.
65. Subramanyam R, Tapia IE, Zhang B, et al. Secondhand smoke exposure and risk of obstructive sleep apnea in children. Int J Pediatr Otorhinolaryngol 2020;130:109807.
66. Zandieh SO, Cespedes A, Ciarleglio A, et al. Asthma and subjective sleep disordered breathing in a large cohort of urban adolescents. J Asthma 2017;54:62–8.
67. Narayanan A, Yogesh A, Mitchell RB, et al. Asthma and obesity as predictors of severe obstructive sleep apnea in an adolescent pediatric population. Laryngoscope 2020;130:812–7.
68. Flegal KM, Carroll MD, Kit BK, et al. Prevalence of obesity and trends in the distribution of body mass index among US adults, 1999-2010. JAMA 2012;307:491–7.
69. Gee GC, Ro A, Gavin A, et al. Disentangling the effects of racial and weight discrimination on body mass index and obesity among Asian Americans. Am J Public Health 2008;98:493–500.
70. Johnson DA, Sofer T, Guo N, et al. A sleep apnea prediction model developed for African Americans, the Jackson Heart Sleep Study. J Clin Sleep Med 2020;16(7):1171–8.
71. Greenberg H, Fleischman J, Gouda HE, et al. Disparities in obstructive sleep apnea and its management between a minority-serving institution and a Voluntary Hospital. Sleep Breath 2004;8:185–92.
72. Billings ME, Auckley D, Benca R, et al. Race and residential socioeconomics as predictors of CPAP adherence. Sleep 2011;34:1653–8.
73. Dunietz GL, Chervin RD, Burke JF, et al. Obstructive sleep apnea treatment disparities among older adults with neurological disorders. Sleep Health 2020;6:534–40.
74. Joo MJ, Herdegen JJ. Sleep apnea in an urban public hospital: assessment of severity and treatment adherence. J Clin Sleep Med : JCSM 2007;3:285–8.
75. Williams NJ, Robbins R, Rapoport D, et al. Tailored approach to sleep health education (TASHE): study protocol for a web-based randomized controlled trial. Trials 2016;17:585.
76. Jean-Louis G, Robbins R, Williams NJ, et al. Tailored Approach to Sleep Health Education (TASHE): a randomized controlled trial of a web-based application. J Clin Sleep Med : JCSM 2020;16:1331–41.
77. Jean-Louis G, Newsome V, Williams NJ, et al. Tailored behavioral intervention among blacks with metabolic syndrome and sleep apnea: results of the metso trial. Sleep 2017;40.
78. Seixas AA, Trinh-Shevrin C, Ravenell J, et al. Culturally tailored, peer-based sleep health education and social support to increase obstructive sleep apnea assessment and treatment adherence among a community sample of blacks: study protocol for a randomized controlled trial. Trials 2018;19:519.
79. Boss EF, Benke JR, Tunkel DE, et al. Public insurance and timing of polysomnography and surgical care for children with sleep-disordered breathing. JAMA Otolaryngol Head Neck Surg 2015;141:106–11.
80. Samuel-Hodge CD, Gizlice Z, Cai J, et al. Family functioning and weight loss in a sample of African Americans and whites. Ann Behav Med 2010;40:294–301.
81. Shah N, Hanna DB, Teng Y, et al. Sex-specific prediction models for sleep apnea from the Hispanic community health study/study of Latinos. Chest 2016;149:1409–18.
82. Khoury MJ, Iademarco MF, Riley WT. Precision public health for the era of precision medicine. Am J Prev Med 2016;50:398–401.
83. Liang J, Cade BE, Wang H, et al. Comparison of heritability estimation and linkage analysis for multiple traits using principal component analyses. Genet Epidemiol 2016;40:222–32.
84. Seixas AA, Moore J, Chung A, et al. Benefits of Community-based approaches in assessing and addressing sleep health and sleep-related cardiovascular disease risk: a precision and personalized population health approach. Curr Hypertens Rep 2020;22:52.
85. Bowleg L. The problem with the phrase women and minorities: intersectionality-an important theoretical framework for public health. Am J Public Health 2012;102:1267–73.
86. Ye L, Pien GW, Ratcliffe SJ, et al. The different clinical faces of obstructive sleep apnoea: a cluster analysis. Eur Respir J 2014;44:1600–7.
87. Zinchuk AV, Jeon S, Koo BB, et al. Polysomnographic phenotypes and their cardiovascular implications in obstructive sleep apnoea. Thorax 2018;73:472–80.
88. Mazzotti DR, Keenan BT, Lim DC, et al. Symptom subtypes of obstructive sleep apnea predict incidence of cardiovascular outcomes. Am J Respir Crit Care Med 2019;200:493–506.
89. Xie J, Sort Kuniyoshi FH, Covassin N, et al. Excessive daytime sleepiness independently predicts increased cardiovascular risk after myocardial infarction. J Am Heart Assoc 2018;7.
90. Azarbarzin A, Sands SA, Taranto-Montemurro L, et al. The sleep apnea-specific hypoxic burden predicts incident heart failure. Chest 2020;158:739–50.

91. Azarbarzin A, Ostrowski M, Younes M, et al. Arousal responses during overnight polysomnography and their reproducibility in healthy young adults. Sleep 2015;38:1313–21.
92. Jackson CL, Umesi C, Gaston SA, et al. Multiple, objectively measured sleep dimensions including hypoxic burden and chronic kidney disease: findings from the Multi-Ethnic Study of Atherosclerosis. Thorax 2021;76:704–13.
93. Bonuck KA, Blank A, True-Felt B, et al. Promoting sleep health among families of young children in head start: protocol for a social-ecological approach. Preventing chronic Dis 2016;13:E121.
94. Alcántara C, Diaz SV, Cosenzo LG, et al. Social determinants as moderators of the effectiveness of health behavior change interventions: scientific gaps and opportunities. Health Psychol Rev 2020; 14:132–44.
95. Bakker JP, Wang R, Weng J, et al. Motivational enhancement for increasing adherence to CPAP: a randomized controlled trial. Chest 2016;150:337–45.
96. Alcántara C, Giorgio Cosenzo L, McCullough E, et al. Cultural adaptations of psychological interventions for prevalent sleep disorders and sleep disturbances: a systematic review of randomized controlled trials in the United States. Sleep Med Rev 2021;56:101455.
97. Damschroder LJ, Aron DC, Keith RE, et al. Fostering implementation of health services research findings into practice: a consolidated framework for advancing implementation science. Implement Sci 2009;4:50.
98. Glasgow RE, Vogt TM, Boles SM. Evaluating the public health impact of health promotion interventions: the RE-AIM framework. Am J Public Health 1999;89:1322–7.

Sleep Deficiency

A Symptoms Perspective: Exemplars from Chronic Heart Failure, Inflammatory Bowel Disease, and Breast Cancer

Nancy S. Redeker, PhD, RN[a,*], Samantha Conley, PhD[b,1], Youri Hwang, MSN, FNP-C[c,1]

KEYWORDS

- Excessive daytime sleepiness • Fatigue • Sleep disorders • Sleep • Heart failure
- Inflammatory bowel disease • Breast cancer

KEY POINTS

- Multiple aspects of sleep deficiency contribute to symptoms of excessive daytime sleepiness and fatigue.
- These sleep deficiency–related symptoms are highly prevalent and associated with poor quality of life and function, and difficulty with cognition and self-management.
- There is a critical need for efficacious sleep interventions that improve sleep deficiency, fatigue, and excessive daytime sleepiness.

INTRODUCTION

Excessive daytime sleepiness (EDS) and fatigue are important and disabling consequences of sleep deficiency. Sleep deficiency includes short, prolonged, fragmented, mistimed, and/or irregular sleep, as well as specific sleep disorders. Both fatigue and EDS are common in the general population and have multiple demographic, social, clinical, environmental, and behavioral determinants, in addition to sleep deficiency.[1–7] Sleep deficiency and sleep disorders, such as sleep-disordered breathing (SDB) and insomnia, are also prevalent among people with common chronic medical and psychiatric conditions (eg, cancer, heart disease, metabolic disease, depression) and may contribute to EDS and fatigue, as well as disease pathology (eg, worsening heart failure [HF], immune function). In turn, EDS[5] and fatigue contribute to decrements in quality of life, cognition, performance, safety, and other aspects of daily function, including the ability to perform self-care, adhere to treatment, and self-manage chronic conditions[5,8]—all of which are important to health and quality of life outcomes among people with chronic conditions. Thus, these symptoms warrant attention to predict the risk of negative health outcomes and serve as targets for intervention. The purpose of this article is to discuss the contributions of sleep deficiency and sleep disorders to fatigue and EDS among people with chronic conditions. We use exemplars from the literature on chronic HF, inflammatory bowel disease (IBD), and breast cancer (BC) to (1) describe the prevalence of fatigue and EDS and their consequences; (2) examine the evidence for the contributions of sleep deficiency and sleep disorders to these symptoms; and (3) recommend implications for future research and practice to address sleep deficiency and sleep-related daytime symptoms.

[a] UCONN School of Nursing, Yale University, University of Connecticut School of Nursing, 231 Glenbrook Road, Unit 4026, Storrs, CT 06269-4026, USA; [b] Nursing Research Division, Department of Nursing, Mayo Clinic, 200 First Street SW, Rochester, MN 55905, USA; [c] Yale School of Nursing, PO Box 27399, West Haven, CT 06516-0972, USA
[1] Present address: Office 400 West Campus Drive, Orange, CT 06477.
* Corresponding author. Office 400 West Campus Drive, Orange, CT 06477.
E-mail address: nancy.redeker@uconn.edu

Clin Chest Med 43 (2022) 217–228
https://doi.org/10.1016/j.ccm.2022.02.006
0272-5231/22/

Fatigue and EDS are highly prevalent and separate, but often overlapping, phenomena that are both consequences of sleep deficiency and sleep disorders, although sleepiness is thought to be a more specific response than fatigue to sleep loss. These symptoms are often conflated in clinical practice and research. However, differentiating them is critical to accurate diagnosis and treatment[9–11] and to addressing their negative effects. For example, people with insomnia are often not sleepy but may report fatigue.[1,10] EDS is considered a cardinal sign of sleep apnea but people with sleep apnea also report fatigue.[10] Interventions for both fatigue and sleepiness may include a focus on sleep deficiency and specific sleep disorders, as well as attention to disease characteristics and other determinants.

Fatigue is a patient-reported outcome that has been defined in various ways (eg, "vital exhaustion," "tiredness") and levels of fatigue do not consistently track with the severity of pathophysiology. The Patient-Reported Outcome System group defined it as "an overwhelming, debilitating and sustained sense of exhaustion that decreases the ability to function and carry out daily activities."[12] However, fatigue may also be characterized by both physical and psychological dimensions and distinguished by its acute versus chronic nature. Fatigue has also been described as central (arising from the central nervous system) and peripheral (arising from the peripheral nervous system or musculature), although there are variations within these conceptualizations.[13] As a patient-reported phenomenon, fatigue is measured with a variety of self-report formats, including questionnaires, visual analog scales, and other methods that use various time frames and dimensions (eg, severity, impact, frequency).

Although data are conflicting because of the wide variety of measurement methods and populations studied, the prevalence of fatigue ranges from about 22% to 32% in adults and older adults in the general population[1,4] Fatigue is more frequently reported by women than men and more prevalent among people with chronic medical and psychiatric conditions. Fatigue also depends on the severity of the disease, trajectory of the condition (eg, remissions vs exacerbations), treatment phase, and other factors, although these physical characteristics do not always correspond with fatigue severity. Chronic fatigue and cancer fatigue are generally considered to be pathologic phenomena that are not relieved by rest or sleep. However, increasing evidence suggests that sleep deficiency is an important and often modifiable contributor to multiple aspects of fatigue, and sleep extension has been shown to improve it.[14]

The International Classification of Sleep Disorders (ICSD)[15] defines EDS as difficulty staying awake and alert during the major waking period. EDS has been operationalized as both a symptom (based on self-report) and a sign (measured with objective testing, such as the multiple sleep latency test), and these measures are often discrepant.[11,13,16] Disorders of hypersomnolence that are primarily characterized by sleepiness represent a separate class of sleep disorders in the ICSD and do not explain the EDS that is a consequence of other forms of sleep deficiency.[17] EDS may also be a disorder of altered consciousness.[18] Sleepiness has been measured as both an acute and chronic phenomenon. It is responsive to acute sleep loss, but also a chronic symptom. Measurement includes both objective (ie, multiple sleep latency test, maintenance of wakefulness test, and psychomotor vigilance) and acute (ie, Stanford Sleepiness test) and chronic (Epworth Sleepiness Scale) self-report approaches. Each may elicit different attributes.[11] EDS is only resolved by obtaining adequate sleep[18] and is considered a specific response to sleep loss, with the exception of sleepiness associated with the use of sedating medications.

EDS is estimated to occur in between 9% and 28% of adults.[3,7] This wide range may be due to the use of a variety of measurement methods and specific characteristics of the populations studied. A recently completed population-based study of over 2000 community-residing adults that used the Epworth Sleepiness Scale, a well-validated self-report measure, revealed that 33% of participants reported EDS at baseline. Short sleep, sleep apnea, insomnia, and chronic medical conditions were statistically significant predictors of EDS. Prevalent EDS, described as "difficulty staying awake and alert during the major waking period," was reported in 23%[5] to 33%[2] of participants in separate studies; 28% of participants had incident sleepiness over 5 years.[2]

SLEEP DISTURBANCE, FATIGUE, AND SLEEPINESS AMONG PEOPLE WITH CHRONIC HF

People with chronic HF, a group of almost 6.5 million Americans[19] and over 26 million people worldwide,[20] often report sleep disturbance, fatigue, and EDS. As many as 75% of people with HF report poor global sleep quality[6,21]; people with HF also have more fragmented sleep and wake after sleep onset, but no shorter sleep duration than a healthy comparison group.[21] About half of the people with HF reported difficulties initiating and maintaining sleep, and wakening too early[22]—

symptoms suggestive of insomnia,[23] and from 40% to 81% of people with HF have significant SDB, including both central and obstructive sleep apnea, with rates varying between those with reduced ejection fraction compared with preserved ejection fraction and depending on measures and cut-offs for levels of the apnea-hypopnea index,[24] as well as stable versus exacerbated HF.

Fatigue is a classic symptom of HF, with rates between 28% and 90%.[25–28] This broad range is likely attributable to differences in measurement, severity, and etiology of HF, uncompensated versus stable disease, comorbidity, medications, and the presence of depression,[29] among other factors. Fatigue often occurs as a component of clustered symptoms[30–32] and may be either central or peripheral.[33] Although it has received less attention than fatigue among people with HF, EDS is also common and experienced by 21% and 44% of people with HF.[6,21,22,28,34] However, these data are generally limited to studies that focused on groups with sleep disorders, and many studies of symptoms among people with HF have not measured EDS because it has not been considered a classic symptom of HF.

Sleep deficiency, insomnia, and SDB contribute to both fatigue and EDS among people with HF, although the contributions of sleep deficiency to fatigue and EDS are often conflicting. For example, self-reported sleep disturbance, poor sleep quality,[28] and insomnia symptoms were associated with both fatigue and EDS.[23] In addition to sleep quality, functional class, nonadherence to diuretics, and lack of physical activity explained EDS, but only sleep quality was associated with fatigue ($P < .001$).[28] Notably, despite high rates of EDS in people in the general population who have SDB, SDB did not explain EDS in several studies of people with HF,[6,35–37] and self-reported EDS is lower among people with HF when compared with other groups with a similar severity of SDB.[38] Although the reasons for this discrepancy are not completely known, it may be explained by the alerting effects of sympathetic arousal associated with both HF and sleep disorders.[39,40] These findings may also be explained by discrepancies between self-reported EDS and objective measures of alertness, such as the psychomotor vigilance test. Patients with HF may not be aware of objective decrements in behavioral alertness.[16,41] Each of these measures may elicit different dimensions of sleepiness,[11] and people with objective decrements may not self-report sleepiness.

Sleep-related fatigue and EDS are important concerns for people with HF as they may signal the presence of sleep disorders, but they also contribute to other HF outcomes, including daytime function, cognition, medication adherence, and self-care related to HF. EDS was associated with physical function, measured with the Kansas City Cardiomyopathy Scale and the Medical Outcomes Study SF-12.[42] A latent variable consisting of sleepiness, fatigue, and depressive symptoms mediated the effects of insomnia and sleep quality on self-report functional performance and 6-minute walk distance among people with stable HF. This relationship was not explained by SDB, comorbidity, or HF severity.[43] However, the cross-sectional nature of these data precludes understanding of the causal or temporal relationships among these phenomena.

EDS was also associated with self-care among people with HF in a small study.[44] Although EDS was associated with cognitive impairment, an important influence on self-care, in middle-aged adults with HF.[45] EDS was independently associated with medication adherence, an important self-care behavior.[46] In contrast, fatigue, but not sleep disturbance, was also associated with self-care behavior in 2 studies,[29,47] and despite the frequent association of depression with fatigue symptoms, depression did not explain this relationship.[47]

Given the prevalence and consequences of both EDS and sleep-related fatigue and the influence of sleep deficiency and specific sleep disorders on these outcomes, treatment of sleep deficiency, including sleep apnea, insomnia, and short sleep, may improve fatigue and sleepiness. However, the data are somewhat conflicting. Among people with HF and central sleep apnea, adaptive servo-ventilation did not improve daytime sleepiness,[48] whereas both exercise and continuous positive airway pressure (CPAP) improved the apnea-hypopnea index and daytime sleepiness in people with HF and obstructive sleep apnea. However, the effects of exercise were larger than CPAP on function.[49] Autotitrating CPAP also improved EDS, but not other outcomes among people with chronic HF and obstructive sleep apnea.[50]

There is also evidence that treatment of insomnia may also improve EDS, fatigue, and functional outcomes in HF. Cognitive behavioral therapy for insomnia (CBT-I) had large effects on fatigue, but not EDS among people with insomnia.[51] Pharmacologic treatment of insomnia may also improve insomnia and in, turn, EDS and fatigue, but benzodiazepines were associated with adverse prognosis in HF,[52] and patients with HF expressed concern about their potential addictive effects.[53] In addition, the negative effects of polypharmacy and drug interactions are important to consider, given the large number of prescribed medications taken by people with HF. A small group of HF patients with insomnia also reported frequent use of over-the-counter diphenhydramine-containing products that produced daytime sedation and functional impairment. Administration of melatonin has beneficial cardiovascular effects[54] and may be cardioprotective for ischemic HF.[55] Although data are not conclusive, melatonin has been effective for sleep-onset insomnia and sleep disturbance,[56] including among older adults.[57] Newer insomnia drugs and wake-promoting agents may also play a role in the treatment of insomnia among people with HF, but data on their safety in this population are not consistently available. Given the widespread efficacy of CBT-I in other groups, including those with chronic conditions, CBT-I alone or in combination with melatonin or other agents may be efficacious.

Considerable attention has been focused by the sleep disorders community on SDB among people with HF. However, increasing evidence suggests that insomnia is also common,[58] frequently comorbid with,[23,51] and not explained by[23] SDB. These findings suggest the importance of treating both conditions together. However, to the best of our knowledge, there has not been a randomized controlled trial among people with HF. This may be beneficial in improving cardiovascular function, as well as EDS, fatigue, and daytime function.

SLEEP DISTURBANCE, EDS, AND FATIGUE AMONG PEOPLE WITH IBD

IBD, a chronic progressive immune-mediated disease that includes Crohn disease and ulcerative colitis, afflicts 1.6 million people in the United States.[59] IBD is characterized by intestinal inflammation and follows an unpredictable course of active and inactive disease. The disease burden in people with IBD is high as most people with IBD are diagnosed in adolescence and young adulthood. People with IBD experience significant life disruptions to education and careers and poor quality of life.[60,61]

Self-reported sleep disturbance is highly prevalent in adults with IBD, with between 55% and 78% reporting poor sleep quality during active disease and 33% to 64% during inactive disease.[62–64] Although fewer data are available on objectively measured sleep characteristics in IBD, polysomnographic and wrist actigraph studies demonstrate that sleep is short and highly fragmented, further supporting that this population faces substantial sleep deficiency.[65–68]

Self-reported sleep disturbance is associated with increased risk for clinically active disease over 6 and 12 months[62,69] and increased risk of hospitalizations and IBD-related surgery over 1 year.[70] These results are supported by mouse models of colitis, in which intermittent sleep deprivation and shifting of sleep timing cause worsening of colonic inflammation.[71,72] Worsening of disease activity may result from the negative effects of sleep deficiency on the immune system as chronic sleep deprivation increases proinflammatory cytokines (eg, IL-6 and IL-1β) in healthy adults. These cytokines are key in regulating the immune response of the gastrointestinal tract.[73] These results suggest that interventions that target sleep deficiency in this population may not only improve sleep but may also improve gastrointestinal and systemic inflammation and possibly daytime consequences, including bowel symptoms and fatigue.

Fatigue continues to be an unmet need for people with IBD, and a key patient-reported outcome.[74] Fatigue is a severe and prevalent symptom in people with IBD and about 55% of people with IBD experience substantial fatigue.[75,76] Although fatigue is often worse during active disease, it persists during inactive phases of IBD.[62] Both self-reported sleep disturbance and evening chronotype were associated with fatigue among people with IBD.[62,77,78] However, how specific aspects of sleep deficiency (eg, duration, timing, fragmentation) are associated with fatigue is unknown.

Despite the apparent high levels of sleep deficiency and fatigue among people with IBD, they do not report substantial EDS measured by the Epworth Sleepiness Scale even during active disease.[66,68] These findings may reflect the conceptual distinction between EDS and fatigue, but it is also possible that objective measurement of EDS may reveal decreased alertness given the high levels of sleep deficiency in this population. Future studies with objective measurements are needed to address this possibility.

As in some other groups with chronic conditions (eg, HF, cancer, chronic obstructive pulmonary disease), fatigue often co-occurs with symptoms of pain, sleep disturbance, and mood disturbance, with symptoms persisting for as long as a year or more.[79] Despite evidence from several studies of self-reported sleep disturbance, little is known about the contributions of specific objective measures of sleep fragmentation, sleep timing, or sleep disorders to fatigue in IBD. Likewise, there are no studies that examined the biological mechanisms that may explain the relationships between sleep deficiency and fatigue, such as potentially common inflammatory pathways (eg, cytokines, gut microbiome) in co-occurring fatigue and sleep deficiency in people with IBD. These foundational studies are needed to illuminate the type and timing of sleep intervention needed to improve sleep deficiency ad sleep-related fatigue in this population.

Despite the prevalence of sleep disturbance among people with IBD, there have been few studies of interventions to improve sleep deficiency and sleep-related fatigue. A 4-week stepped care brief behavioral therapy (BBT) for IBD, with the addition of bupropion for some individuals, improved both fatigue and sleep disturbance in young adults ages 15 to 30 years with IBD.[80] However, although fatigue improved, it did not fully resolve for any of the participants and the addition of the bupropion did not improve on BBT alone. The follow-up for this study was only 12 weeks, and improvements in fatigue may require a longer duration follow-up duration to be seen. In addition, although sleep disturbance improved, objective sleep characteristics were not elicited; thus, it is unclear which specific characteristics of sleep may have improved after the intervention. A second study of an 8-week aerobic exercise intervention for children and adolescents with IBD improved polysomnographic-measured deep sleep and wake after sleep onset but not self-report sleep disturbance.[81] Notably, fatigue outcomes were not assessed. These studies suggest the importance of symptom management among people with IBD, but studies are needed that examine the extent to which improvements in sleep lead to improved daytime symptoms, such as EDS and fatigue.

Biologic therapy for IBD with vedolizumab and antitumor necrosis factor α agents also improved sleep disturbance over 6 weeks.[82] However, the effects on sleep may be related to improvement in disease activity, reduction of systemic cytokines, and/or nighttime symptoms (eg, nocturnal diarrhea) rather than direct effects on sleep. Although these interventions show promise, additional research is needed to determine the types and timing of sleep interventions that improve not only sleep deficiency but also reduce the risk of active disease and fatigue.

SLEEP DISTURBANCE, FATIGUE, AND EDS AMONG WOMEN WITH BC

BC is the most common cancer in women around the world. In the United States, there are 3.8 million women with a history of BC.[83] Women treated for BC are at risk for persistent physical and psychological comorbid symptoms before, during, and after cancer treatment, including sleep disturbance, fatigue, and EDS. These symptoms may vary over the trajectory of treatment, but they persist long after treatment for many women.

Fatigue is the most common, persistent symptom in adults with cancer in general, and cancer-related fatigue is distinguished from the broader concept of fatigue as it does not improve with sleep or rest. It is characterized by long duration and high severity and a consequence of cancer or its treatment.[84,85] Before adjuvant chemotherapy, 72% of patients report mild fatigue and 27% reported moderate fatigue.[86] As many as 99% of women undergoing chemotherapy and/or radiation therapy report some degree of fatigue.[84] A meta-analysis of 68 studies involving 12,125 women revealed that the prevalence of severe self-reported fatigue is 27% in women with BC across stages 0 to IIII.[87] Although studies suggest that fatigue improves after the first 6 months following the last cancer treatment,[87,88] approximately 34% of women with BC report fatigue after 10 years of cancer survivorship.[89]

Patients with BC frequently report sleepiness with fatigue, but these terms are not well differentiated.[84] During chemotherapy, 38% of women reported EDS measured by the Epworth Sleepiness Scale.[90] Among recently diagnosed women, physical and attentional fatigue predicted the trajectory of daytime sleepiness, assessed by the General Sleep Disturbance Scale, over the continuum of treatment.[91] Women with more education and those who did not receive neoadjuvant chemotherapy had higher levels of EDS over time.[91] Younger age and more acute pain were also significantly associated with EDS.[92] Future studies are needed to investigate the relationship between fatigue and EDS to better distinguish these symptoms and to focus interventions among oncology patients.[10]

Sleep deficiency is closely associated with fatigue through inflammatory processes in patients with cancer.[93] Before breast surgery, interleukin-6, interleukin-13, and tumor necrosis factor α were associated with greater level of a symptom cluster of self-reported sleep disturbance, fatigue, pain, and depressive mood.[94] However, the exact mechanism has not been clearly determined,[95,96] and more studies are needed to confirm the underlying mechanisms that explain these linkages, as well as the causal directions as sleep deficiency may also contribute to inflammation.

Although fatigue and EDS have multiple determinants, self-reported sleep disturbance is among the most common debilitating symptoms in women with BC[97] and contributes to these outcomes. Self-reported sleep disturbance refers to a symptom caused by sleep deficiency defined as deficiency in the quantity or quality of sleep to maintain optimal health.[98] Sleep disorders, insufficient sleep duration, and fragmented sleep can cause sleep deficiency.[98] Overall, 67% to 90% of women report sleep disturbance and up to 70% of women experience insomnia symptoms (eg, difficulty falling asleep, staying asleep).[91,99,100] Before adjuvant chemotherapy, 36% to 66% report sleep disturbance as measured with the Pittsburgh Sleep Quality (PSQI),[86,101–104] and these rates may change over the course of treatment and recovery. During chemotherapy, 49% to 58% report sleep disturbance.[101,103] Sleep disturbance persists after completion of cancer treatment, with 38% report poor sleep quality assessed by the PSQI at 5 years after cancer treatment and continues to worsen over the course of cancer survivorship.[91,101,105,106]

Although symptoms of sleep disturbance, as a result of sleep deficiency, are widely studied in women with BC, few studies specifically determined the presence of specific sleep disorders, with the exception of insomnia.[107] The prevalence rate of insomnia in patients with BC is over 30% and it is higher than patients of other cancer types.[108,109] Possible contributing factors to insomnia in women with BC include female sex, stress related to the cancer diagnosis and treatment, psychological symptoms of anxiety and depression, and chronic maladaptive sleep behaviors that may lead to chronic insomnia.[93] In post-treatment women diagnosed with stage 0 to III BC, 98% reported symptoms of chronic insomnia and 79% reported symptoms suggestive of SDB.[97] Although the reasons for risk for SDB are not completely clear, weight gain is common in patients with BC,[110–112] and the relationship between high body mass index (BMI) and SDB is well established.[113] There is also evidence of a positive relationship between BMI and daytime sleepiness and difficulty falling asleep in women with BC.[91,114] Given that EDS is one of the common symptoms reported with SDB, the increased incidence of SDB with menopause, and the high prevalence of chemotherapy-induced menopause following BC treatment, there is a need for more study on SDB in patients with BC, given the limited body of research or consideration of SDB in this population.

Numerous studies assessed the effects of physical exercise and mind-body interventions on sleep deficiency and CBT-I among women with BC.[115–117] Based on a meta-analysis of 14 randomized controlled trials of CBT-I on insomnia in patients with BC, CBT-I has medium to large intervention effects on improving insomnia symptoms among women with BC.[115] Although this meta-analysis did not report the pooled effect size of CBT-I on fatigue, 9 of 14 studies measured fatigue with various fatigue measures (eg, Multidimensional Fatigue Symptom Inventory, Piper Fatigue Scale) in addition to insomnia symptoms.[115] There is evidence that CBT-I also improves fatigue in post-treatment patients with BC.[118,119] CBT-I also significantly improved daytime sleepiness, assessed by the Epworth Sleepiness Scale, among post-treatment patients with various cancer types (70% or more BC).[120]

Mind-body interventions, such as mindfulness-based stress reduction intervention, improve sleep and fatigue in women with BC, although effects were small and measured only over the short term.[117] With regards to cancer-related fatigue, physical exercise and psychological interventions are clinical recommendations in practice because they have shown a significant benefit over pharmaceutical interventions in improving fatigue.[121] These interventions may also improve sleep, although the extent to which improvements in fatigue are associated with reducing sleep deficiency is understudied. Although the results of studies were not consistent, a meta-analysis suggested that oral administration of melatonin may also improve insomnia and sleep disturbance in cancer.[122] Taken together, these studies suggest that intervention may be effective in improving sleep deficiency and fatigue–significant problems in the BC population. However, future research is needed.

There is a need for research to assess the relationship between sleep deficiency and sleep-related daytime symptoms and shared underlying biological and behavioral mechanisms, as well as the differential effects of interventions over the course of treatment, recovery, and survivorship. The relationship between fatigue and EDS needs to be clearly defined and investigated to develop effective interventions. In addition, identifying sleep disorders, such as SDB, and their associations with EDS would enhance our understanding of sleep deficiency in patients with BC. The effect of CBT-I and mind-body interventions on sleep deficiency and sleep-related daytime symptoms requires further investigation.

IMPLICATIONS FOR PRACTICE AND FUTURE RESEARCH

Sleep deficiency, EDS, and fatigue are important phenomena experienced by people with chronic conditions that influence the quality of life, function, safety, and the ability to self-manage. Sleep deficiency also contributes to pathophysiologic processes that may also lead to fatigue, EDS, and poor function. We discussed exemplars from 3 specific chronic conditions, but adults with other chronic conditions also suffer from the negative effects of sleep deficiency, fatigue, and EDS.[123,124] As with the other exemplars provided, these people demonstrate improvement in symptoms and function with appropriate treatment of sleep deficiency, including insomnia,[125] SDB,[126] and fragmented or irregular sleep. Thus, focused assessment and intervention for sleep deficiency and associated daytime symptoms should be an important component of chronic disease management. Although this may seem obvious, patients have reported that despite their high levels of concern about their sleep quality and its negative daytime effects, non-sleep specialist clinicians often do not elicit this information.[53] Although the reasons for this are likely factorial, inclusion of specific questions in the health history regarding sleep and providing referral for sleep assessment and treatment may improve chronic disease management for these patients and should be an important component of the standard of care, especially for people at high risk for sleep deficiency.

Despite growing reports of the contributions of sleep disturbance to fatigue and EDS among people with chronic conditions, additional research is needed to define the contributions of specific sleep characteristics and disorders to daytime symptoms, as well as disease pathology, given that many studies focused on global self-reported sleep quality. This measure does not provide information to guide understanding of specific sleep mechanisms or targets for interventions focused on specific sleep characteristics (eg, duration, timing, regularity, fragmentation, or specific sleep disorders).

Although interventions such as cognitive behavioral therapy for insomnia have shown efficacy for some chronic conditions, others might focus on sleep variability or circadian regulation but have seldom been considered in these populations. Given the close interrelationships between sleep deficiency, EDS, and fatigue, sleep-promoting interventions for people with chronic conditions should also address these outcomes. Mechanistic studies that address multiple levels, including biological, psychological, clinical, and environmental factors are also needed to improve understanding of the contributions of sleep deficiency to EDS and fatigue. For example, studies of inflammation[127] and the microbiome[128] are beginning to provide useful information.

SUMMARY

Fatigue and EDS are often consequences of sleep deficiency, and these phenomena are common among people with chronic conditions among whom sleep deficiency and sleep disorders are prevalent. There is a need for careful clinical assessment and intervention for these phenomena because of their influences on health outcomes in this large and growing population of adults. Although research remains needed, efficacious interventions are available to improve these disabling symptoms.

CLINICS CARE POINTS

- Fatigue and excessive daytime sleepiness are common and disabling symptoms among people with chronic heart failure, inflammatory bowel disease, and breast cancer.
- These symptoms may warrant further assessment and treatment of sleep deficiency and sleep.
- Treatment of sleep deficiency and specific sleep disorders may improve these daytime symptoms.

DISCLOSURE

The authors have nothing to disclose.

REFERENCES

1. Galland-Decker C, Marques-Vidal P, Vollenweider P. Prevalence and factors associated with fatigue in the Lausanne middle-aged population: a population-based, cross-sectional survey. BMJ open 2019;9(8):e027070.
2. Jaussent I, Morin CM, Ivers H, et al. Natural history of excessive daytime sleepiness: a population-based 5-year longitudinal study. Sleep 2020; 43(3):zsz249.
3. Jaussent I, Morin CM, Ivers H, et al. Incidence, worsening and risk factors of daytime sleepiness in a population-based 5-year longitudinal study. Scientific Rep 2017;7(1):1372.
4. Meng H, Hale L, Friedberg F. Prevalence and predictors of fatigue in middle-aged and older adults: evidence from the health and retirement study. J Am Geriatr Soc 2010;58(10):2033–4.
5. Kolla BP, He JP, Mansukhani MP, et al. Excessive sleepiness and associated symptoms in the U.S. adult population: prevalence, correlates, and comorbidity. Sleep Health 2020;6(1):79–87.
6. Redeker NS, Muench U, Zucker MJ, et al. Sleep disordered breathing, daytime symptoms, and functional performance in stable heart failure. Sleep 2010;33(4):551–60.
7. Berger M, Hirotsu C, Haba-Rubio J, et al. Risk factors of excessive daytime sleepiness in a

prospective population-based cohort. J Sleep Res 2021;30(2):e13069.

8. Riegel B, Lee CS, Ratcliffe SJ, et al. Predictors of objectively measured medication nonadherence in adults with heart failure. Circ Heart Fail 2012; 5(4):430–6.
9. Singareddy R, Bixler EO, Vgontzas AN. Fatigue or daytime sleepiness? J Clin Sleep Med 2010;6(4): 405.
10. Pigeon WR, Sateia MJ, Ferguson RJ. Distinguishing between excessive daytime sleepiness and fatigue: toward improved detection and treatment. J Psychosom Res 2003;54(1):61–9.
11. Trotti LM. Characterizing sleepiness: are we drawing the right line in the sand? J Clin Sleep Med 2017;13(12):1369–70.
12. Cella D, Yount S, Rothrock N, et al. The patient-reported outcomes measurement information system (PROMIS): progress of an NIH Roadmap cooperative group during its first two years. Med Care 2007;45(5 Suppl 1):S3–11.
13. Shen J, Barbera J, Shapiro CM. Distinguishing sleepiness and fatigue: focus on definition and measurement. Sleep Med Rev 2006;10(1):63–76.
14. Mantua J, Skeiky L, Prindle N, et al. Sleep extension reduces fatigue in healthy, normally-sleeping young adults. Sleep Sci 2019;12(1):21–7.
15. Medicine AAoS. International classification of sleep disorders. 3rd edition. Darien, IL: American Academy of Sleep Medicine; 2014.
16. Mehra R, Wang L, Andrews N, et al. Dissociation of objective and subjective daytime sleepiness and biomarkers of systemic inflammation in sleep-disordered breathing and systolic heart failure. J Clin Sleep Med 2017;13(12):1411–22.
17. Gandhi KD, Mansukhani MP, Silber MH, et al. Excessive daytime sleepiness: a clinical review. Mayo Clin Proc 2021;96(5):1288–301.
18. Hitchcott PK, Menicucci D, Frumento S, et al. The neurophysiological basis of excessive daytime sleepiness: suggestions of an altered state of consciousness. Sleep Breath 2020;24(1):15–23.
19. Virani SS, Alonso A, Benjamin EJ, et al. Heart disease and stroke statistics-2020 update: a report from the american heart association. Circulation 2020;141(9):e139–596.
20. Savarese G, Lund LH. Global public health burden of heart failure. Card Fail Rev 2017;3(1): 7–11.
21. Redeker NS, Stein S. Characteristics of sleep in patients with stable heart failure versus a comparison group. Heart Lung 2006;35(4):252–61.
22. Johansson P, Alehagen U, Svensson E, et al. Determinants of global perceived health in community-dwelling elderly screened for heart failure and sleep-disordered breathing. J Cardiovasc Nurs 2010;25(5):E16–26.
23. Redeker NS, Jeon S, Muench U, et al. Insomnia symptoms and daytime function in stable heart failure. Sleep 2010;33(9):1210–6.
24. Khattak HK, Hayat F, Pamboukian SV, et al. Obstructive sleep apnea in heart failure: review of prevalence, treatment with continuous positive airway pressure, and prognosis. Tex Heart Inst J 2018;45(3):151–61.
25. Williams BA. The clinical epidemiology of fatigue in newly diagnosed heart failure. BMC Cardiovasc Disord 2017;17(1):122.
26. Evangelista LS, Moser DK, Westlake C, et al. Correlates of fatigue in patients with heart failure. Prog Cardiovasc Nurs 2008;23(1):12–7.
27. Ishida H, Makaya M. Fatigue in patients with heart failure: results from a systematic review. J Card Fail 2017;23(10):S47.
28. Riegel B, Ratcliffe SJ, Sayers SL, et al. Determinants of excessive daytime sleepiness and fatigue in adults with heart failure. Clin Nurs Res 2012; 21(3):271–93.
29. Fink AM, Gonzalez RC, Lisowski T, et al. Fatigue, inflammation, and projected mortality in heart failure. J Card Fail 2012;18(9):711–6.
30. Park J, Moser DK, Griffith K, et al. Exploring symptom clusters in people with heart failure. Clin Nurs Res 2019;28(2):165–81.
31. Yu DS, Li PW, Chong SO. Symptom cluster among patients with advanced heart failure: a review of its manifestations and impacts on health outcomes. Curr Opin Support Palliat Care 2018;12(1):16–24.
32. Smith OR, Gidron Y, Kupper N, et al. Vital exhaustion in chronic heart failure: symptom profiles and clinical outcome. J Psychosom Res 2009;66(3): 195–201.
33. Matura LA, Malone S, Jaime-Lara R, et al. A systematic review of biological mechanisms of fatigue in chronic illness. Biol Res Nurs 2018; 20(4):410–21.
34. Brostrom A, Stromberg A, Dahlstrom U, et al. Sleep difficulties, daytime sleepiness, and health-related quality of life in patients with chronic heart failure. J Cardiovasc Nurs 2004;19(4):234–42.
35. Wang HQ, Chen G, Li J, et al. Subjective sleepiness in heart failure patients with sleep-related breathing disorder. Chin Med J (Engl) 2009; 122(12):1375–9.
36. Johansson P, Arestedt K, Alehagen U, et al. Sleep disordered breathing, insomnia, and health related quality of life – a comparison between age and gender matched elderly with heart failure or without cardiovascular disease. Eur J Cardiovasc Nurs 2010;9(2):108–17.
37. Pak VM, Strouss L, Yaggi HK, et al. Mechanisms of reduced sleepiness symptoms in heart failure and obstructive sleep apnea. J Sleep Res 2019;28(5): e12778.

38. Arzt M, Young T, Finn L, et al. Sleepiness and sleep in patients with both systolic heart failure and obstructive sleep apnea. Arch Intern Med 2006; 166(16):1716–22.
39. Taranto Montemurro L, Floras JS, Millar PJ, et al. Inverse relationship of subjective daytime sleepiness to sympathetic activity in patients with heart failure and obstructive sleep apnea. Chest 2012;142(5): 1222–8.
40. Atalla A, Carlisle TW, Simonds AK, et al. Sleepiness and activity in heart failure patients with reduced ejection fraction and central sleep-disordered breathing. Sleep Med 2017;34:217–23.
41. Masterson Creber R, Pak VM, Varrasse M, et al. Determinants of behavioral alertness in adults with heart failure. J Clin Sleep Med 2016;12(4): 589–96.
42. Piamjariyakul U, Shapiro AL, Wang K, et al. Impact of sleep apnea, daytime sleepiness, comorbidities, and depression on patients' heart failure health status. Clin Nurs Res 2021;30(8):1222–30.
43. Jeon S, Redeker NS. Sleep disturbance, daytime symptoms, and functional performance in patients with stable heart failure: a mediation analysis. Nurs Res 2016;65(4):259–67.
44. Riegel B, Vaughan Dickson V, Goldberg LR, et al. Factors associated with the development of expertise in heart failure self-care. Nurs Res 2007;56(4): 235–43.
45. Byun E, Kim J, Riegel B. Associations of subjective sleep quality and daytime sleepiness with cognitive impairment in adults and elders with heart failure. Behav Sleep Med 2017;15(4):302–17.
46. Riegel B, Moelter ST, Ratcliffe SJ, et al. Excessive daytime sleepiness is associated with poor medication adherence in adults with heart failure. J Card Fail 2011;17(4):340–8.
47. Kessing D, Denollet J, Widdershoven J, et al. Fatigue and self-care in patients with chronic heart failure. Eur J Cardiovasc Nurs 2016;15(5):337–44.
48. Yang H, Sawyer AM. The effect of adaptive servo ventilation (ASV) on objective and subjective outcomes in Cheyne-Stokes respiration (CSR) with central sleep apnea (CSA) in heart failure (HF): a systematic review. Heart Lung 2016;45(3): 199–211.
49. Servantes DM, Javaheri S, Kravchychyn ACP, et al. Effects of exercise training and cpap in patients with heart failure and OSA: a preliminary study. Chest 2018;154(4):808–17.
50. Smith LA, Vennelle M, Gardner RS, et al. Auto-titrating continuous positive airway pressure therapy in patients with chronic heart failure and obstructive sleep apnoea: a randomized placebo-controlled trial. Eur Heart J 2007;28(10):1221–7.
51. Redeker NS, Jeon S, Andrews L, et al. Feasibility and Efficacy of a self-management intervention for insomnia in stable heart failure. J Clin Sleep Med 2015;11(10):1109–19.
52. Sato Y, Yoshihisa A, Hotsuki Y, et al. Associations of benzodiazepine with adverse prognosis in heart failure patients with insomnia. J Am Heart Assoc 2020;9(7):e013982.
53. Andrews LK, Coviello J, Hurley E, et al. I'd eat a bucket of nails if you told me it would help me sleep:" perceptions of insomnia and its treatment in patients with stable heart failure. Heart Lung 2013;42(5):339–45.
54. Pandi-Perumal SR, BaHammam AS, Ojike NI, et al. Melatonin and human cardiovascular disease. J Cardiovasc Pharmacol Ther 2017;22(2):122–32.
55. Sehirli AO, Koyun D, Tetik S, et al. Melatonin protects against ischemic heart failure in rats. J Pineal Res 2013;55(2):138–48.
56. Baglioni C, Bostanova Z, Bacaro V, et al. A systematic review and network meta-analysis of randomized controlled trials evaluating the evidence base of melatonin, light exposure, exercise, and complementary and alternative medicine for patients with insomnia disorder. J Clin Med 2020;9(6):1949.
57. Pierce M, Linnebur SA, Pearson SM, et al. Optimal melatonin dose in older adults: a clinical review of the literature. Sr Care Pharm 2019;34(7):419–31.
58. Javaheri S, Redline S. Insomnia and risk of cardiovascular disease. Chest 2017;152(2):435–44.
59. Shivashankar R, Tremaine WJ, Harmsen WS, et al. Incidence and prevalence of Crohn's disease and ulcerative colitis in Olmsted County, Minnesota from 1970 through 2010. Clin Gastroenterol Hepatol 2017;15(6):857–63.
60. Blue Cross Blue S. The health of millennials. Available at: https://www.bcbs.com/the-health-of-america/reports/the-health-of-millennials. 2019. Accessed August 20, 2021.
61. Jones JL, Nguyen GC, Benchimol EI, et al. The impact of inflammatory bowel disease in Canada 2018: quality of life. J Can Assoc Gastroenterol 2019;2(Suppl 1):S42–8.
62. Graff LA, Vincent N, Walker JR, et al. A population-based study of fatigue and sleep difficulties in inflammatory bowel disease. Inflamm Bowel Dis 2011;17(9):1882–9.
63. Hood MM, Wilson R, Gorenz A, et al. Sleep quality in ulcerative colitis: associations with inflammation, psychological distress, and quality of life. Int J Behav Med 2018;25(5):517–25.
64. Marinelli C, Savarino EV, Marsilio I, et al. Sleep disturbance in Inflammatory bowel disease: prevalence and risk factors - a cross-sectional study. Scientific Rep 2020;10(1):507.
65. Bar-Gil Shitrit A, Chen-Shuali C, Adar T, et al. Sleep disturbances can be prospectively observed in patients with an inactive inflammatory bowel disease. Dig Dis Sci 2018;63(11):2992–7.

66. Bazin T, Micoulaud Franchi JA, Terras N, et al. Altered sleep quality is associated with Crohn's disease activity: an actimetry study. Sleep Breath 2020;24(3):971–7.
67. Conley S, Jeon S, Lehner V, et al. Sleep characteristics and rest-activity rhythms are associated with gastrointestinal symptoms among adults with inflammatory bowel disease. Dig Dis Sci 2021; 66(1):181–9.
68. Qazi T, Verma R, Hamilton MJ, et al. The use of actigraphy differentiates sleep disturbances in active and inactive Crohn's disease. Inflamm Bowel Dis 2019;25(6):1044–53.
69. Ananthakrishnan AN, Long MD, Martin CF, et al. Sleep disturbance and risk of active disease in patients with Crohn's disease and ulcerative colitis. Clin Gastroenterol Hepatol 2013;11(8): 965–71.
70. Sofia MA, Lipowska AM, Zmeter N, et al. Poor Sleep quality in crohn's disease is associated with disease activity and risk for hospitalization or surgery. Inflamm Bowel Dis 2020;26(8):1251–9.
71. Preuss F, Tang Y, Laposky AD, et al. Adverse effects of chronic circadian desynchronization in animals in a "challenging" environment. Am J Physiol Regul Integr Comp Physiol 2008;295(6):2034.
72. Tang Y, Preuss F, Turek FW, et al. Sleep deprivation worsens inflammation and delays recovery in a mouse model of colitis. Sleep Med 2009;10(6): 597–603.
73. Irwin MR. Sleep and inflammation: partners in sickness and in health. Nat Rev Immunol 2019;19(11): 702–15.
74. Hindryckx P, Laukens D, D'Amico F, et al. Unmet needs in IBD: the case of fatigue. Clin Rev Allergy Immunol 2018;55(3):368–78.
75. Schreiner P, Biedermann L, Valko PO, et al. Fatigue in inflammatory bowel disease and its impact on daily activities. Aliment Pharmacol Ther 2021; 53(1):138–49.
76. Villoria A, Garcia V, Dosal A, et al. Fatigue in outpatients with inflammatory bowel disease: prevalence and predictive factors. PLoS One 2017; 12(7):e0181435.
77. Chrobak AA, Nowakowski J, Zwolinska-Wcislo M, et al. Associations between chronotype, sleep disturbances and seasonality with fatigue and inflammatory bowel disease symptoms. Chronobiol Int 2018;35(8):1142–52.
78. Hashash JG, Ramos-Rivers C, Youk A, et al. Quality of sleep and coexistent psychopathology have significant impact on fatigue burden in patients with inflammatory bowel disease. J Clin Gastroenterol 2018;52(5):423–30.
79. Conley S, Proctor DD, Jeon S, et al. Symptom clusters in adults with inflammatory bowel disease. Res Nurs Health 2017;40(5):424–34.
80. Hashash JG, Knisely MR, Germain A, et al. Brief behavioral therapy and bupropion for sleep and fatigue in young adults with crohn's disease: an exploratory open trial study. Clin Gastroenterol Hepatol 2022;20(1):96–104.
81. Mählmann L, Gerber M, Furlano RI, et al. Aerobic exercise training in children and adolescents with inflammatory bowel disease: influence on psychological functioning, sleep and physical performance – an exploratory trial. Ment Health Phys activity 2017;13:30–9.
82. Stevens BW, Borren NZ, Velonias G, et al. Vedolizumab therapy is associated with an improvement in sleep quality and mood in inflammatory bowel diseases. Dig Dis Sci 2017;62(1):197–206.
83. ACS. Cancer. Treatment & survivorship: facts & figures 2019-2021. Atlanta, GA: American Cancer Society; 2019.
84. Bardwell WA, Ancoli-Israel S. Breast cancer and fatigue. Sleep Med Clin 2008;3(1):61–71.
85. Berger AM, Mooney K, Alvarez-Perez A, et al. Cancer-related fatigue, version 2.2015. J Natl Compr Canc Netw 2015;13(8):1012–39.
86. Berger AM, Farr LA, Kuhn BR, et al. Values of sleep/wake, activity/rest, circadian rhythms, and fatigue prior to adjuvant breast cancer chemotherapy. J Pain Symptom Manage 2007;33(4):398–409.
87. Abrahams HJG, Gielissen MFM, Schmits IC, et al. Risk factors, prevalence, and course of severe fatigue after breast cancer treatment: a meta-analysis involving 12 327 breast cancer survivors. Ann Oncol 2016;27(6):965–74.
88. Biering K, Frydenberg M, Pappot H, et al. The long-term course of fatigue following breast cancer diagnosis. J Patient Rep Outcomes 2020;4(1):37.
89. Bower JE, Ganz PA, Desmond KA, et al. Fatigue in long-term breast carcinoma survivors. Cancer 2006;106(4):751–8.
90. Eldin EST, Younis SG, El Aziz LMA, et al. Evaluation of sleep pattern disorders in breast cancer patients receiving adjuvant treatment (chemotherapy and/or radiotherapy) using polysomnography. J BUON 2019;24(2):529–34.
91. Van Onselen C, Paul SM, Lee K, et al. Trajectories of sleep disturbance and daytime sleepiness in women before and after surgery for breast cancer. J Pain Symptom Manage 2013;45(2):244–60.
92. Klyushnenkova EN, Sorkin JD, Gallicchio L. Association of obesity and sleep problems among breast cancer survivors: results from a registry-based survey study. Support Care Cancer 2015;23(12):3437–45.
93. Palesh O, Aldridge-Gerry A, Ulusakarya A, et al. Sleep disruption in breast cancer patients and survivors. J Natl Compr Cancer Netw 2013;11(12): 1523–30.
94. Doong S-H, Dhruva A, Dunn LB, et al. Associations between cytokine genes and a symptom cluster of

pain, fatigue, sleep disturbance, and depression in patients prior to breast cancer surgery. Biol Res Nurs 2015;17(3):237–47.
95. Bower JE. Behavioral symptoms in patients with breast cancer and survivors. J Clin Oncol 2008; 26(5):768–77.
96. Bower JE, Ganz PA, Desmond KA, et al. Fatigue in breast cancer survivors: occurrence, correlates, and impact on quality of life. J Clin Oncol 2000; 18(4):743–53.
97. Otte JL, Davis L, Carpenter JS, et al. Sleep disorders in breast cancer survivors. Support Care Cancer 2016;24(10):4197–205.
98. Czeisler CA. Impact of sleepiness and sleep deficiency on public health–utility of biomarkers. J Clin Sleep Med 2011;7(5 Suppl):S6–8.
99. Otte JL, Carpenter JS, Russell KM, et al. Prevalence, severity, and correlates of sleep-wake disturbances in long-term breast cancer survivors. J Pain Symptom Manage 2010;39(3):535–47.
100. Ancoli-Israel S, Liu L, Marler MR, et al. Fatigue, sleep, and circadian rhythms prior to chemotherapy for breast cancer. Support Care Cancer 2006;14(3):201–9.
101. Sanford SD, Wagner LI, Beaumont JL, et al. Longitudinal prospective assessment of sleep quality: before, during, and after adjuvant chemotherapy for breast cancer. Support Care Cancer 2013;21(4): 959–67.
102. Liu L, Fiorentino L, Natarajan L, et al. Pre-treatment symptom cluster in breast cancer patients is associated with worse sleep, fatigue and depression during chemotherapy. Psychooncology 2009; 18(2):187–94.
103. Fakih R, Rahal M, Hilal L, et al. Prevalence and severity of sleep disturbances among patients with early breast cancer. Indian J Palliat Care 2018;24(1):35–8.
104. Beck SL, Berger AM, Barsevick AM, et al. Sleep quality after initial chemotherapy for breast cancer. Support Care Cancer 2010;18(6):679–89.
105. Beverly CM, Naughton MJ, Pennell ML, et al. Change in longitudinal trends in sleep quality and duration following breast cancer diagnosis: results from the Women's Health Initiative. NPJ Breast Cancer 2018;4(1):15.
106. Lowery-Allison AE, Passik SD, Cribbet MR, et al. Sleep problems in breast cancer survivors 1–10 years posttreatment. Palliat Support Care 2018; 16(3):325–34.
107. Otte JL, Carpenter JS, Manchanda S, et al. Systematic review of sleep disorders in cancer patients: can the prevalence of sleep disorders be ascertained? Cancer Med 2015;4(2):183–200.
108. Davidson JR, MacLean AW, Brundage MD, et al. Sleep disturbance in cancer patients. Soc Sci Med 2002;54(9):1309–21.
109. Savard J, Simard S, Blanchet J, et al. Prevalence, clinical characteristics, and risk factors for insomnia in the context of breast cancer. Sleep 2001;24(5):583–90.
110. Vance V, Mourtzakis M, McCargar L, et al. Weight gain in breast cancer survivors: prevalence, pattern and health consequences. Obes Rev 2011;12(4):282–94.
111. Gordon AM, Hurwitz S, Shapiro CL, et al. Premature ovarian failure and body composition changes with adjuvant chemotherapy for breast cancer. Menopause 2011;18(11):1244–8.
112. Makari-Judson G, Braun B, Jerry DJ, et al. Weight gain following breast cancer diagnosis: implication and proposed mechanisms. World J Clin Oncol 2014;5(3):272–82.
113. Ogilvie RP, Patel SR. The epidemiology of sleep and obesity. Sleep Health 2017;3(5):383–8.
114. Imayama I, Alfano CM, Neuhouser ML, et al. Weight, inflammation, cancer-related symptoms and health-related quality of life among breast cancer survivors. Breast Cancer Res Treat 2013; 140(1):159–76.
115. Ma Y, Hall DL, Ngo LH, et al. Efficacy of cognitive behavioral therapy for insomnia in breast cancer: a meta-analysis. Sleep Med Rev 2021;55:101376.
116. Kreutz C, Schmidt ME, Steindorf K. Effects of physical and mind–body exercise on sleep problems during and after breast cancer treatment: a systematic review and meta-analysis. Breast Cancer Res Treat 2019;176(1):1–15.
117. Haller H, Winkler MM, Klose P, et al. Mindfulness-based interventions for women with breast cancer: an updated systematic review and meta-analysis. Acta Oncol 2017;56(12):1665–76.
118. Dirksen SR, Epstein DR. Efficacy of an insomnia intervention on fatigue, mood and quality of life in breast cancer survivors. J Adv Nurs 2008;61(6): 664–75.
119. Savard J, Ivers H, Savard MH, et al. Is a video-based cognitive behavioral therapy for insomnia as efficacious as a professionally administered treatment in breast cancer? Results of a randomized controlled trial. Sleep 2014;37(8):1305–14.
120. Garland SN, Roscoe JA, Heckler CE, et al. Effects of armodafinil and cognitive behavior therapy for insomnia on sleep continuity and daytime sleepiness in cancer survivors. Sleep Med 2016;20: 18–24.
121. Mustian KM, Alfano CM, Heckler C, et al. Comparison of pharmaceutical, psychological, and exercise treatments for cancer-related fatigue: a meta-analysis. JAMA Oncol 2017;3(7):961–8.
122. Jafari-Koulaee A, Bagheri-Nesami M. The effect of melatonin on sleep quality and insomnia in patients with cancer: a systematic review study. Sleep Med 2021;82:96–103.

123. Ebadi Z, Goertz YMJ, Van Herck M, et al. The prevalence and related factors of fatigue in patients with COPD: a systematic review. Eur Respir Rev 2021;30(160):200298.
124. Nobeschi L, Zangirolami-Raimundo J, Cordoni PK, et al. Evaluation of sleep quality and daytime somnolence in patients with chronic obstructive pulmonary disease in pulmonary rehabilitation. BMC Pulm Med 2020;20(1):14.
125. Kapella MC, Herdegen JJ, Perlis ML, et al. Cognitive behavioral therapy for insomnia comorbid with COPD is feasible with preliminary evidence of positive sleep and fatigue effects. Int J Chron Obstruct Pulmon Dis 2011;6:625–35.
126. Wang TY, Lo YL, Lee KY, et al. Nocturnal CPAP improves walking capacity in COPD patients with obstructive sleep apnoea. Respir Res 2013;14(1):66.
127. Ji YB, Bo CL, Xue XJ, et al. Association of inflammatory cytokines with the symptom cluster of pain, fatigue, depression, and sleep disturbance in Chinese patients with cancer. J Pain Symptom Manage 2017;54(6):843–52.
128. Gonzalez-Mercado VJ, Henderson WA, Sarkar A, et al. Changes in gut microbiome associated with co-occurring symptoms development during chemo-radiation for rectal cancer: a proof of concept study. Biol Res Nurs 2021;23(1):31–41.

Sleep Deficiency in Young Children

Monica Roosa Ordway, PhD, APRN, PPCNP-BC*, Sarah Logan, PhD, RN,
Eloise Hannah Sutton, MS

KEYWORDS

• Sleep • Children • Infant • Sleep deficiency • Health disparities • Sleep inequities

KEY POINTS

- Sleep deficiency in early childhood is a growing public health concern.
- Sleep in early childhood is influenced by social and ecological variables that are unique to those that influence adolescents and adults.
- Behavioral sleep interventions hold great promise in improving children's sleep health.
- Studies on behavioral sleep interventions lack inclusive sampling, and more research is needed to develop and test multilevel interventions that can be personalized and tailored to meet the diverse population of young children.

INTRODUCTION

As early as the prenatal period, sleep is vital to the health and development of all children. Amid the epidemic of insufficient sleep in adulthood, there is growing public health concern in response to the evidence that 25% to 40% of children are reported to have sleep insufficiency before they are school-age,[1–3] placing them at risk for sleep-associated poor health outcomes, including metabolic,[4] cardiovascular,[5] and mental health.[6] In addition, when sleep problems develop in early life, they often are persistent,[3,7] contributing to long-term problems with school performance, quality of life, risk of injury, and mental health.[8–13] Adding to the public health concern is the increasing evidence that minoritized children have higher levels of sleep deficiency[14–17] and are at increased risk of associated health disparities[18–20] compared with non-Hispanic White children. Moreover, there is emerging evidence that sleep health disparities emerge as early as 1 year of age.[16,21,22] The purpose of this review is to summarize the key advances in our understanding of sleep health in early childhood (ie, birth through school age) and the possible role of sleep deficiency during early childhood in the development of health disparities.

Sleep and Health in Children

Recently there has been a sharp growth in the research attention given to childhood sleep patterns, development, and disorders.[23] Notably, the official statement on the importance of healthy sleep by the American Thoracic Society included recommendations to increase our understanding of how sleep health and sleep disorders develop from early life and across the lifespan as a priority in future research.[24] Moreover, the statement highlighted that the physiologic and clinical basis for approaches to sleep health need to be tailored differently when considering pediatric sleep.

Historically, research on sleep and sleep-related disorders has focused on sleep as an outcome, rather than a predictor of health.[19] As such, sleep health promotion messaging has been largely absent in public health messaging.[25] The shift in research to examining sleep as a predictor of health has prompted the characterization of sleep health as a multidimensional construct that includes sleep duration, efficiency, satisfaction, alertness/sleepiness, and timing[25]; this was recently reevaluated as it applies to childhood; importantly, an additional dimension, sleep-related behaviors, was added to the child-specific definition in order to capture bedtime

Yale School of Nursing, PO Box 27399, West Haven, CT 06516-7399, USA
* Corresponding author.
E-mail address: Monica.ordway@yale.edu

Clin Chest Med 43 (2022) 229–237
https://doi.org/10.1016/j.ccm.2022.02.007
0272-5231/22/

routines and the consistency of sleep timing and duration that may influence child sleep.[26]

Sleep-related behaviors include the actions and activities that may promote or inhibit sleep health in children before bedtime and the regularity of those actions and activities. The establishment of a consistent routine that occurs in the hour preceding bedtime has been associated with earlier bedtimes, shorter sleep onset latency, fewer night awakenings, and longer sleep duration.[27] The addition of sleep-related behaviors to the pediatric-specific definition of sleep health brings important awareness of the influence of parental control on the sleep health of young children.[26] This relationship is highlighted in Sadeh's transactional model of infant sleep that highlights parenting as the most proximal influence on children's sleep in the early years.[28,29] The model describes how the relationship between parenting and early childhood sleep is influenced by parent's beliefs, expectations, and behaviors related to their child's sleep.

Regarding the other 5 dimensions of sleep, sleep duration has been the most extensively studied in connection with adverse outcomes. Sleep duration refers to the total duration of sleep within a 24-hour period. Shorter night sleep duration in children has been associated with lower levels of social interaction, cooperation, and peer acceptance[6,30,31] and increased likelihood of aggressive behavior, anxiety,[32] and depression. In children between 29 and 72 months of age, children with persistent short sleep duration showed a heightened risk for a low vocabulary receptive score in comparison with children with greater than 10 hours of sleep.[33] Studies have shown a link between adiposity and sleep health, primarily a negative correlation between sleep duration and adiposity, with shorter sleep duration predicting both concurrent and future increased adiposity.[34–36] Shorter sleep duration was also associated with greater time spent using the computer or television, which may also contribute to adiposity.[37] Increased total sleep duration was associated with better emotional response regulation[38,39] and greater capacity for receptive vocabulary.[6,40] However, shorter sleep duration has not consistently been shown to result in anxiety and depression across all studies,[41] and a prospective study found that nighttime sleep duration at 30 months was not predictive of receptive vocabulary when measuring subjects at 60 months,[42] warranting a need for further studies and reporting of potential confounding factors. Interestingly, it is important to consider that there can be a discrepancy between parental and teacher perspectives on the association between sleep duration and attention; parents reported a positive association between sleep duration and attention, whereas teachers did not.[43] These results highlight an important angle for continued study and touch on the importance of involving both parents and teachers in the child's sleep and related outcomes.

Apart from sleep duration, sleep efficiency is perhaps the next most studied sleep health dimension with respect to overall health outcomes. Children's ability to fall asleep and stay asleep during the night is a major contributor to their sleep efficiency. Numerous health outcomes are associated with sleep efficiency, including conduct problems, anxiety, depression, and cognitive abilities, including memory and recognition.[44] For example, conduct problems have been associated with a longer sleep onset latency and greater nighttime wakefulness in 57- and 68-month-old children.[30,45] Mixed or nonsignificant results were shown when examining bedtime, sleep efficiency, sleep onset latency, or total sleep duration and prosocial behavior.[6,30,31] Greater duration of nighttime wakefulness was associated with anxiety and depression.[32] In a separate study, sleep problems were also associated with literacy and numeracy abilities, but no relationship with receptive vocabulary was found.[46]

Although recommendations for pediatric sleep duration exist,[47] age- and sex-based recommendations for other dimensions of sleep health such as alertness and sleep satisfaction are still lacking. These dimensions have received less research attention in pediatrics than the other dimensions of sleep health such as duration and efficiency. Sleep satisfaction is characterized by the subjective perception of sleep as "good" or "poor." As such, measurement of sleep satisfaction and alertness in young children depend on parent report. Parental reports of children's sleep satisfaction commonly differ from objective measurement of children's sleep[48] and are influenced by parents' mental health and their own sleep health.[49] Furthermore, sleep satisfaction is the most difficult dimension of sleep health to measure in children, adolescents, and adults,[25,26] and few validated measures of pediatric sleep satisfaction/quality are available.[26,50] There is emerging evidence that sleep satisfaction/quality over a 7-day period significantly predicted psychological stress and general health among 5- to 9-year-old children.[51]

Important maturational changes to the circadian and sleep homeostatic processes during childhood are critical to the assessment of children's alertness/sleepiness. Perhaps most notably, early childhood is marked by a higher homeostatic sleep pressure that underlies children's need for naps.[52] Napping decreases with age as the homeostatic sleep process decreases throughout childhood.[52] However, there is evidence that racial and ethnic differences exist in napping among 2- to 8-year-old children, and this finding warrants further investigation.[53] Children's alertness or sleepiness during the daytime also has implications for many dimensions of their life, from education to health and development. Recent evidence suggests that sleepiness in childhood is related to some, but not all, cognitive and academic performances. Specifically, the effects of sleepiness were more profound on verbal than nonverbal abilities and on higher cognitive functions such as executive function and divergent thinking than on more automatic, less complex cognitive functioning.[54] More research in this area is needed to understand the relationship between sleepiness and learning in childhood.

In summary, clear associations have been established between sleep duration and behavioral, cognitive, and mental and physical health outcomes. However, according to a recent systematic review, there remains a paucity of research on the other sleep domains and varied health outcomes.[19] Moving forward, research on pediatric sleep outcomes should work toward examining sleep as a multidimensional construct including sleep-related behaviors. In addition, high-quality research on the biological need for sleep and barriers and facilitators of good sleep health is also needed.[24]

Sleep Health Inequities in Early Childhood

There are critical socioecological factors that are now recognized as relevant to the study of sleep health. Placing sleep health within a social-environmental conceptual framework may clarify the relationship between sleep and race, ethnicity, racism, and socioeconomic disadvantage.[55] Following the evidence of race and ethnicity differences in adult sleep, studies have emerged describing similar differences in children's sleep patterns. More research is needed to examine the role of the personal, interpersonal, community, and societal influences on sleep health in early childhood (**Fig. 1**).[56] The complexity of elucidating the mechanism behind ethnic and racial sleep differences in sleep health includes such factors as the physical home (eg, crowded homes, availability of sleep space), community (eg, noise, violence, light pollution), and society (eg, parent work schedules and reliance on public transportation to childcare that may require additional commute time and earlier awakening).[57] These factors are different across the developmental stages of childhood. For example, among older children, environmental conditions (eg, noise, temperature) and presleep worries (eg, about family, friends) explained 29% of the association between socioeconomic status (SES) and sleep/wake problems.[58] Ultimately, it is vital that clinicians consider the complex interplay between sleep health dimensions and environmental exposures when assessing children's sleep.

Multiple studies on sleep in early childhood have found non-Hispanic White children's nighttime sleep duration is on average 20 to 88 minutes longer than Hispanic and Black children.[53,59,60] Non-Hispanic White children are also 1.4 to 1.8 times more likely to have a bedtime routine compared with Hispanic and Black children.[61,62] Although there is compelling evidence that race and ethnic disparities exist in obtaining recommended sleep duration and timing, the mechanisms are less understood.[57] A recent systematic review of racial disparities in early childhood sleep suggested that cultural attitudes, acceptability of bedtimes, regular naps, and sleep practices are among the most common mechanisms supported in the literature.[57] Although many of these mechanisms are likely modifiable with tailored sleep education and intervention programs, more research is needed to develop and test such approaches in early childhood.

There is limited research on sleep characteristics among young children living with socioeconomic adversity. However, shorter sleep duration and disrupted sleep patterns are more prevalent among socioeconomically disadvantaged children,[63] rendering these children more vulnerable to adverse health problems.[21,64–66] Most of the existing research has focused on adolescents and adults with higher SES. However, there is emerging evidence that decreased sleep duration and sleep efficiency occurs as early as 1 year of age among children living with socioeconomic adversity.[21,63,64]

Sleep Health and Adverse Childhood Experiences

Although it is well known that sleep deficiency contributes to many health problems, less is known about how adversity contributes to sleep deficiency and how sleep deficiency, in turn, contributes to the activation of children's stress response systems.[67] Over the past decade, advances in the fields of neuroscience, molecular biology, genomics, developmental psychology, epidemiology and sociology have supported a paradigm shift in understanding the root of many poor health outcomes in adulthood. As such,

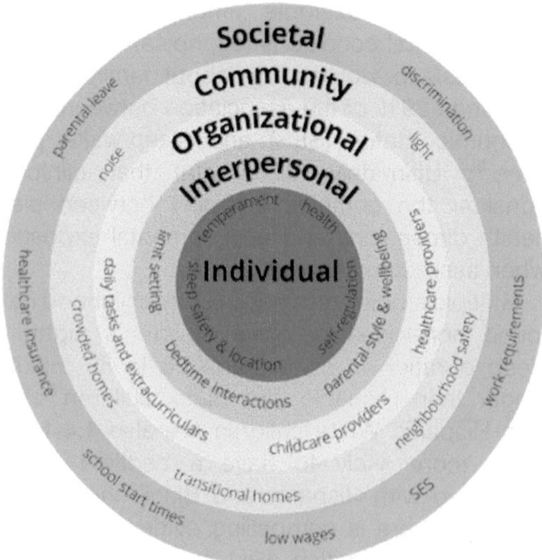

Fig. 1. Social ecological influences of sleep health in childhood.

disorders exhibited in adulthood can be traced back to adverse experiences early in life that resulted in a prolonged stress response, termed toxic stress, with negative health consequences across the lifespan.[68] Again, more prospective research is needed with inclusive sampling of young children to understand how adverse childhood experiences and sleep health in early childhood influence sleep problems in adulthood, but the evidence from retrospective adult studies is strong. According to a systematic review, most of these studies have documented statistically significant associations between sleep problems in adulthood and adverse early childhood experiences, as well as a dose-response relationship wherein the higher the number and severity of the adverse experiences reported by adults during their childhood, the stronger the association with their current sleep problems.[69] Furthermore, there is strong evidence that adults' sleep health is associated with objectively measured physiologic biomarkers within the stress response system.[5,70–72] Thus, prospective examination of the associations between children's sleep, stress response, and health may help understand how sleep deficiency in early childhood may contribute to the biological embedding of adverse childhood experiences or, conversely, may buffer the risk of developing toxic stress.[73] There are a growing number of studies currently underway to advance the science in this area.[67,74]

Approaches to Improve Sleep of Children

Interventions aimed at promoting healthy sleep duration and efficiency early in life may be important to reducing the sleep disparities among very young children living with adversity and preventing some of the negative short- and long-term sequelae. Although the research on young children's sleep and their health lags behind the studies of adolescents and adults, there is a consensus that health care providers should be trained in the importance of sleep health and how to effectively promote sleep health with their patients.[24] There are considerable differences between child and adult sleep that are important to understand before sleep training recommendations are presented to parents; to begin with, sleep in the first 3 months of life characterized by equal time in nonrapid eye movement (NREM) and rapid eye movement (REM) sleep.[75] The lack of sleep cycles before age 3 months is the reason why sleep training is not effective and therefore not recommended before this age. As infants progress through the first year of life, they begin to develop 3 stages of NREM sleep, and REM sleep continues to be longer than that of adults. Daytime napping is also important for infant sleep, but this need decreases with age. In particular, a drastic reduction in napping duration occurs between 18 months and 4 years of age.[76] It is not until the age of 4 to 5 years that children's sleep architecture resembles that of adults.[77] However, as with adult sleep patterns, it is important to acknowledge that the specific patterns are individually variable.

Interventions to promote healthy sleep habits, including parent education,[78] positive bedtime routines (eg, reading, bathing),[79,80] and extinction techniques to address bedtime resistance and nocturnal awakenings[81] are efficacious from late infancy into the preschool years.[81,82] Studies on behavioral sleep interventions (BSIs) in early childhood have demonstrated modest effects on the improvement of sleep duration and sleep quality with parent-reported sleep measures.[83–87] However, few studies included racially and ethnically diverse families who live with socioeconomic adversity and in socioecological contexts described earlier that may limit the feasibility and efficacy of previously developed BSIs.[88–91]

Because health disparities are generally embedded in social or structural determinants of health, multilevel interventions that concomitantly examine influences on health at the individual, interpersonal, organizational, community, and/or societal levels are best suited to improve sleep health in childhood.[92–94] Existing BSIs focus primarily at a single level (eg, individual or interpersonal).[95,96] The lack of tailored education and multilevel approaches among existing BSIs along with the lack of inclusion of diverse, multiethnic families in BSI studies suggests a critical gap in pediatric sleep research. This gap is of concern because children from marginalized families have a higher prevalence of sleep deficiency[14–17] and are at increased risk for other health disparities that have been associated with sleep deficiency,[19,97] suggesting that sleep health promotion may play an important role in reducing health disparities.

It should be noted, however, that inclusive sampling in BSI studies may not be adequate, and existing BSIs should be evaluated for their appropriateness and acceptability across diverse cultures. The development of tailored BSIs that meet the needs of diverse families requires interdisciplinary collaboration between scientists, providers, educators, and parents, followed by thorough testing of the efficacy of these interventions using protocols that include inclusive sampling. A recent study of real-world implementation of BSIs among a racially and ethnically diverse sample of families found no differences in the initiation of BSIs between Hispanic, non-Hispanic Black, and non-Hispanic families, yet non-Hispanic Black families were significantly more likely to be informed about BSIs by pediatric providers and nearly 5 times more likely to discontinue a BSI before completion.[98]

The interdependent dyadic relationship between parents and children is intrinsically linked with sleep health in early childhood. Poor sleep health in children results in stress and worsening mood in parents.[99,100] Parental well-being, including stress, distress, and depressive symptoms, generally improve concurrently with improvements in child sleep deficiency in BSI studies.[85,89,101–103]

DISCUSSION

Although adults have historically been the primary focus when examining sleep health, the critical importance of also investigating sleep in early childhood has more recently been identified.[1,3] The purpose of this review was to summarize the key advances in our understanding of sleep health in early childhood and the possible role of sleep deficiency during early childhood in the development of health disparities. Discussion of the current literature highlights the importance of assessing the multiple dimensions of children's sleep health and conceptualizing sleep health within a social-ecological framework, understand how and when sleep may contribute to the development of health disparities, and the proposition that multilevel interventions are needed to combat the epidemic of sleep insufficiency in early childhood. The hope is that this paper may serve as a resource for sleep education, future research, and clinical consideration.

In addition to pediatric sleep deficiency being a problem in and of itself, the intersection of sleep insufficiency and physiologic development poses a permanent risk in contributing to future health problems as highlighted in recent systematic and meta-reviews.[19,67,104,105] Children who experience sleep insufficiency are predicted to suffer from a myriad of other disease states; pediatric sleep problems have been identified as a risk for future health outcomes, and scientists and clinicians are more aware of approaches to address pediatric sleep insufficiency.

With the emerging concept of sleep as a multidimensional construct, multilevel interventions are also essential. When focusing on the individual, their immediate environment is considered, including a child's education and care, relationship with parents and other individuals, home environment and exposures, and community.[106] At the community and, furthermore, the societal level, it has become undeniable that there are significant socioeconomic disparities that play a role in sleep health.[55] Despite a relatively reduced availability of information in how to combat socioeconomic disparities and sleep, it is encouraging that there is further effort in studying and intervening in all populations, especially the most vulnerable.

Future interventions and areas of interest include continuing to focus on and define sleep as a pillar of health; this includes an all-encompassing scope of contributing factors to sleep health. It is critical to acknowledge the inextricable role of parental control and that socioecological influences on sleep health in early childhood are likely to be distinct from those in adolescence and adulthood. From an intervention standpoint, the home, childcare/schools, health care visits, and community resources all play an invaluable role in identification/diagnosis, education, and support for children and their families. Caring for children and families of all ethnicities, educational levels, and SES is a crucial step, regardless of financial means, physical location, and access to resources. In the future, a movement toward standardizing education and care related to sleep may reduce this gap that occurs across individuals of varying populations.

Overall, all children and their families should have the means to recognize the importance of sleep health, and this will require collaboration from parents, educators, researchers, and clinicians; this is driven by continued focus to further knowledge in pediatric sleep health. The connection between increasing health care burdens and sleep has become more evident. Addressing this health disparity in the pediatric stage may prove to be critical in improving health and quality of life, both presently and in the future.

CLINICS CARE POINTS

- Sleep health is a low-cost, modifiable construct that may contribute to the development of health disparities early in life.
- History taking must include questions to assess the multidimensional constructs of sleep health to accurately develop a full understanding of children's sleep deficiency.
- SES is a significant contributor to poor sleep outcomes and health of children and their families.
- Behavioral sleep interventions in childhood should consider individual, familial, educational, clinical, community, and societal influences.

DISCLOSURE

The authors have nothing to disclose.

ACKNOWLEDGMENTS

This work was supported by the National Institutes of Health (NIH) and the National Institute of Nursing Research 1R34NR019283 to 01A1. We would like to thank Dr Samantha Conley for her feedback and edits to this review.

REFERENCES

1. Owens J. Classification and epidemiology of childhood sleep disorders. Prim Care 2008;35(3):533–46.
2. Knutson KL. Sociodemographic and cultural determinants of sleep deficiency: implications for cardiometabolic disease risk. Soc Sci Med 2013;79(1):7–15.
3. Byars KC, Yolton K, Rausch J, et al. Prevalence, patterns, and persistence of sleep problems in the first 3 years of life. Pediatrics 2012;129(2):e276–84.
4. Cappuccio FP, Taggart FM, Kandala N-B, et al. Meta-Analysis of short sleep duration and obesity in children and adults. Sleep 2008;31(5):619–26.
5. Meier-Ewert HK, Ridker PM, Rifai N, et al. Effect of sleep loss on C-Reactive protein, an inflammatory marker of cardiovascular risk. J Am Coll Cardiol 2004;43(4):678–83. https://doi.org/10.1016/j.jacc.2003.07.050.
6. Vaughn BE, Elmore-Staton L, Shin N, et al. Sleep as a support for social Competence, peer relations, and cognitive functioning in preschool children. Behav Sleep Med 2014;13(2):92–106.
7. Kataria S, Swanson MS, Trevathan GE. Persistence of sleep disturbances in preschool children. J Pediatr 1987;110(4):642–6.
8. Magee CA, Gordon R, Caputi P. Distinct developmental trends in sleep duration during early childhood. Pediatrics 2014;133(6):e1561–7.
9. Keller PS, Kouros CD, Erath SA, et al. Longitudinal relations between maternal depressive symptoms and child sleep problems: the role of parasympathetic nervous system reactivity. J Child Psychol Psychiatry 2014;55(2):172–9.
10. Scharf RJ, Demmer RT, Silver EJ, et al. Nighttime sleep duration and externalizing behaviors of preschool children. J Dev Behav Pediatr 2013;34(6):384–91.
11. Reid GJ, Hong RY, Wade TJ. The relation between common sleep problems and emotional and behavioral problems among 2- and 3-year-olds in the context of known risk factors for psychopathology. J Sleep Res 2009;18(1):49–59.
12. Spruyt K, Gozal D. The underlying interactome of childhood obesity: the potential role of sleep. Child Obes 2012;8(1):38–42.
13. Owens JA, Fernando S, Mc Guinn M. Sleep disturbance and injury risk in young children. Behav Sleep Med 2005;3(1):18–31.
14. Combs D, Goodwin JL, Quan SF, et al. Longitudinal differences in sleep duration in Hispanic and Caucasian children. Sleep Med 2016;18:61–6.
15. Guglielmo D, Gazmararian JA, Chung J, et al. Racial/ethnic sleep disparities in US school-aged children and adolescents: a review of the literature. Rev *Sleep Health* 2018;4(1):68–80.
16. Doane LD, Breitenstein RS, Beekman C, et al. Early life socioeconomic disparities in children's sleep: the Mediating role of the current home environment. Article in press. J Youth Adolesc 2018. https://doi.org/10.1007/s10964-018-0917-3.
17. Yip T, Cheon YM, Wang Y, et al. Racial disparities in sleep: associations with Discrimination among ethnic/racial minority adolescents. Article. Child Dev 2019. https://doi.org/10.1111/cdev.13234.
18. Flores G. Racial and ethnic disparities in the health and health care of children. Pediatrics 2010;125(4):e979.
19. Matricciani L, Paquet C, Galland B, et al. Children's sleep and health: a meta-review. Review. Sleep Med Rev 2019;46:136–50.
20. Laposky AD, Van Cauter E, Diez-Roux AV. Reducing health disparities: the role of sleep deficiency and sleep disorders. Sleep Med 2016;18:3–6.
21. Cronin A, Halligan SL, Murray L. Maternal Psychosocial adversity and the longitudinal development of infant sleep. Infancy 2008;13(5):469–95.

22. Ordway MR, Sadler LS, Jeon S, et al. Early emergence of race/ethnicity differences in sleep health in a sample of economically marginalized toddlers. Behav Sleep Med. under review;
23. Bruni O, Ferri R. The Discovery of pediatric sleep Medicine. In: Nevšímalová S, Bruni O, editors. Sleep disorders in children. Springer International Publishing; 2017. p. 31–51.
24. Mukherjee S, Patel SR, Kales SN, et al. An official American Thoracic society statement: the importance of healthy sleep. Recommendations and future Priorities. Am J Respir Crit Care Med 2015; 191(12):1450–8.
25. Buysse DJ. Sleep Health: Can We define it? Does it Matter? Sleep 2014;37(1):9–17.
26. Meltzer LJ, Williamson AA, Mindell JA. Pediatric sleep health: it matters, and so does how we define it. Sleep Med Rev 2021;57:101425.
27. Mindell JA, Williamson AA. Benefits of a bedtime routine in young children: sleep, development, and beyond. Review. Sleep Med Rev 2018;40: 93–108.
28. Sadeh A, Anders TF. Infant sleep problems: Origins, assessment, interventions. Infant Ment Health J 1993;14(1):17–34.
29. Sadeh A, Tikotzky L, Scher A. Parenting and infant sleep. Sleep Med Rev 2010;14(2):89–96.
30. Quach J, Hiscock H, Wake M. Sleep problems and mental health in primary school new entrants: cross-sectional community-based study. J Paediatr Child Health 2012;48(12):1076–81.
31. Zheng M, Rangan A, Olsen NJ, et al. Longitudinal association of nighttime sleep duration with emotional and behavioral problems in early childhood: results from the Danish Healthy Start Study. Article. *Sleep*. 2021;44(1). https://doi.org/10.1093/sleep/zsaa138. zsaa138.
32. Jansen PW, Saridjan NS, Hofman A, et al. Does disturbed sleeping precede symptoms of anxiety or depression in toddlers? The generation R study. Psychosom Med 2011;73(3):242–9.
33. Touchette E, Petit D, Séguin JR, et al. Associations between sleep duration patterns and behavioral/cognitive functioning at school entry. Sleep 2007; 30(9):1213–9.
34. Cespedes EM, Rifas-Shiman SL, Redline S, et al. Longitudinal associations of sleep curtailment with metabolic risk in mid-childhood. Obesity 2014;22(12):2586–92.
35. Chaput JP, Lambert M, Gray-Donald K, et al. Short sleep duration is independently associated with overweight and obesity in Quebec children. Can J Public Health 2011;102(5):369–74.
36. Zhou M, Lalani C, Banda JA, et al. Sleep duration, timing, variability and measures of adiposity among 8- to 12-year-old children with obesity. Obes Sci Pract 2018;4(6):535–44.
37. Magee C, Caputi P, Iverson D. Lack of sleep could increase obesity in children and too much television could be partly to blame. Acta Paediatr Int J Paediatrics 2014;103(1):e27–31.
38. Miller AL, Seifer R, Crossin R, et al. Toddler's self-regulation strategies in a challenge context are nap-dependent. J Sleep Res 2015;24(3):279–87.
39. Berger RH, Miller AL, Seifer R, et al. Acute sleep restriction effects on emotion responses in 30- to 36-month-old children. J Sleep Res 2012;21(3): 235–46.
40. Lam JC, Mahone EM, Mason TBA, et al. The effects of napping on cognitive function in preschoolers. J Dev Behav Pediatr 2011;32(2):90–7.
41. Becker SP, Sidol CA, Van Dyk TR, et al. Intraindividual variability of sleep/wake patterns in relation to child and adolescent functioning: a systematic review. Review. Sleep Med Rev 2017;34:94–121.
42. Dionne G, Touchette E, Forget-Dubois N, et al. Associations between sleep-wake consolidation and language development in early childhood: a longitudinal twin study. Sleep 2011;34(8):987–95. https://doi.org/10.5665/SLEEP.1148. http://europepmc.org/abstract/MED/21804661. https://www.ncbi.nlm.nih.gov/pmc/articles/pmid/21804661/pdf/?tool=EBI. https://www.ncbi.nlm.nih.gov/pmc/articles/pmid/21804661/?tool=EBI. https://europepmc.org/articles/PMC3138173. https://europepmc.org/articles/PMC3138173?pdf=render.
43. Kohler MJ, Kennedy JD, Martin AJ, et al. Parent versus teacher report of daytime behavior in snoring children. Article. Sleep and Breath 2013; 17(2):637–45.
44. Giganti F, Arzilli C, Conte F, et al. The effect of a daytime nap on priming and recognition tasks in preschool children. Sleep 2014;37(6):1087–93. https://doi.org/10.5665/sleep.3766. http://europepmc.org/abstract/MED/24882903. https://europepmc.org/articles/PMC4015382. https://europepmc.org/articles/PMC4015382?pdf=render.
45. Martin J, Hiscock H, Hardy P, et al. Adverse associations of infant and child sleep problems and parent health: an Australian population study. Pediatrics 2007;119(5):947–55.
46. Hiscock H, Canterford L, Ukoumunne OC, et al. Adverse associations of sleep problems in Australian preschoolers: national population study. Pediatrics 2007;119(1):86–93.
47. Paruthi S, Brooks LJ, D'Ambrosio C, et al. Recommended Amount of sleep for pediatric populations: a consensus statement of the American Academy of sleep Medicine. J Clin Sleep Med 2016;12(6): 785–6.
48. Holley S, Hill CM, Stevenson J. A comparison of Actigraphy and parental report of sleep habits in

Typically developing children aged 6 to 11 Years. Behav Sleep Med 2010;8(1):16–27.
49. Rönnlund H, Elovainio M, Virtanen I, et al. Poor parental sleep and the reported sleep quality of their children. Pediatrics 2016;137(4). https://doi.org/10.1542/peds.2015-3425.
50. Forrest CB, Meltzer LJ, Marcus CL, et al. Development and validation of the PROMIS pediatric sleep disturbance and sleep-related Impairment item banks. Sleep 2018;41(6). https://doi.org/10.1093/sleep/zsy054.
51. Blackwell CK, Hartstein LE, Elliott AJ, et al. Better sleep, better life? How sleep quality influences children's life satisfaction. Article. Qual Life Res 2020; 29(9):2465–74.
52. Jenni OG, LeBourgeois MK. Understanding sleep–wake behavior and sleep disorders in children: the value of a model. Curr Opin Psychiatry 2006;19(3).
53. Crosby B, LeBourgeois MK, Harsh J. Racial differences in reported napping and nocturnal sleep in 2- to 8-year-old children. Pediatrics 2005;115(1 Suppl):225–32.
54. Macchitella L, Marinelli CV, Signore F, et al. Sleepiness, Neuropsychological Skills, and Scholastic learning in children. Brain Sci 2020;10(8):529.
55. Grandner MA, Williams NJ, Knutson KL, et al. Sleep disparity, race/ethnicity, and socioeconomic position. Sleep Med 2016;18:7–18.
56. Owens J, Ordway MR. Sleep among children. In: DT D I K S. R, editor. The social epidemiology of sleep. Oxford University Press; 2019.
57. Smith JP, Hardy ST, Hale LE, et al. Racial disparities and sleep among preschool aged children: a systematic review. Article. Sleep Health 2019;5(1): 49–57.
58. Bagley EJ, Kelly RJ, Buckhalt JA, et al. What keeps low-SES children from sleeping well: the role of presleep worries and sleep environment. Article. Sleep Med 2015;16(4):496–502.
59. Wilson KE, Miller AL, Lumeng JC, et al. Sleep environments and sleep durations in a sample of low-income preschool children. J Clin Sleep Med 2014;10(3):299–305.
60. Patrick KE, Millet G, Mindell JA. Sleep differences by race in preschool children: the roles of parenting behaviors and socioeconomic status. Article. Behav Sleep Med 2016;14(5):467–79.
61. Hale L, Berger LM, Lebourgeois MK, et al. Social and demographic predictors of preschoolersâ€™ bedtime routines. Article. J Dev Behav Pediatr 2009;30(5):394–402.
62. Burnham MM, Gaylor EE, Wei X. Toddler naps in child care: associations with demographics and developmental outcomes. Article. Sleep Health 2016;2(1):25–9.
63. Gellis LA. Children's sleep in the context of socioeconomic status, race, and ethnicity. In: El-Sheikh M, editor. *Sleep and development: Sleep and development: Familial and Socio-cultural considerations* Oxford Scholarship Online. 2011.
64. El-Sheikh M, Bagley EJ, Keiley M, et al. Economic adversity and children's sleep problems: multiple indicators and moderation of effects. Health Psychol 2013;32(8):849–59.
65. Spruyt K, Alaribe CU, Nwabara OU. To sleep or not to sleep: a Repeated Daily challenge for African American children. CNS Neurosci Ther 2015; 21(1):23–31.
66. Hirshkowitz M, Whiton K, Albert SM, et al. National Sleep Foundation's sleep time duration recommendations: methodology and results summary. Sleep Health 2015;1(1):40–3.
67. Ordway MR, Condon EM, Ibrahim BB, et al. A systematic review of the association between sleep health and stress biomarkers in children. Sleep Med Rev 2021. https://doi.org/10.1016/j.smrv.2021.101494.
68. Shonkoff JP, Garner AS, Siegel BS, et al. The lifelong effects of early childhood adversity and toxic stress. Pediatrics 2012;129(1):e232–46.
69. Kajeepeta S, Gelaye B, Jackson CL, et al. Adverse childhood experiences are associated with adult sleep disorders: a systematic review. Sleep Med 2015;16(3):320–30.
70. Motivala SJ, Sarfatti A, Olmos L, et al. Inflammatory markers and sleep disturbance in major depression. Psychosom Med 2005;67(2):187–94.
71. Ferrie JE, Kivimaki M, Akbaraly TN, et al. Associations between change in sleep duration and inflammation: findings on C-reactive protein and interleukin 6 in the Whitehall II Study. Am J Epidemiol 2013;178(6):956–61.
72. Bei B, Seeman TE, Carroll JE, et al. Sleep and physiological Dysregulation: a Closer Look at sleep Intraindividual variability. Sleep 2017;40(9):zsx109.
73. Bourchtein E, Langberg JM, Eadeh HM. A review of pediatric Nonpharmacological sleep interventions: effects on sleep, Secondary outcomes, and populations with Co-occurring mental health conditions. Article. Behav Ther 2019. https://doi.org/10.1016/j.beth.2019.04.006.
74. Ordway MR, Sadler LS, Canapari CA, et al. Sleep, biological stress, and health among toddlers living in socioeconomically disadvantaged homes: a research protocol. Res Nurs Health 2017. https://doi.org/10.1002/nur.21832. Article in Press.
75. Daftary Ameet S, Jalou Hasnaa E, Shively L, et al. Polysomnography reference values in healthy Newborns. J Clin Sleep Med. 15(03):437-443.
76. Iglowstein I, Jenni OG, Molinari L, et al. Sleep duration from infancy to adolescence: reference values and generational trends. *Pediatr* Feb 2003;111(2):302–7.
77. Ohayon MM, Carskadon MA, Guilleminault C, et al. Meta-analysis of quantitative sleep parameters

from childhood to old age in healthy individuals: developing normative sleep values across the human lifespan. Sleep 2004;27(7):1255–73.
78. Eckerberg B. Treatment of sleep problems in families with small children: is written information enough? Acta Paediatr 2002;91(8):952–9.
79. Hale L, Berger LM, LeBourgeois MK, et al. A longitudinal study of preschoolers' language-based bedtime routines, sleep duration, and well-being. J Fam Psychol 2011;25(3):423–33.
80. Mindell JA, Li AM, Sadeh A, et al. Bedtime routines for young children: a dose-dependent association with sleep outcomes. Sleep 2015;38(5):717–22.
81. Morgenthaler TI, Owens J, Alessi C, et al. Practice parameters for behavioral treatment of bedtime problems and night wakings in infants and young children. Sleep 2006;29(10):1277–81.
82. Mindell JA, Kuhn B, Lewin DS, et al. Behavioral treatment of bedtime problems and night wakings in infants and young children. Sleep 2006;29(10): 1263–76.
83. Mindell JA, Du Mond CE, Sadeh A, et al. Long-term efficacy of an internet-based intervention for infant and toddler sleep disturbances: one year follow-up. J Clin Sleep Med 2011;7(5):507–11.
84. Mindell JA, Du Mond CE, Sadeh A, et al. Efficacy of an internet-based intervention for infant and toddler sleep disturbances. Sleep 2011;34(4): 451–8.
85. Hall WA, Hutton E, Brant RF, et al. A randomized controlled trial of an intervention for infants' behavioral sleep problems. Article. BMC Pediatr 2015; 15(1):181.
86. Paul IM, Savage JS, Anzman-Frasca S, et al. INSIGHT responsive parenting intervention and infant sleep. Article *Pediatr* 2016;138(1):e20160762.
87. Meltzer LJ, Mindell JA. Systematic review and meta-analysis of behavioral interventions for pediatric Insomnia. J Pediatr Psychol 2014;39(8): 932–48.
88. Gradisar M, Jackson K, Spurrier NJ, et al. Behavioral interventions for infant sleep problems: a randomized controlled trial. Article. Pediatrics 2016; 137(6):e20151486.
89. Hall WA, Clauson M, Carty EM, et al. Effects on parents of an intervention to resolve infant behavioral sleep problems. Pediatr Nurs 2006;32(3):243–50.
90. Wilson KE, Miller AL, Bonuck K, et al. Evaluation of a sleep education program for low-income preschool children and their families. Sleep 2014; 37(6):1117–25.
91. Schwichtenberg AJ, Abel EA, Keys E, et al. Diversity in pediatric behavioral sleep intervention studies. Sleep Med Rev 2019;47:103–11.
92. Gorin SS, Badr H, Krebs P, et al. Multilevel interventions and racial/ethnic health disparities. J Natl Cancer Inst Monogr 2012;2012(44):100–11.
93. Paskett E, Thompson B, Ammerman AS, et al. Multilevel interventions to address health disparities Show promise in improving population health. Health Aff (Project Hope) 2016;35(8):1429–34.
94. Reifsnider E, Gallagher M, Forgione B. Using ecological models in research on health disparities. J Prof Nurs 2005;21(4):216–22.
95. Allen SL, Howlett MD, Coulombe JA, et al. ABCs of SLEEPING: a review of the evidence behind pediatric sleep practice recommendations. Sleep Med Rev 2016;29:1–14.
96. McDowall PS, Galland BC, Campbell AJ, et al. Parent knowledge of children's sleep: a systematic review. Sleep Med Rev 2017;31:39–47. https://doi.org/10.1016/j.smrv.2016.01.002.
97. Braveman PA, Kumanyika S, Fielding J, et al. Health disparities and health equity: the issue is justice. Am J Public Health 2011;101(SUPPL. 1): S149–55.
98. Honaker SM, Mindell JA, Slaven JE, et al. Implementation of infant behavioral sleep intervention in a diverse sample of Mothers. Behav Sleep Med 2021;19(4):547–61.
99. Meltzer LJ, Montgomery-Downs HE. Sleep in the family. Pediatr Clin North Am 2011;58(3):765–74.
100. Meltzer LJ, Mindell JA. Relationship between child sleep disturbances and maternal sleep, mood, and parenting stress: a pilot study. J Fam Psychol 2007; 21(1):67–73.
101. Moore M, Mindell JA. The impact of behavioral interventions for sleep problems on secondary outcomes in young children and their families. The Oxford handbook of infant, child, and adolescent sleep and behavior. Oxford University Press; 2013. p. 547–58. Oxford library of psychology.
102. Mindell JA, Telofski LS, Wiegand B, et al. A nightly bedtime routine: Impact on sleep in young children and maternal mood. Sleep 2009;32(5):599–606.
103. Eckerberg B. Treatment of sleep problems in families with young children: effects of treatment on family well-being. Article. Acta Paediatr Int J Paediatrics 2004;93(1):126–34.
104. Miller MA, Bates S, Ji C, et al. Systematic review and meta-analyses of the relationship between short sleep and incidence of obesity and effectiveness of sleep interventions on weight gain in preschool children. Obes Rev 2021;22(2):e13113. https://doi.org/10.1111/obr.13113 (no pagination.
105. Zhang Z, Sousa-Sá E, Pereira JR, et al. Correlates of sleep duration in early childhood: a systematic review. Review. Behav Sleep Med 2021;19(3): 407–25.
106. Grandner MA. Chapter 5 - social-ecological model of sleep health. In: Grandner MA, editor. Sleep and health. Academic Press; 2019. p. 45–53.

Sleep Deficiency in Adolescents

The School Start Time Debate

Olufunke Afolabi-Brown, MBBS[a,*], Melisa E. Moore, PhD[a,b], Ignacio E. Tapia, MD[a]

KEYWORDS

• Teenager • Insufficient sleep • Teen sleep • School start times • Insomnia • Daytime sleepiness

KEY POINTS

- Physiologic, psychological, and social factors contribute to sleep deficiency in adolescents.
- Adolescent sleep deprivation is a public health crisis, and early school start times contribute to the harmful outcomes seen in this age group.
- Implementing delayed school start times can be an effective strategy for increasing total sleep duration in adolescents, thereby improving their overall health and performance.

INTRODUCTION

Adolescence is commonly accepted as a challenging and tumultuous time for sleep. There are multiple changes in adolescent sleep, both intrinsically and extrinsically driven, and the consequences of sleep deprivation are both common and impactful. In 2014, the American Academy of Pediatrics issued a statement addressing the public health crisis of adolescent sleep deprivation and recommending later school start times to improve overall sleep duration.[1] This article reviews the causes and consequences of adolescent sleep deficiency and examines the potential impact of later school start times on adolescent sleep and overall functioning.

Changes in sleep architecture during adolescence

Adolescence, a dynamic transition process from childhood to adulthood, is characterized by simultaneous and asynchronous development that starts with puberty and ends with adulthood.[2] The brain and sleep are also subject to significant changes during adolescence.[3] One of the most important changes in sleep architecture and physiology occurring during adolescence is a higher density of sleep spindles,[4] reflecting the continuous development of thalamocortical networks.[5] In addition, adolescence is characterized by extensive white matter development and increased white matter diffusion along axons, resulting in higher spindle density.[6] Considering the thalamocortical origin of sleep spindles, the increase in spindle density and frequency likely reflects advanced myelination in thalamocortical circuits, shaping a more mature and effective network.[7] Spindles have been associated with several cognitive functions, such as learning and memory,[8,9] intelligence,[10] synaptic plasticity,[11] and sleep-dependent memory consolidation.[12,13] Hence, these domains may be affected by sleep deficiency.

The development of spindle density is also linked to an increase in the percentage of total sleep time spent in stage N2 and a subsequent decrease in stage N3 during adolescence. The authors and other investigators have shown that stage N3 is inversely correlated with Tanner stage as shown in **Fig. 1**.[14,15] Arousal index directly

[a] Division of Pulmonary and Sleep Medicine, Children's Hospital of Philadelphia, 3401 Civic Center Boulevard, Philadelphia, PA 19104, USA; [b] Department of Children and Adolescent Psychiatry and Behavioral Sciences, Children's Hospital of Philadelphia, Philadelphia, PA, USA
* Corresponding author.
E-mail address: afolabibro@chop.edu

Clin Chest Med 43 (2022) 239–247
https://doi.org/10.1016/j.ccm.2022.02.008

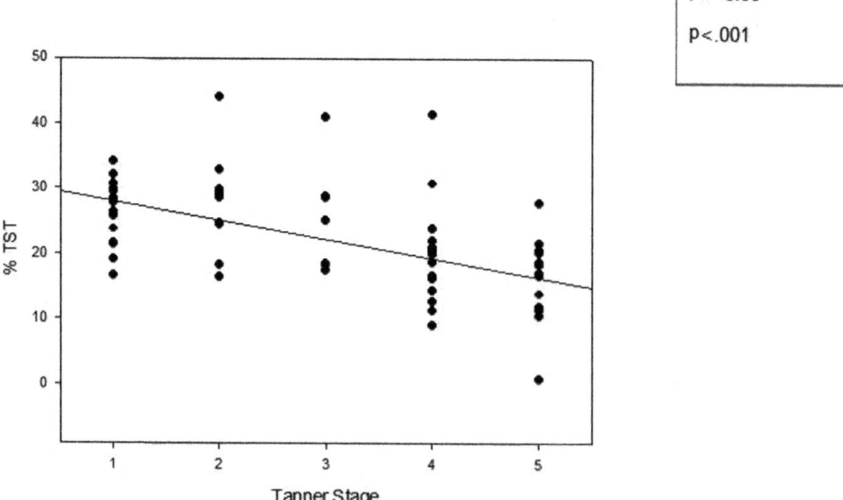

Legend: Scatter plot of stage N3 (expressed as percentage of total sleep time) according to Tanner stage

Fig. 1. Tanner stage versus N3.

correlates with age, increasing from childhood to adulthood,[16] implying that adolescents are more susceptible to interrupted sleep and hence shorter sleep, compared with younger children.

Changes in circadian rhythm during adolescence

The 2-process model of sleep regulation proposed by Borbely and colleagues[17] postulates that 2 separate and interacting processes influence sleep: the circadian and sleep homeostatic processes (process C and process S). The circadian process oscillates with an approximately 24-hour length, whereas sleep homeostasis is sleep-wake dependent. Hence, it exhibits across wake an exponentially saturating increase in sleep pressure that exponentially decreases during sleep.[18] Homeostatic sleep pressure decreases with age,[19] thus contributing to reduced sleep time observed from childhood to adulthood.[20] Indeed, studies have shown that there is a 14-minute decrease per year in sleep duration during adolescence.[21,22] Similarly, older adolescents seem to tolerate sleep restriction better compared with younger adolescents.[23] In contrast to popular beliefs, however, adolescents do not exhibit adaptation to sleep restriction.[24] Therefore, they will sleep longer if given the opportunity.

Melatonin release is also delayed during adolescence, favoring later bedtimes. Cross-sectional and longitudinal studies have implied this by analyzing actigraphy and sleep diary data.[25,26] For example, Crowley and colleagues[27] demonstrated this shift longitudinally when they studied thirty-eight 9- to 10-year-old children and fifty-six 15- to 16-year-old adolescents and followed them for 2.5 years.[27] Participants completed actigraphy, sleep diaries, and salivary dim light melatonin onset (DLMO) measurements every 6 months. They found out that DLMO shifted to later times with age. This delayed shift makes it challenging for teens to fall asleep until later, affecting their ability to wake up early in the morning. With the presence of early school start times in adolescents, the constraints between their physiologic changes and societal demands create a short sleep duration and chronic sleep deprivation.

SLEEP DISORDERS IN ADOLESCENTS

Although biological factors certainly contribute to poor sleep in adolescents, it is imperative to acknowledge the potential additive influence of sleep disorders. The following section summarizes sleep problems often encountered in adolescents and young adults and frequently resulting in sleep deficiency based on the third edition of The International Classification of Sleep Disorders.[28]

Inadequate sleep hygiene

Sleep hygiene encompasses having consistent sleep schedules (eg, regular, appropriate sleep times), healthy habits (eg, bedtime routine and avoiding electronics and caffeine before bedtime), and conducive sleep environments (eg, cool, dark, and quiet room).[29] With the increased use of media and technology, adolescents are spending more time on their electronic devices. Based on the 2006 National Sleep Foundation's poll of Sleep in America, 97% of adolescents had at least one electronic device in the bedroom.[30] Having these devices in the room is associated with problems falling asleep and staying asleep.[31,32] Electronic media disrupts sleep through various postulated mechanisms.[33] Commonly, the time spent enjoying media-related activities such as texting, playing video games, or interacting on social media displaces sleep or other activities that promote good sleep hygiene. In addition, the light produced from these devices tends to suppress nocturnal melatonin production, further disrupting the circadian rhythm.[34] Finally, the use of media causes increased psychological and mental arousal, further affecting sleep quality.[35]

Caffeine use also interferes with sleep duration and sleep quantity, and up to 75% of adolescents consume caffeinated beverages.[36] Studies have shown a dose-dependent relationship with shortened sleep duration, increased sleep latency, and daytime sleepiness among children with higher caffeine intake.[37] In addition, caffeine causes REM and non-REM sleep distribution changes, with potential impact on learning and memory consolidation.[38]

Addressing inadequate sleep hygiene involves focusing on educating the adolescents and parents on healthy sleep habits and the effect of insufficient sleep on all aspects of function. Practical strategies can be provided, such as helping the family set a consistent sleep schedule and routine, reinforcing healthy sleep practices, and minimizing electronic and caffeine use around bedtime. These strategies should be conducted with a collaborative approach, engaging the adolescent as much as possible while ensuring appropriate parental supervision.[29]

Insomnia

Insomnia is the most common and persistent sleep disorder in adolescents, with prevalence rates between 13.6% and 23.6%.[39] Components of insomnia definition include (1) difficulty initiating and maintaining sleep or early morning awakening, (2) subjective dissatisfaction with sleep quantity, (3) presence of significant daytime impairment, and (4) symptoms that occur despite adequate opportunity and circumstances for sleep.[28] In addition, insomnia often occurs with other comorbid conditions such as psychiatric, medical, and behavioral problems. Deleterious effects of insomnia include excessive daytime sleepiness (EDS), fatigue, psychopathology, and neurocognitive deficits.

Targeted behavioral interventions, sleep education, and sometimes medications have been implemented to treat insomnia in adolescents. Cognitive behavioral therapy for insomnia (CBT-I), the first-line treatment of insomnia in adults, can be successfully adapted in adolescents.[40] However, more studies on the efficacy of CBT-I in this age group are needed. In addition to these specific interventions, it is critical to address other underlying comorbid conditions such as major depression, anxiety, and other perpetuating factors.

Delayed sleep-wake phase disorder

A perpetual delay in the sleep-wake time of greater than 2 hours relative to social norms leading to disrupted daily activities[28] (eg, school, work, and extracurricular activities) characterizes delayed sleep-wake phase disorder (DSWPD). This disorder is estimated to occur in 3% of adolescents.[41] With the onset of puberty, there is a physiologic shift in the sleep cycle, and most adolescents have a propensity toward an evening-type circadian phase.Typically, patients with DSWPD present with complaints of difficulty falling asleep and awakening in the morning. Although there is an overlap between DSWPD and the physiologic shift seen the adolescents' circadian rhythm, these 2 entities are distinctly different. Even though most adolescents are required to sleep and wake earlier than they would naturally choose, they are able to adapt with some changes to their routines. In contrast, patients with DSWPD have extreme difficulties adjusting to socially required schedules such as at work or school. With earlier school start times, there is a significant impact on adolescents' function and performance with this disorder. When adolescents with DSWPW are allowed to sleep at their desired bedtime and wake time, they report no difficulties falling asleep and can obtain the recommended sleep hours.[42]

The focus of treatment of DSWPD aims at resynchronizing the circadian system while maintaining a rigid sleep/wake schedule.[42] Treatment starts with adolescents going to bed at their actual bedtime and gradually moving this earlier. Increasing bright light exposure in the morning and limiting daytime naps are typically recommended. Melatonin can also promote a phase shift and induce sleep[42]; however, there are no clinical trials on the appropriate dosage, effectiveness, or long-term use in adolescents. Adherence to DSWPD treatment is often challenging and requires a committed and highly motivated adolescent.

Obstructive Sleep Apnea

The prevalence of obstructive sleep apnea (OSA) is as high as 5.7% in children[43]; the precise prevalence in adolescents is unknown. There is, however, an increased likelihood of OSA in adolescents, particularly with obesity.[44] Adolescents with OSA have subcortical arousal during upper airway obstruction events, resulting in sleep fragmentation and nonrestorative sleep. Similar to adults, adolescents may present with daytime sleepiness. If left untreated, adolescents with OSA can develop cardiac complications such as hypertension, endothelial dysfunction, and left ventricular dysfunction.[45] Other manifestations of metabolic dysregulation such as insulin resistance, dyslipidemia, and liver disease can occur.[46] Currently, the gold standard for diagnosing OSA is a polysomnogram (PSG). Although home sleep apnea testing is an alternative option for diagnosis in adults with OSA and is of growing interest in younger children and adolescents, the evidence in this age group is limited. Management of OSA includes surgical interventions such as adenotonsillectomy, continuous positive airway pressure, and weight loss (through dietary and exercise measures and bariatric surgery).[47]

Narcolepsy

Narcolepsy is a rare neurologic disorder that affects an estimated one in every 2000 people in the United States.[48] Typically characterized by sudden onset EDS beginning between ages 10 and 20 years, narcolepsy affects daytime function, school, and work activities. In addition to EDS, other symptoms of narcolepsy are sudden loss of muscle tone triggered by strong emotion (cataplexy), hypnagogic and/hypnopompic hallucination, sleep paralysis, and fragmented sleep.[28] Type 1 narcolepsy (with cataplexy) is less common than narcolepsy type 2 (narcolepsy without cataplexy).[49] The diagnosis is based on findings on a polysomnogram and multiple sleep latency tests (MSLT). Specifically, a mean sleep latency of less than 8 minutes, as well as 2 or more sleep-onset REM periods (attaining REM sleep within 15 minutes of sleep onset) highly suggest narcolepsy in the proper clinical setting.[28] However, clinicians should interpret MSLT findings in adolescents with caution. For example, adolescents with chronic sleep deprivation, on medications that affect sleep, or with underlying sleep disorders such as OSA, may have MSLT results that mimic narcolepsy.[28]Additionally, a comprehensive drug screen is recommended before testing. Narcolepsy treatment includes both pharmacologic and behavioral approaches, such as improving sleep hygiene and incorporating scheduled naps. Stimulant medications including methylphenidate, (dextro) amphetamines, and wake promoting agents such as (ar) modafinil improve EDS. Cataplexy symptoms respond well to sodium oxybate (which also improves sleep consolidation), tricyclic antidepressants, and serotonin reuptake inhibitors. Education, counseling, and close collaboration with the school are essential in supporting learning accommodations.

Restless Leg Syndrome and Periodic Limb Movement Disorder

Restless legs syndrome (RLS) and periodic limb movement disorder (PLMD), common conditions in adults, frequently occur in adolescents. Although the most common presenting complaints are difficulties falling asleep and daytime sleepiness, patients report a negative mood, low energy, and impaired concentration at school/work.[50] RLS is a clinical diagnosis made based on the adolescent's report of the following criteria: an urge to move the legs that (1) is due to an uncomfortable and unpleasant sensation; (2) begins or worsens with inactivity such as sitting or lying down; (3) is partially or relieved by movement such as walking or stretching, and (4) worsens in the evening or night than during the day.[28]

Periodic limb movement disorder (PLMD) is clinically distinct from RLS, and a PSG is required to make this diagnosis. The diagnostic criteria include (1) an elevated number of periodic limb movements per hour (>5/h); (2) clinically significant sleep disturbance and other essential areas of daytime function; and (3) not better explained by other underlying sleep, medical, neurologic, or mental disorder.[28] PLMDs may occur before the sensory symptoms of RLS present.[51]

Iron deficiency, genetic factors, and dopamine dysregulation are known pathophysiologic mechanisms for RLS/PLMD. Precipitating factors are neuropathies, pregnancy, renal failure, and certain medications.[50] In addition, RLS/PLMD is frequently comorbid with ADHD, depression, and anxiety disorders.[51] RLS/PLMD treatment approaches include education on proper sleep habits and physical countermeasures such as physical relaxation, massage/stretching exercises, and warm baths. Iron supplementation is recommended in children with RLS when serum ferritin is less than 50 ng/mL.[52] Other forms of pharmacotherapy may be needed if symptoms persist despite iron replacement. Some of these medications include clonidine, benzodiazepines, gabapentin, and dopaminergic agents.[52] However, well-controlled trials in adolescents are lacking.

CONSEQUENCES OF SLEEP DEFICIENCY IN ADOLESCENTS

Adolescents are more biologically susceptible to sleep loss due to the combination of internal (physiologic) and external (environmental and social) factors (**Fig. 2**). The following section will highlight the impact of this loss on mood, risk behaviors, obesity, and academic performance.

Mood disturbances

There is likely a bidirectional relationship between sleep deficiency and mood disturbances in adolescents. In a survey of more than 10,000 US adolescents, decreased total sleep time on weeknights and oversleeping on the weekends were associated with increased odds of mood, anxiety, substance abuse, and behavioral disorders.[53] In a cross-sectional study of a nationally based population sample, 9.4% of the adolescents with a history of depression, suicidality, alcohol, cannabis, and other drug use reported insomnia symptoms.[54] Given the widespread impact of this bidirectional relationship, research is needed to determine the effect of interventions targeting sleep while examining these associations.[55]

Drowsy Driving

Insufficient sleep is a recognized risk factor for motor vehicle crashes in all age groups.[56] Because of sleep loss, there is a delay in reaction times, decreased executive functioning, and poor decision-making skills, all of which are associated with increased crash risk.[57] Drowsy driving in adolescents and young adults is a leading cause of death in this age group.[58] Studies have attributed these observations to insufficient sleep as well as circadian misalignment in adolescents.[59] In a population-based study of teen drivers, shorter school-night sleep duration and an evening chronotype were associated with self-reported drowsy driving, suggesting that circadian misalignment, in addition to chronic sleep loss, poses an increased risk of car crashes.[60]

Obesity

The prevalence of obesity worldwide, particularly over the last 3 decades, has tripled in adolescents.[61] Although several lifestyle factors (such as increased food intake, snacking, and decreased physical activity) contribute to these public health concerns, sleep deficiency plays a significant role. Based on experimental studies, changes in metabolic profiles seen with insufficient sleep include increased insulin resistance, decreased glucose tolerance, increased cortisol secretion, increased ghrelin, and decreased leptin.[62] These changes may manifest as increased hunger and decreased satiety, resulting in increased caloric intake.[62] In addition, these metabolic changes are associated with an increased risk of type 2 diabetes in obese adolescents. The increased prevalence of OSA in obese adolescents further complicates the inflammatory and metabolic consequences in these individuals.[63]

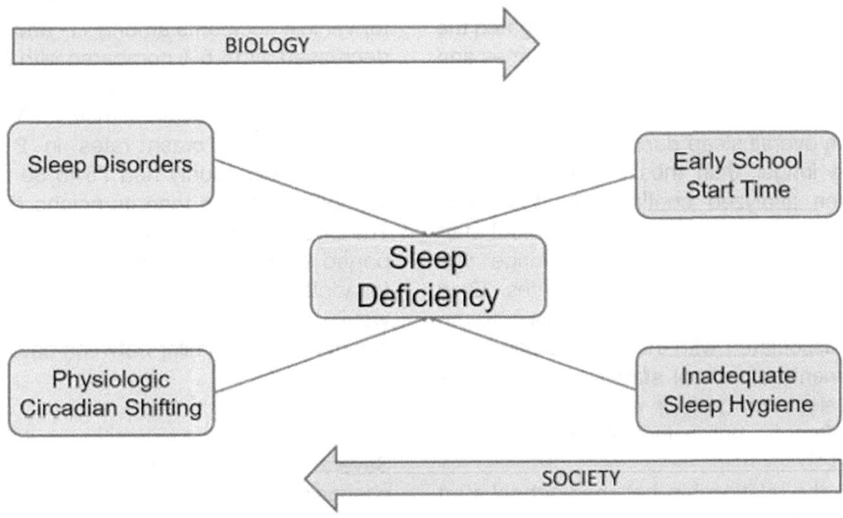

Fig. 2. Factors contributing to sleep deficiency in adolescents.

The underlying mechanism between sleep deficiency and obesity in adolescents needs to be further elucidated.[64]

Academic Performance

Over time, sleep deficiency leads to cumulative impairment with increased daytime sleepiness. These effects have been measured objectively using MSLT.[65,66] With increased sleepiness, there is a decline in cognitive function, leading to an increased likelihood of errors and lower grades. In addition, EDS significantly affects attention and concentration in school, resulting in poor school performance.[67] Adolescents tend to combat the EDS, and sleep debt accrued over the school week by oversleeping on the weekends. Increased weekend sleep of more than 2 hours has been reported in this age group and is associated with poor academic performance.[68]

SCHOOL START TIMES

Sleep deprivation in adolescents has many harmful consequences, which affect almost all domains of functioning. One option for remediating these effects is to increase overall sleep duration by moving school start times later. Resistance to later school start times is common in many school districts across the United States. Yet, robust research foundation demonstrates that (1) later school start times relate to increased sleep duration in adolescents and (2) increased sleep duration in adolescents is associated with better health, executive functions, and performance.[69]

Although most research has focused on specific school districts, at least one study investigated the relationships between high school start times and sleep duration via actigraphy across 20 cities.[70] Adolescents with school start times at 8:30 AM or later had an overall sleep duration that was 21 to 34 minutes longer than those with earlier start times. When analyzed continuously, the study found that for every 1-hour delay in school start times, sleep duration was 21 minutes longer due to later wake times of 32 to 64 minutes. Even modest delays in high school start times (>10 minutes) are associated with increased sleep duration. Opponents of school start time delays cite increased electronic use or decreased physical activity as factors, but in fact, the opposite has been found.[71]

Although the relationship between school start times and nonsleep outcomes is generally mediated by overall sleep duration, several studies have looked at the impact of school start times on domains such as health, performance, and academics. Each of these studies investigated a population where school start times were later.

Health encompasses multiple domains of functioning, and school start times have been associated with several factors. Later school start times have been associated with fewer visits to the school health office for fatigue or rest.[72] At least 3 studies have found later school start times are associated with fewer symptoms of depression[73–75] and anxiety.[74] In terms of substance use, delayed start times have been associated with decreased daily and weekly caffeine use.[73,74] Teens with later school start times are also 1.37 times less likely to use tobacco, 1.51 times less likely to use alcohol, and 1.45 times less likely to use drugs.[74]

Later school start times have also been implicated in increased attention and reaction time, 2 processes that affect performance. Two critical examples of performance in adolescents are academic functioning and driving. School start times have been associated with overall attention levels,[76] number of lapses, and better median reaction time[77] and psychomotor speed.[78]

Later school start times have been associated with better academic performance as measured by scores on school-based standardized tests.[78] They have also been shown to improve several practical measures, including lateness,[73,74,78,79] falling asleep in class, and feeling too tired to do schoolwork.[73,80]

Finally, 2 naturalistic studies have investigated the association between school start times and motor vehicle accidents in adolescents.[81,82] During the 2 years in which a school in Kentucky implemented a start time delay of 1 hour, teen motor vehicle accidents among 17- and 18-year-olds decreased by 16.5% compared with an increase in teen motor vehicle accidents of 8.0% in the 2 years before the later start times.[82] Another study compared teen crash rates in 2 SE Virginia counties: one county had 75 to 80 minutes later school start times than its neighboring county.[81] The county with the later school start times reported statistically significantly fewer crash rates for adolescents, especially at the times most teens would be driving to school.[83] Adult motor vehicle accidents were similar between counties.

SUMMARY

Several physiologic, psychological, and social changes occur during adolescence. These changes significantly affect sleep and contribute to sleep deficiency in this age group. All aspects of an adolescent's life are affected by sleep deficiency, ranging from decreased academic performance, poor executive function, and decision-making to increased risk of obesity and other health consequences, increased risk of mood disorders, suicidality, and higher rates of car crashes. Sleep disorders, including obstructive sleep apnea, narcolepsy, and restless legs syndrome, affect daytime function, resulting in sleep disruption manifested as sleep deficiency. Sleep deficiency management in adolescents involves addressing various underlying medical causes of sleep disruptors and proper healthy sleep education while addressing other psychophysiological contributors to poor sleep. Implementing delayed school start times is an effective strategy to ensure adolescents get sufficient sleep and decrease known morbidity and burden of adolescent sleep loss.

CLINICS CARE POINTS

- Sleep problems in adolescents are multifactorial. A detailed evaluation of medical, psychological and social contributors should be conducted to determine the appropriate intervention.
- Given the deleterious health and mental consequences of insufficient sleep in adolescents, there is a need for a multidisciplinary approach to addressing these issues.

DISCLOSURE

The authors have no financial or commercial conflicts of interest.

REFERENCES

1. Owens JA, Allison M, Ancona R, et al. School start times for adolescents. Pediatrics 2014;134(3):642–9.
2. Rosen DS. Physiologic growth and development during adolescence. Pediatr Rev 2004;25(6):194–200.
3. Dustman RE, Shearer DE, Emmerson RY. Life-span changes in EEG spectral amplitude, amplitude variability and mean frequency. Clin Neurophysiol 1999;110(8):1399–409.
4. Hahn M, Joechner A-K, Roell J, et al. Developmental changes of sleep spindles and their impact on sleep-dependent memory consolidation and general cognitive abilities: a longitudinal approach. Dev Sci 2019;22(1):e12706.
5. Goldstone A, Willoughby AR, de Zambotti M, et al. Sleep spindle characteristics in adolescents. Clin Neurophysiol 2019;130(6):893–902.
6. Piantoni G, Poil S-S, Linkenkaer-Hansen K, et al. Individual differences in white matter diffusion affect sleep oscillations. J Neurosci 2013;33(1):227–33.
7. Tarokh L, Carskadon MA, Achermann P. Trait-like characteristics of the Sleep EEG across adolescent development. J Neurosci 2011;31(17):6371–8.
8. Fogel SM, Smith CT. Learning-dependent changes in sleep spindles and Stage 2 sleep. J Sleep Res 2006;15(3):250–5.
9. Sulkamo S, Hagstrom K, Huupponen E, et al. Sleep spindle features and neurobehavioral performance in healthy school-aged children. J Clin Neurophysiol 2021;38(2):149–55.
10. Geiger A, Huber R, Kurth S, et al. Sleep electroencephalography topography and children's intellectual ability. Neuroreport 2012;23(2):93–7.
11. Dickey CW, Sargsyan A, Madsen JR, et al. Travelling spindles create necessary conditions for spike-timing-dependent plasticity in humans. Nat Commun 2021;12(1):1027.
12. Clemens Z, Fabo D, Halasz P. Overnight verbal memory retention correlates with the number of sleep spindles. Neuroscience 2005;132(2):529–35.
13. Gais S, Mölle M, Helms K, et al. Learning-dependent increases in sleep spindle density. J Neurosci 2002;22(15):6830–4.
14. Tapia IE, Karamessinis L, Bandla P, et al. Polysomnographic values in children undergoing puberty: pediatric vs. adult respiratory rules in adolescents. Sleep 2008;31(12):1737–44.
15. Jenni OG, Carskadon MA. Spectral analysis of the sleep electroencephalogram during adolescence. Sleep 2004;27(4):774–83.
16. Boselli M, Parrino L, Smerieri A, et al. Effect of age on EEG arousals in normal sleep. Sleep 1998;21(4):351–7.
17. Borbely AA. A two process model of sleep regulation. Hum Neurobiol 1982;1(3):195–204.
18. Borbely AA, Daan S, Wirz-Justice A, et al. The two-process model of sleep regulation: a reappraisal. J Sleep Res 2016;25(2):131–43.
19. Carskadon MA. Sleep in adolescents: the perfect storm. [Review]. Pediatr Clin North Am 2011;58(3):637–47. https://doi.org/10.1016/j.pcl.2011.03.003.
20. Ohayon MM, Carskadon MA, Guilleminault C, et al. Meta-analysis of quantitative sleep parameters from childhood to old age in healthy individuals: developing normative sleep values across the human life-span.[see comment]. Sleep 2004;27(7):1255–73.
21. Owens J. Insufficient sleep in adolescents and young adults: an update on causes and consequences. Pediatrics 2014;134(3):e921–32.
22. Olds T, Blunden S, Petkov J, et al. The relationships between sex, age, geography and time in bed in

adolescents: a meta-analysis of data from 23 countries. Sleep Med Rev 2010;14(6):371–8.
23. Jenni OG, Achermann P, Carskadon MA. Homeostatic sleep regulation in adolescents. Sleep 2005;28(11):1446–54.
24. Skorucak J, Weber N, Carskadon MA, et al. Homeostatic response to sleep restriction in adolescents. Sleep 2021;44(9):zsab106.
25. Wolfson AR, Carskadon MA, Acebo C, et al. Evidence for the validity of a sleep habits survey for adolescents. Sleep 2003;26(2):213–6.
26. Sadeh A, Dahl RE, Shahar G, et al. Sleep and the transition to adolescence: a longitudinal study. Sleep 2009;32(12):1602–9.
27. Crowley SJ, Van Reen E, LeBourgeois MK, et al. A longitudinal assessment of sleep timing, circadian phase, and phase angle of entrainment across human adolescence. PLoS One 2014;9(11):e112199.
28. American Academy of Sleep Medicine. International classification of sleep disorders. 3rd edition. Darien, IL: American Academy of Sleep Medicine; 2014.
29. Moore M. Behavioral sleep problems in children and adolescents. J Clin Psychol Med Settings 2012;19(1):77–83.
30. C Drake MK, Phillips B. National Sleep Foundation. 2005 sleep in America poll: summary of findings. 2005. www.sleepfoundation.org.
31. Calamaro CJ, Mason TBA, Ratcliffe SJ. Adolescents living the 24/7 lifestyle: effects of caffeine and technology on sleep duration and daytime functioning. Pediatrics 2009;123(6):E1005–10.
32. Hysing M, Pallesen S, Stormark KM, et al. Sleep and use of electronic devices in adolescence: results from a large population-based study. BMJ Open 2015;5(1):e006748.
33. Cain N, Gradisar M. Electronic media use and sleep in school-aged children and adolescents: a review. Sleep Med 2010;11(8):735–42.
34. Crowley SJ, Cain SW, Burns AC, et al. Increased sensitivity of the circadian system to light in early/mid-puberty. J Clin Endocrinol Metab 2015;100(11):4067–73.
35. Weaver E, Gradisar M, Dohnt H, et al. The effect of presleep video-game playing on adolescent sleep. J Clin Sleep Med 2010;6(2):184–9.
36. Carskadon MA, Mindell J, Drake C. Contemporary sleep patterns of adolescents in the USA: results of the 2006 national sleep foundation sleep in America poll. J Sleep Res 2006;15:42.
37. Pollak CP, Bright D. Caffeine consumption and weekly sleep patterns in US seventh-, eighth-, and ninth-graders. Pediatrics 2003;111(1):42–6.
38. Orbeta RL, Overpeck MD, Ramcharran D, et al. High caffeine intake in adolescents: associations with difficulty sleeping and feeling tired in the morning. J Adolesc Health 2006;38(4):451–3.
39. Hysing M, Pallesen S, Stormark KM, et al. Sleep patterns and insomnia among adolescents: a population-based study. J Sleep Res 2013;22(5):549–56.
40. Dewald-Kaufmann J, de Bruin E, Michael G. Cognitive behavioral therapy for insomnia (CBT-i) in school-aged children and adolescents. Sleep Med Clin 2019;14(2):155.
41. Sivertsen B, Pallesen S, Stormark KM, et al. Delayed sleep phase syndrome in adolescents: prevalence and correlates in a large population based study. BMC Public Health 2013;13:1163.
42. Crowley SJ, Acebo C, Carskadon MA. Sleep, circadian rhythms, and delayed phase in adolescence. Sleep Med 2007;8(6):602–12.
43. Marcus CL, Brooks LJ, Draper KA, et al. Diagnosis and management of childhood obstructive sleep apnea syndrome. Pediatrics 2012;130(3):576–84.
44. Schwab RJ, Kim C, Bagchi S, et al. Understanding the anatomic basis for obstructive sleep apnea syndrome in adolescents. Am J Respir Crit Care Med 2015;191(11):1295–309.
45. Khan MA, Mathur K, Barraza G, et al. The relationship of hypertension with obesity and obstructive sleep apnea in adolescents. Pediatr Pulmonol 2020;55(4):1020–7.
46. Patinkin ZW, Feinn R, Santos M. Metabolic consequences of obstructive sleep apnea in adolescents with obesity: a systematic literature review and meta-analysis. Child Obes 2017;13(2):102–10.
47. Amin R, Simakajornboon N, Szczesniak R, et al. Early improvement in obstructive sleep apnea and increase in orexin levels after bariatric surgery in adolescents and young adults. Surg Obes Relat Dis 2017;13(1):95–100.
48. Thorpy MJ, Krieger AC. Delayed diagnosis of narcolepsy: characterization and impact. Sleep Med 2014;15(5):502–7.
49. Goldbart A, Peppard P, Finn L, et al. Narcolepsy and predictors of positive MSLTs in the Wisconsin sleep cohort. Sleep 2014;37(6):1043–51.
50. Picchietti D, Allen RP, Walters AS, et al. Restless legs syndrome: prevalence and impact in children and adolescents - the Peds REST study. Pediatrics 2007;120(2):253–66.
51. Picchietti DL, Stevens HE. Early manifestations of restless legs syndrome in childhood and adolescence. Sleep Med 2008;9(7):770–81.
52. Sharon D, Walters AS, Simakajornboon N. Restless legs syndrome and periodic limb movement disorder in children. J Child Sci 2019;9(1):E38–49.
53. Zhang JH, Paksarian D, Lamers F, et al. Sleep patterns and mental health correlates in US adolescents. J Pediatr 2017;182:137–43.
54. Roane BM, Taylor DJ. Adolescent insomnia as a risk factor for early adult depression and substance abuse. Sleep 2008;31(10):1351–6.

55. Dodor BA, Shelley MC, Hausafus CO. Adolescents' health behaviors and obesity: does race affect this epidemic? Nutr Res Pract 2010;4(6):528–34.
56. Connor J, Norton R, Ameratunga S, et al. Driver sleepiness and risk of serious injury to car occupants: population based case control study. BMJ 2002;324(7346):1125–1128A.
57. Czeisler CA, Wickwire EM, Barger LK, et al. Sleep-deprived motor vehicle operators are unfit to drive: a multidisciplinary expert consensus statement on drowsy driving. Sleep Health 2016;2(2):94–9.
58. Pizza F, Contardi S, Antognini AB, et al. Sleep quality and motor vehicle crashes in adolescents. J Clin Sleep Med 2010;6(1):41–5.
59. Millman RP, Working Grp Sleepiness A, Adolescence AAPC. Excessive sleepiness in adolescents and young adults: causes, consequences, and treatment strategies. Pediatrics 2005;115(6): 1774–86.
60. Owens JA, Dearth-Wesley T, Herman AN, et al. Drowsy driving, sleep duration, and chronotype in adolescents. J Pediatr 2019;205:224–9.
61. Ogden CL, Carroll MD, Kit BK, et al. Prevalence of childhood and adult obesity in the United States, 2011-2012 2014;311(8):806–14.
62. Van Cauter E, Splegel K, Tasali E, et al. Metabolic consequences of sleep and sleep loss. Sleep Med 2008;9:S23–8.
63. Andersen IG, Holm JC, Homoe P. Obstructive sleep apnea in children and adolescents with and without obesity. Eur Arch Otorhinolaryngol 2019;276(3): 871–8.
64. Buzek T, Poulain T, Vogel M, et al. Relations between sleep duration with overweight and academic stress-just a matter of the socioeconomic status? Sleep Health 2019;5(2):208–15.
65. Dinges DF, Pack F, Williams K, et al. Cumulative sleepiness, mood disturbance, and psychomotor vigilance performance decrements during a week of sleep restricted to 4-5 hours per night. Sleep 1997;20(4):267–77.
66. Doran SM, Van Dongen HPA, Dinges DF. Sustained attention performance during sleep deprivation: evidence of state instability. Arch Ital Biol 2001;139(3): 253–67.
67. Wolfson AR, Carskadon MA. Sleep schedules and daytime functioning in adolescents. Child Dev 1998;69(4):875–87.
68. Knutson KL, Lauderdale DS. Sociodemographic and behavioral predictors of bed time and wake time among US adolescents aged 15 to 17 years. J Pediatr 2009;154(3):426–30.
69. Minges KE, Redeker NS. Delayed school start times and adolescent sleep: a systematic review of the experimental evidence. Sleep Med Rev 2016;28: 86–95.
70. Nahmod NG, Lee S, Master L, et al. Later high school start times associated with longer actigraphic sleep duration in adolescents. Sleep 2019;42(2): zsy212.
71. Patte KA, Qian W, Cole AG, et al. School start time changes in the COMPASS study: associations with youth sleep duration, physical activity, and screen time. Sleep Med 2019;56:16–22.
72. Whitaker RC, Dearth-Wesley T, Herman AN, et al. A quasi-experimental study of the impact of school start time changes on adolescents' mood, self-regulation, safety, and health. Sleep Health 2019; 5(5):466–9.
73. Boergers J, Gable CJ, Owens JA. Later school start time is associated with improved sleep and daytime functioning in adolescents. J Dev Behav Pediatr 2014;35(1):11–7.
74. Wahlstrom KL, Owens JA. School start time effects on adolescent learning and academic performance, emotional health and behaviour. Curr Opin Psychiatry 2017;30(6):485–90.
75. Owens JA, Belon K, Moss P. Impact of delaying school start time on adolescent sleep, mood, and behavior. Arch Pediatr Adolesc Med 2010;164(7): 608–14.
76. Lufi D, Tzischinsky O, Hadar S. Delaying school starting time by one hour: some effects on attention levels in adolescents. J Clin Sleep Med 2011;7(2): 137–43.
77. Vedaa O, Saxvig IW, Wilhelmsen-Langeland A, et al. School start time, sleepiness and functioning in Norwegian adolescents. Scand J Educ Res 2012;56(1): 55–67.
78. Alfonsi V, Palmizio R, Rubino A, et al. The association between school start time and sleep duration, sustained attention, and academic performance. Nat Sci Sleep 2020;12:1161–72.
79. Wahlstrom KL, Berger AT, Widome R. Relationships between school start time, sleep duration, and adolescent behaviors. Sleep Health 2017;3(3):216–21.
80. Li SH, Arguelles L, Jiang F, et al. Sleep, school performance, and a school-based intervention among school-aged children: a sleep series study in China. Plos One 2013;8(7):e67928.
81. Vorona RD, Szklo-Coxe M, Lamichhane R, et al. Adolescent crash rates and school start times in two central Virginia counties, 2009-2011: a follow-up study to a southeastern Virginia study, 2007-2008. J Clin Sleep Med 2014;10(11):1169–77.
82. Danner F, Phillips B. Adolescent sleep, school start times, and teen motor vehicle crashes. J Clin Sleep Med 2008;4(6):533–5.
83. Vorona RD, Szklo-Coxe M, Wu A, et al. Dissimilar teen crash rates in two neighboring southeastern Virginia cities with different high school start times. J Clin Sleep Med 2011;7(2):145–U181.

Work Around the Clock

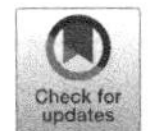

How Work Hours Induce Social Jetlag and Sleep Deficiency

Joseph T. Hebl, BA[a], Josie Velasco, BS[b,c], Andrew W. McHill, PhD[b,c,*]

KEYWORDS

• Shift work • Circadian misalignment • Chronic disease • Sleep hygiene
• Sleep and circadian medicine • Chronotherapy

KEY POINTS

- The endogenous circadian time-keeping system influences human physiology in healthy and in diseased states.
- Misalignment between behaviors and the circadian clock (ie, circadian misalignment) disrupts optimal functioning of physiologic processes, predisposing individuals to cardiovascular, metabolic, and respiratory disease.
- Working during biologic nighttime hours (ie, shift work) and weekly changes in sleep and subsequent circadian timing (ie, social jetlag) are common causes of circadian misalignment and are associated with impaired health profiles.
- Countermeasures, such as improving sleep hygiene, maintaining consistent sleep schedules, and scheduling work timing to match endogenous circadian timing, have been shown to be effective in combating circadian misalignment.

INTRODUCTION

As much as the understanding of human health and disease is predicated on behaviors and exposures during wakefulness, several decades of research have begun to uncover the importance of sleep and its impacts on physiology and pathology. From an evolutionary perspective, sleep places humans in a state of vulnerability, and yet this behavior is shared universally by mammals.[1] However, it is now understood that sleep duration and timing are essential for optimal cognitive and physiologic functioning.[2–4] Sleep and wakefulness are impacted by several external and internal factors, but none are more important than the endogenous circadian system.

The term circadian is derived from Latin meaning “about a day” and the circadian “clock” is an endogenous, self-sustaining, biologic time-keeping system with a period of approximately 24 hours in humans.[5] This system is extremely precise, with a standard deviation of 12 minutes within mice models and 8 minutes in humans, yet

Support: This work was supported by National Institutes of Health grants K01HL146992, R56 HL156948, R35 HL155681, and U19OH010154; and by the Oregon Institute of Occupational Health Sciences at Oregon Health & Science University via funds from the Division of Consumer and Business Services of the State of Oregon (ORS 656.630).

[a] Oregon Health and Sciences University, School of Medicine, 3455 SW US Veterans Hospital Road, Mailcode: SN-ORD, Portland, OR 97239, USA; [b] Sleep, Chronobiology, and Health Laboratory, School of Nursing, Oregon Health & Science University, 3455 SW US Veterans Hospital Road, Mailcode: SN-ORD, Portland, OR 97239, USA; [c] Oregon Institute of Occupational Health Sciences, Oregon Health & Science University, 3455 SW US Veterans Hospital Road, Mailcode: SN-ORD, Portland, OR 97239, USA

* Corresponding author. Sleep, Chronobiology, and Health Laboratory, School of Nursing, Oregon Health & Science University, 3455 SW US Veterans Hospital Road, Mailcode: SN-ORD, Portland, OR 97239.
E-mail address: mchill@ohsu.edu

Clin Chest Med 43 (2022) 249–259
https://doi.org/10.1016/j.ccm.2022.02.003
0272-5231/22/

chestmed.theclinics.com

entrainable to external and behavioral stimuli known as "zeitgebers" (ie, time givers).[5–7] Mechanistically, the precision of the circadian clock is established by a transcriptional autoregualtory loop that exists centrally within the suprachiasmatic nucleus of the hypothalamus, and in peripheral tissues.[8,9] The suprachiasmatic nucleus further supports the system's pliability by modulating the pineal gland's secretion of the hormone melatonin in response to changes in light-timing exposure.[7–10] Circadian "rhythms" are the physiologic outputs of the circadian clock, such as the circadian-based variations in hormone secretion, enzyme activity, and organ function, among others.[11,12]In the laboratory, the circadian clock is measured via oscillations in these physiologic processes (ie, core body temperature, cortisol, or melatonin concentrations).[11]

Much of what is known about the circadian clock and its impacts on physiology has come from studies where the clock is desynchronized from confounding behaviors (ie, sleep, wakefulness, eating, and physical activity) and from external stimuli (eg, light exposure), which can influence physiologic rhythms. This desynchronization is also understood as circadian misalignment, a behavioral pattern in which sleep and activity occur during conflicting circadian phases (eg, sleeping during the day, eating and activity during the night). Circadian misalignment can also be observed naturally in individuals experiencing irregular sleep either resulting from endogenous factors, such as sleep disorders, or from exogenous factors, such as work and social schedules (**Fig. 1**). We review the fundamental relationships between the circadian timing system and biologic processes, considering how common practices, such as shift work and variations in sleep timing on work/school versus work/school-free days (ie, social jetlag), disrupt circadian alignment and predispose individuals to cardiovascular, metabolic, and pulmonary disease.

CIRCADIAN IMPACTS ON PHYSIOLOGY

The self-regulatory genes that define the circadian clock can themselves directly impact the transcription of genes involved in biologically relevant pathways. Research into mouse models has shown that nearly half of all transcripts in the genome are under circadian control.[13] This is true even within complex tissues, such as the liver and heart, which both demonstrate circadian variations in gene expression, although the expression profile varies significantly between the two.[14] This variation in gene expression ultimately manifests in circadian dynamics of macroscopic physiology.

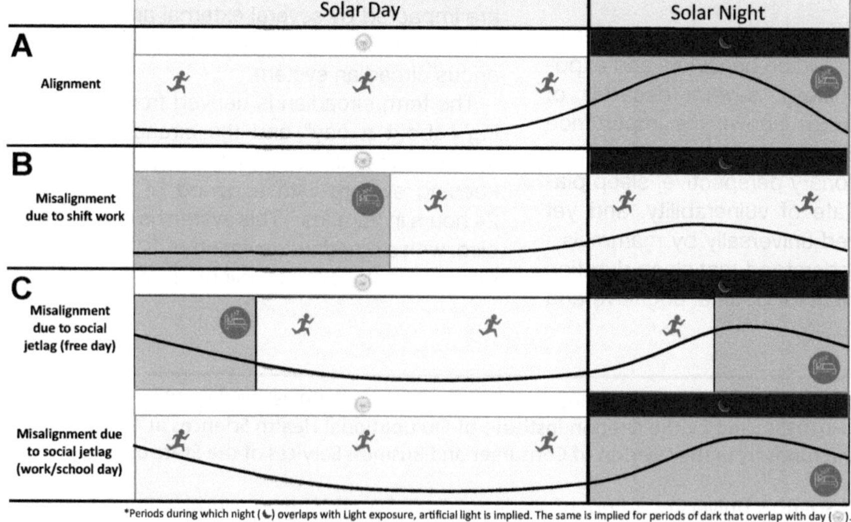

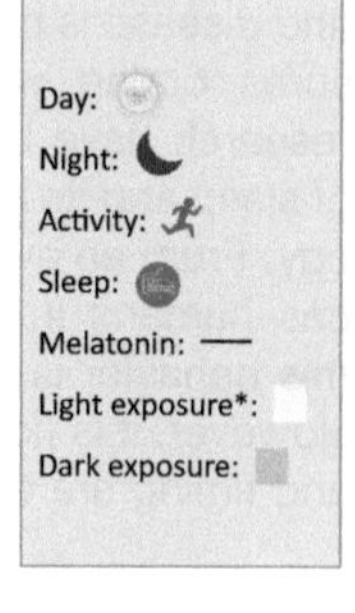

Fig. 1. Relationships between light exposure, activity/rest patterns, and the melatonin rhythm during circadian alignment, shift work, and social jetlag. (*A*) An alignment in which activity/rest, the internal biologic circadian day/night (represented by the circadian melatonin rhythm), and light exposure are synchronized. (*B*) Demonstration of how work hours (ie, shift work) create a misalignment by altering light exposure and activity patterns that dampen the melatonin peak at night. (*C*) Misalignment resulting from social jetlag on the weekend. Specifically, social jetlag is a phenomenon in which individuals delay bedtime (thereby exposed to light later) on free days resulting in a free day delay in the circadian clock (*C, top row*), which subsequently causes a misalignment when an individual must return to work/school schedules (*C, bottom row*).

Cardiovascular System

Within the cardiovascular system, many processes are influenced by circadian timing. Under tightly controlled in-laboratory environments, blood pressure displays circadian rhythmicity with a predictable zenith and nadir even in the absence of sleep.[15] However, sleep induces an additional "dip" in blood pressure in most healthy individuals.[16] Although, in the heart, this is likely the result of cortisol and vagal modulation, variation in blood pressure can also be attributed to the influence of circadian timing in the kidney, mediated by the renin-angiotensin-aldosterone system, and via blood flow dynamics within the vasculature.[17–19] Circadian timing, in addition to diurnal variation, may also play a role in cardiovascular dysfunction, as evidenced by the observed increase in major cardiovascular events during the morning.[20,21] Several factors have been implicated in this epidemiologic phenomenon and evidence suggests that the circadian-based variation in cortisol, a stress hormone that is elevated during the morning and impacts cardiovascular and metabolic functioning, may play a role.[22] Thus, these factors place a predisposed heart at increased risk.

Metabolism

Many rate-limiting enzymes involved in metabolic pathways, such as in fatty acid and sterol biosynthesis, are under circadian control.[23,24] Moreover, many metabolic hormones and subsequent metabolites demonstrate circadian rhythmicity.[25] Glucose homeostasis appears to depend on circadian influences, with one study finding that ablation of circadian genes in the pancreas triggers poor glucose control and the onset of diabetes mellitus in mice.[26] In a seminal study investigating the impact of circadian timing on postprandial glucose, insulin, and cortisol, healthy participants were given isocaloric meals every 6 or 12 hours over a 36-hour period, with both scenarios involving a "morning" (0600h) and "evening" (2000h) meal. Results showed that postprandial glucose response was greater following evening meals but, interestingly, was not associated with a commensurate increase in insulin secretion.[12] This latter finding suggests possible circadian variation in β-cell function in the pancreas (ie, variation in insulin production in response to increased blood glucose). The dawn phenomena, a symptom of diabetes in which an increased dosage of insulin in type 2 diabetics is required in the morning for what is believed to be the result of decreased insulin sensitivity, may also exemplify how circadian timing impacts physiology in the diseased state.[27] The circadian variation in insulin sensitivity and β-cell function, specifically as it relates to circadian misalignment, is discussed later.

The process of respiration displays circadian rhythmicity during controlled in-laboratory settings, with increased and decreased respiratory rates observed in the morning and evening, respectively.[28] Moreover, this variation observed in the laboratory persists even as the circadian clock is dissociated from behaviors, such as sleep, wakefulness, eating, and activity.[28,29] The decrease in apparent respiratory drive at night is believed to play a major role in the pathophysiology of sleep disorders and to contribute to increased rates of respiratory failure at night.[30] Chronic respiratory diseases, such as asthma, are also affected by circadian timing. Most notably, it has long been observed that asthma symptoms increase at night, likely reflecting the injurious affects that circadian variation can have on predisposed individuals.[31–34]

SHIFT WORK AND SOCIAL JETLAG

Sleep deficiency and dysregulation can result from several mechanisms involving endogenous and/or exogenous factors. We consider how human behaviors, such as shift work and social jet lag (see **Fig. 1**), affect sleep behavior, induce circadian misalignment, and impact health.[35–38]

Shift Work

An estimated 17% to 20% of the US workforce engages in some form of shift work, which typically involves periods of work that occur during normal sleep time.[39] In this way shift work can precipitate circadian misalignment, which manifests most directly in irregular sleep schedules, less overall sleep, and poorer sleep hygiene when compared with a daytime work schedule.[40] The American Academy of Sleep Medicine has developed the shift work sleep disorder diagnosis in response to this robust finding of sleep deficiency among shift workers.[41] Contrary to what is commonly believed, adjustment to night shift work, as measured via melatonin phase, seems minimal even among chronic night shift workers with one report finding that less than a quarter of these individuals demonstrate "substantial" circadian adjustment.[42,43] Without the capacity to sufficiently shift the circadian clock, many shift workers are exposed to extended episodes of circadian misalignment, which is linked to a multitude of adverse health outcomes.[40,43–48]

Regarding chronic disease, shift workers have up to a 40% increased risk of cardiovascular disease, a 25% to 45% increased risk in obesity, a

10% to 16% increased risk of diabetes, and up to a 55% increase in odds of having asthma.[44,45,47,49] Given these epidemiologic findings, recent work has been done in laboratory settings to understand the degree to which these adverse health trends are explained by circadian misalignment versus other factors, such as food intake, activity level, sleep, and light exposure.

Cardiovascular System

In investigating the impacts of shift work on cardiovascular biomarkers, one study exposed chronic shift workers to two 3-day protocols, one of which simulated night work (12-hour inverted behavioral and environmental schedule) and the other simulated day work. Circadian misalignment, as represented by a simulated night shift, was significantly correlated with increased blood pressure and increased C-reactive protein, a non-specific inflammatory marker implicated in the progression of heart disease.[50,51] Exposure to similar protocols has revealed that circadian misalignment significantly increases the serum concentration of other non-specific inflammatory markers, including interleukin-6 and tumor necrosis factor-α, which are themselves risk factors for cardiovascular disease.[52] Blood pressure, which can represent a risk factor for cardiovascular disease, is also impacted by shift work. Blood pressure "dipping" ($\geq$10% reduction in blood pressure as compared with daytime levels) during sleep is a typical phenomenon in healthy individuals, whereas "nondippers" (<10% reduction in blood pressure as compared with daytime levels) have been found to have increased mortality and cardiovascular disease risk.[53,54] A study investigating how shift work impacts "dipping" status found that among newly hired transit operators who began working the early morning shift and who were considered "dippers" before employment, 62% were converted to a "nondipper" status at 90 days of working early morning shifts.[55] This is in comparison with those who began working the day shift, all of whom were found to have healthy blood pressure dipping at the 90-day mark, and 50% of whom had converted to a dipping status during the study monitoring period.[55] Similar studies have been conducted to understand how shift work predisposes individuals to metabolic disease.

Metabolism

Shift work is associated with increased rates of obesity and metabolic disease.[46,49,56] To elucidate probable mechanisms, researchers using rodent models have shown that restricting feeding to only the rest phase (as is similar with night shift workers who consume a major portion of their calories during the circadian rest phase) results in significant increases in body weight, fat deposits, and body mass index.[57,58] This was true even though there was no statistical difference with control mice regarding total caloric intake and physical activity. Similar findings in human studies suggest that the mechanism of weight gain secondary to circadian misalignment is partly caused by changes in energy expenditure that are not explained by variations in physical activity and caloric intake.[59] In one study, researchers used an 8-day crossover protocol in which participants were exposed to either 5 days of simulated night shifts or day shifts, which was then repeated later using the same 8-day protocol with the alternative simulated schedule (night versus day shift). The study found that diet-induced thermogenesis, which represents a major component of daily energy expenditure, was 44% lower following evening as compared with morning meals and was primarily explained by circadian influence rather than behavioral pattern.[60] Surprisingly, circadian misalignment did not significantly impact diet-induced thermogenesis in this study, although a similar study using a 6-day protocol with 3 days of inverted sleep and wakefulness (circadian misalignment) found a 3% to 4% decrease in overall energy expenditure, with a 4% decrease in diet-induced thermogenesis following meals consumed later in the evening.[61] This research suggests that food intake during the evening hours (ie, during the circadian rest phase) is metabolized differently than during the circadian daytime. For shift workers, food intake at night is often a necessity, which considering this research may help explain the increased body weight seen in epidemiologic studies.

Underlying these links between adverse changes in body composition and simulated shift work is the change observed in insulin sensitivity and glucose tolerance under circadian misalignment. In a direct experiment looking into the impacts of melatonin on glucose tolerance, participants given an oral dose of melatonin in either the evening or morning had subsequent impairment in glucose tolerance.[62] This is relevant because mealtimes for shift workers often coincide with episodes of increased melatonin (ie, at night during the circadian rest phase). In a more thorough in-laboratory examination of shift work pattern and glucose control, participants in an extended circadian disruption study were subjected to 3 weeks of sleep restriction and extended days (ie, >24 hours).[63] The study found that there was an increase in fasting glucose and postprandial glucose levels of 8% and 14%, respectively, with corresponding decreases in insulin levels of 12% to 27% compared with baseline.[63] The study also found that a 9-day recovery phase following misalignment restored insulin and glucose ranges to baseline levels in most participants, implying that the system is rectifiable.

Insulin dysfunction seen in circadian misalignment highlights the interplay between the function and/or reactivity of pancreatic β cells and insulin sensitivity in peripheral tissues. In normal circadian alignment, β-cell function is decreased during evening hours, resulting in decreased serum insulin relative to blood glucose levels.[12] This may explain why those who eat later tend to have poorer metabolic profiles.[35,64,65] However, the mechanism changes when the circadian system is misaligned.[64] In a study of chronic shift workers exposed to a 12-hour inverted behavioral schedule to mimic shift work, researchers found misalignment to result in a 10% increase in late phase postprandial insulin even while postprandial glucose remained elevated.[43] These results suggest that glucose tolerance diminishes secondarily to decreased insulin sensitivity in peripheral tissues. This may help explain the increased incidence in type 2 diabetes among shift workers because this disease is partly defined by insulin insensitivity.[66]

Shift work is not the only behavioral pattern to impact sleep, circadian rhythms, and health. Social jetlag is a similar phenomenon with a less drastic effect on sleep patterns but with the potential to have equally deleterious health consequences.

Social Jetlag

Social jetlag is defined as a sleep pattern that varies between work/school days and free days (**Fig. 2**). During consecutive work or school days, many individuals are unable to obtain sufficient sleep, or sleep at unpreferred times, and thus resort to "sleeping-in" on free days to recover. Typically, sleep is increased by 2 to 3 hours during this "weekend recovery" sleep, which subsequently shifts the individual's wakefulness schedule in a manner similar to travel-related jetlag.[67] Social jetlag is most common among late chronotypes, colloquially known as "night owls," whose biologic waking time is at odds with work hours.[68] Late chronotypes, in comparison with early chronotypes who fall asleep early and wake early, are more common and represent a growing demographic in industrialized nations likely because of societal selection for prolonged social/work schedules with increased light exposure at night.[68,69]

Poor health is more commonly observed in late chronotypes, who are 2.5 times more likely than early chronotypes to report their general health to be poor or fair.[70] Late chronotypes who are more likely to experience severe social jetlag are also more likely to smoke, participate in sleep-interfering behaviors, are less physically active,

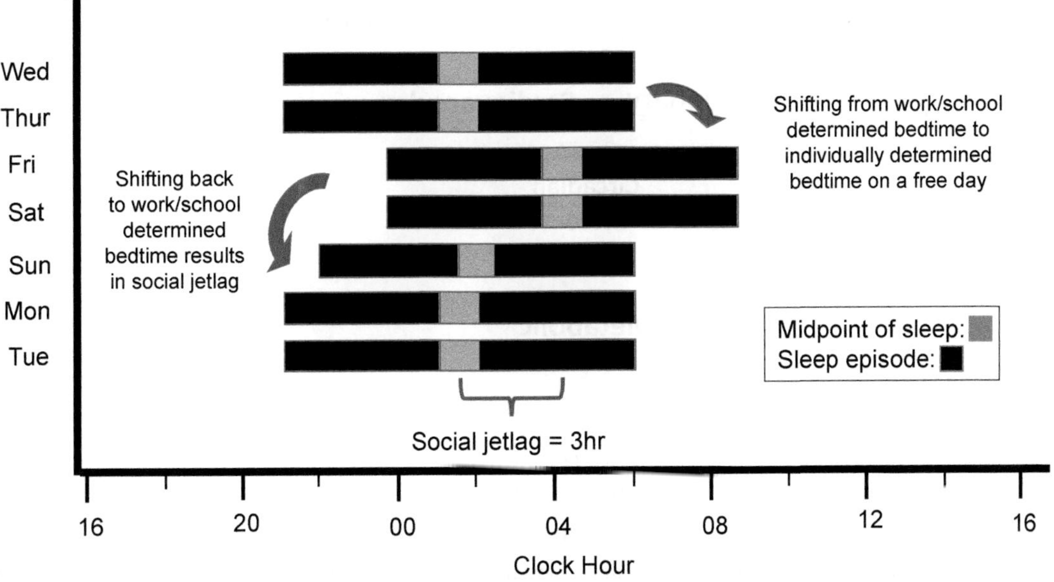

Fig. 2. Example of a social jetlag schedule. Delayed sleep onset on weekends because of individually preferred bedtimes results in later sleep and light exposure timing. Return to work/school-determined sleep pattern abruptly advances sleep timing in a way similar to air travel–associated jetlag.

and report increased rates of sleep disturbance.[71] Objectively speaking, late chronotypes have a 2.5-fold increase in type 2 diabetes mellitus, 1.2-fold increase in obesity, and a 1.3-fold increase in metabolic syndrome, the odds of which increase by 30% for every additional hour of "oversleep" on free days.[72,73] Late chronotypes are also at increased risk of developing asthma.[72] In terms of cardiovascular health, late chronotypes have 1.3-fold increase in hypertension and those experiencing social jetlag have a 20% increase in cardiovascular risk, which increases by 30% for each additional hour of "oversleep."[72,74] Some have linked increased cardiovascular-related deaths on Mondays to the impacts of social jetlag, although others cite a lack of sufficient evidence for the epidemiologic phenomenon.[75,76] Laboratory research into social jetlag has found similar underlying pathologic processes to that of shift work. Regarding insulin sensitivity changes, a study using healthy participants found there to be a 20% reduction in early morning oral and intravenous insulin sensitivity following 5 days of sleep restriction (5 hours per night), with the magnitude of insulin sensitivity directly correlated with the magnitude of circadian misalignment.[77] An investigation into the chronic impacts of social jetlag in mice found that shifting the 12-hour light exposure schedule by 6 hours every 7 days resulted in decreased lifespan and survival rates.[38]

Although shift work is a more severe form of circadian misalignment, social jetlag is linked to a degree of misalignment sufficient to generate similar adverse trends in cardiovascular, metabolic, and respiratory health. From a population health standpoint, social jetlag is more widely experienced in industrialized nations and its consequences more broadly felt, as in one study that found social jetlag induced by time zones to associate not only with poorer health trends, but also poorer economic performance.[78] The adverse impacts of social jetlag are not experienced exclusively by working adults. In fact, social jetlag seems to be an epidemic among adolescent populations.[79]

The physiologic changes occurring during adolescence, in conjunction with the psychosocial factors related to this phase of early life, represents a "perfect storm" that predisposes this population to social jetlag.[79,80] Melatonin release is delayed during adolescence in part because of normal physiologic changes, but also because of increased light sensitivity.[81,82] Furthermore, adolescence represents a phase of increased social

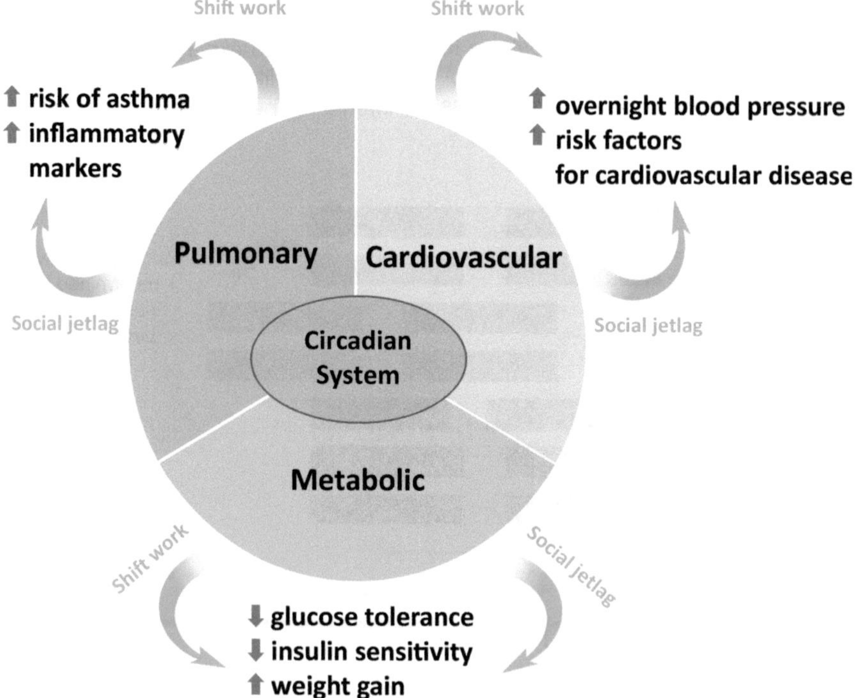

Fig. 3. Cardiometabolic impacts when the circadian system is disrupted by social jetlag and shift work. A typically well-functioning network between the circadian system and major physiologic systems is disrupted by social jetlag and shift work, resulting in adverse health patterns that predispose to disease development and progression. *Blue arrows* point to examples of the disruptive sequelae of social jetlag and shift work.

responsibility and independence (ie, sleep-time autonomy; academic scheduling and pressure; and increased screen time).[83] These factors place adolescents at increased risk of experiencing social jetlag, which is positively associating with anxiety symptoms, poorer eating habits, and body mass index percentile.[69,83–85] Delaying school start times has been shown to mitigate some of these issues related to adolescent sleep deprivation and social jetlag. However, adoption of such measures comes with significant sociopolitical hurdles.[86]

COUNTERMEASURES

The most salient physiologic symptoms of shift work and social jetlag are sleep disruption and decreased alertness while awake. Symptom management has largely centered around the latter via the use of stimulants. Caffeine has for centuries been used to increase awareness and has been shown to improve psychomotor vigilance and wakefulness, particularly during times of circadian misalignment.[87,88] Periodic naps, in conjunction with caffeine, have been found to further augment wakefulness, alertness, and psychomotor vigilance testing on simulated night shifts.[87] However, caffeine can diminish the quality of daytime sleep recovery, thus making the balance between increasing alertness and maintaining sleep quality difficult to achieve.[89] Modafinil, a psychostimulant used to treat excessive daytime sleepiness in patients with narcolepsy and obstructive sleep apnea, has been shown to decrease sleepiness in laboratory settings, and improve tests of memory and attention when compared with placebo.[90–92] However, there is no improvement in duration or quality of daytime recovery sleep, indicating that long-term use may likewise be less effective.[90] Although capable of improving performance measures during the short term, stimulants diminish the duration and quality of recovery sleep, which is essential to restoring and/or adjusting the circadian clock while also being protective against disease. Therefore, approaches to improve sleep recovery have also been tested, including the use of melatonin, which has been shown to improve sleep duration during daytime sleep.[93] However, there is minimal effect on performance measures assessed during subsequent evening shifts.[93]

Alternatively, changes in shift scheduling and other environmental measures may help in diminishing the degree of circadian misalignment. Human circadian rhythms have been shown to respond more quickly to phase delay (ie, going to bed and waking up later), than phase advance (ie, going to bed and waking up earlier).[94] Thus, establishing shift schedules to rotate clockwise (day to afternoon, afternoon to night) and also to involve smaller magnitudes in transition (<6 hours) may mitigate misalignment.[94,95] Controlling for other variables, such as light exposure (eg, wearing sunglasses before day-recovery sleep, or "pulses" of bright light during work), room temperature during sleep and work, and food intake can also improve overall perception of sleepiness and be protective against adverse health effects of shift work.[94,96,97]

For those working permanent night shifts, the goal is to allow for alertness and productivity during the night shift, while also preserving some degree of daytime wakefulness to be used socially on free days. Without a medicinal quick-fix, a "compromised" shift schedule in the circadian clock has been proposed (ie, permanent shift in the circadian-phase positions).[98] By using bright light pulses during simulated shift work, dark sunglasses for use outside to block blue-enriched light, adherence to scheduled sleep times in dark rooms, and outdoor afternoon light exposures to mitigate extreme rhythm delay, researchers have been able to delay participants' circadian clock to have a nadir in alertness at approximately 10:00.[99] In comparison with control subjects who had a circadian nadir of approximately 6:00, the treatment group was found to have increased overall sleep (sufficient sleep during daytime following night shifts and late nighttime on days off), and improved performance during night shifts.[99] As with all attempts at circadian entrainment, the challenge with a compromised circadian-phase shift is adherence to the sleep-behavior regimen.

SUMMARY

The circadian timing system is a powerful biologic system that, when in sync with daily habits, aids in optimal physiologic functioning. However, when exposed to environments that induce misalignment, research demonstrates not only acute, but also long-term impacts on cardiovascular, metabolic, and respiratory health (**Fig. 3**). This is not restricted to those working night shifts, because the adoption of prolonged work and social schedules, and increased light exposure at night have led many in industrialized countries to suffer from varying degrees of circadian misalignment. This social jetlag has also been shown to contribute to worsening health trends. Several modalities have been researched to address the symptoms of sleep deficiency induced by shift work and social jetlag, yet it seems conservative measures, most notably that of consistent sleep schedules in addition to proper sleep hygiene (light exposure, room temperatures, food intake), are the most protective and cost effective.

CLINICS CARE POINTS

- Assessment of sleep patterns, behaviors, and hygiene is an essential component of a thorough medical history.
- Understand that chronic diseases are significantly impacted by and often develop within a context of poor sleep hygiene; therefore, sleep health should be addressed in care planning and disease management.
- Encourage proper sleep hygiene beyond the usual "try to sleep more."
- Establishing and adhering to consistent sleep schedule on work and off days.
- Control light exposure leading up to and during sleep (ie, no cellphones in bed).
- Moderate use of stimulants.
- Recovery days following periods of sleep deficiency are effective at rectifying the circadian system.
- Minimize large meals during evening periods when one is typically sleeping.
- Advocate for your patients with their employers, highlighting not just the health benefits of consistent work and sleep schedules, but also the improved productivity.
- Ensure you yourself practice proper sleep hygiene; before you can take care of others, you must take care of yourself.

DISCLOSURE

The authors have nothing to disclose.

REFERENCES

1. Capellini I, Barton RA, McNamara P, et al. Phylogenetic analysis of the ecology and evolution of mammalian sleep. Evolution 2008;62(7):1764–76.
2. Besedovsky L, Lange T, Haack M. The sleep-immune crosstalk in health and disease. Physiol Rev 2019;99(3):1325–80.
3. Walker MP. The role of sleep in cognition and emotion. Ann N Y Acad Sci 2009;1156:168–97.
4. Cappuccio FP, Miller MA. Sleep and cardio-metabolic disease. Curr Cardiol Rep 2017;19(11):110.
5. Czeisler CA, Duffy JF, Shanahan TL, et al. Stability, precision, and near-24-hour period of the human circadian pacemaker. Science 1999;284(5423):2177–81.
6. Herzog ED, Aton SJ, Numano R, et al. Temporal precision in the mammalian circadian system: a reliable clock from less reliable neurons. J Biol Rhythms 2004;19(1):35–46.
7. VanderLeest HT, Houben T, Michel S, et al. Seasonal encoding by the circadian pacemaker of the SCN. Curr Biol 2007;17(5):468–73.
8. Mohawk JA, Green CB, Takahashi JS. Central and peripheral circadian clocks in mammals. Annu Rev Neurosci 2012;35:445–62.
9. Stratmann M, Schibler U. Properties, entrainment, and physiological functions of mammalian peripheral oscillators. J Biol Rhythms 2006;21(6):494–506.
10. Roenneberg T, Daan S, Merrow M. The art of entrainment. J Biol Rhythms 2003;18(3):183–94.
11. Benloucif S, Guico MJ, Reid KJ, et al. Stability of melatonin and temperature as circadian phase markers and their relation to sleep times in humans. J Biol Rhythms 2005;20(2):178–88.
12. Van Cauter E, Shapiro ET, Tillil H, et al. Circadian modulation of glucose and insulin responses to meals: relationship to cortisol rhythm. Am J Physiol 1992;262(4 Pt 1):E467–75.
13. Zhang R, Lahens NF, Ballance HI, et al. A circadian gene expression atlas in mammals: implications for biology and medicine. Proc Natl Acad Sci 2014;111(45):16219–24.
14. Storch KF, Lipan O, Leykin I, et al. Extensive and divergent circadian gene expression in liver and heart. Nature 2002;417(6884):78–83.
15. Shea SA, Hilton MF, Hu K, et al. Existence of an endogenous circadian blood pressure rhythm in humans that peaks in the evening. Circ Res 2011;108(8):980–4.
16. Lo K, Woo B, Wong M, et al. Subjective sleep quality, blood pressure, and hypertension: a meta-analysis. J Clin Hypertens (Greenwich) 2018;20(3):592–605.
17. Scheer FAJL, Hu K, Evoniuk H, et al. Impact of the human circadian system, exercise, and their interaction on cardiovascular function. Proc Natl Acad Sci 2010;107(47):20541–6.
18. Thosar SS, Rueda JF, Berman AM, et al. Separate and interacting effects of the endogenous circadian system and behaviors on plasma aldosterone in humans. Am J Physiol Regul Integr Comp Physiol 2019;316(2):R157–64.
19. Thosar SS, Berman AM, Herzig MX, et al. Circadian rhythm of vascular function in midlife adults. Arterioscler Thromb Vasc Biol 2019;39(6):1203–11.
20. Willich SN, Levy D, Rocco MB, et al. Circadian variation in the incidence of sudden cardiac death in the Framingham Heart Study population. Am J Cardiol 1987;60(10):801–6.

21. Muller JE, Stone PH, Turi ZG, et al. Circadian variation in the frequency of onset of acute myocardial infarction. N Engl J Med 1985;313(21):1315–22.
22. Crawford AA, Soderberg S, Kirschbaum C, et al. Morning plasma cortisol as a cardiovascular risk factor: findings from prospective cohort and Mendelian randomization studies. Eur J Endocrinol 2019; 181(4):429–38.
23. Bass J, Takahashi JS. Circadian integration of metabolism and energetics. Science 2010;330(6009): 1349–54.
24. Le Martelot G, Claudel T, Gatfield D, et al. REV-ERBalpha participates in circadian SREBP signaling and bile acid homeostasis. Plos Biol 2009;7(9): e1000181.
25. Shea SA, Hilton MF, Orlova C, et al. Independent circadian and sleep/wake regulation of adipokines and glucose in humans. J Clin Endocrinol Metab 2005;90(5):2537–44.
26. Marcheva B, Ramsey KM, Buhr ED, et al. Disruption of the clock components CLOCK and BMAL1 leads to hypoinsulinaemia and diabetes. Nature 2010; 466(7306):627–31.
27. Campbell PJ, Bolli GB, Cryer PE, et al. Pathogenesis of the dawn phenomenon in patients with insulin-dependent diabetes mellitus. N Engl J Med 1985; 312(23):1473–9.
28. Zitting KM, Vujovic N, Yuan RK, et al. Human resting energy expenditure varies with circadian phase. Curr Biol 2018;28(22):3685–90.e3.
29. Spengler CM, Czeisler CA, Shea SA. An endogenous circadian rhythm of respiratory control in humans. J Physiol 2000;526 Pt 3(Pt 3):683–94.
30. Schäfer T. Respiratory pathophysiology: sleep-related breathing disorders. GMS Curr Top Otorhinolaryngol Head Neck Surg 2006;5:Doc01.
31. Turner-Warwick M. Epidemiology of nocturnal asthma. Am J Med 1988;85(1b):6–8.
32. Hetzel MR, Clark TJ. Comparison of normal and asthmatic circadian rhythms in peak expiratory flow rate. Thorax 1980;35(10):732–8.
33. Spiro SG. Nocturnal asthma and sudden death. Am Fam Physician 1976;14(6):62–71.
34. Scheer F, Hilton MF, Evoniuk HL, et al. The endogenous circadian system worsens asthma at night independent of sleep and other daily behavioral or environmental cycles. Proc Natl Acad Sci U S A 2021;(37):118. https://doi.org/10.1073/pnas.2018486118.
35. McHill AW, Czeisler CA, Phillips AJK, et al. Caloric and macronutrient intake differ with circadian phase and between lean and overweight young adults. Nutrients 2019;11(3). https://doi.org/10.3390/nu11030587.
36. Emens J, Lewy A, Kinzie JM, et al. Circadian misalignment in major depressive disorder. Psychiatry Res 2009;168(3):259–61.
37. Merikanto I, Lahti T, Kronholm E, et al. Evening types are prone to depression. Chronobiol Int 2013;30(5): 719–25.
38. Davidson AJ, Sellix MT, Daniel J, et al. Chronic jet-lag increases mortality in aged mice. Curr Biol 2006;21:R914–6.
39. McMenamin TM. A time to work: recent trends in shift work and flexible schedules. Monthly LabRev 2007;130(3):3–15.
40. Costa G. Sleep deprivation due to shift work. Handb Clin Neurol 2015;131:437–46.
41. Sateia MJ. International classification of sleep disorders-third edition: highlights and modifications. Chest 2014;146(5):1387–94.
42. Folkard S. Do permanent night workers show circadian adjustment? A review based on the endogenous melatonin rhythm. Chronobiol Int 2008;25(2): 215–24.
43. Morris CJ, Purvis TE, Mistretta J, et al. Effects of the internal circadian system and circadian misalignment on glucose tolerance in chronic shift workers. J Clin Endocrinol Metab 2016;101(3):1066–74.
44. Vetter C, Dashti HS, Lane JM, et al. Night shift work, genetic risk, and type 2 diabetes in the UK Biobank. Diabetes Care 2018;41(4):762–9.
45. Maidstone RJ, Turner J, Vetter C, et al. Night shift work is associated with an increased risk of asthma. Thorax 2021;76(1):53–60.
46. Vetter C, Devore EE, Wegrzyn LR, et al. Association between rotating night shift work and risk of coronary heart disease among women. JAMA 2016; 315(16):1726–34.
47. Brown DL, Feskanich D, Sánchez BN, et al. Rotating night shift work and the risk of ischemic stroke. Am J Epidemiol 2009;169(11):1370–7.
48. Akerstedt T, Wright KP Jr. Sleep loss and fatigue in shift work and shift work disorder. Sleep Med Clin 2009;4(2):257–71.
49. Karlsson B, Knutsson A, Lindahl B. Is there an association between shift work and having a metabolic syndrome? Results from a population based study of 27,485 people. Occup Environ Med 2001; 58(11):747–52.
50. Morris CJ, Purvis TE, Mistretta J, et al. Circadian misalignment increases C-reactive protein and blood pressure in chronic shift workers. J Biol Rhythms 2017;32(2):154–64.
51. Castro AR, Silva SO, Soares SC. The use of high sensitivity C-reactive protein in cardiovascular disease detection. J Pharm Occupy Sci 2018;21(1): 496–503.
52. Morris CJ, Purvis TE, Hu K, et al. Circadian misalignment increases cardiovascular disease risk factors in humans. Proc Natl Acad Sci U S A 2016; 113(10):E1402–11.
53. Fagard RH, Celis H, Thijs L, et al. Daytime and night-time blood pressure as predictors of death and

cause-specific cardiovascular events in hypertension. Hypertension 2008;51(1):55–61.
54. Ohkubo T, Hozawa A, Yamaguchi J, et al. Prognostic significance of the nocturnal decline in blood pressure in individuals with and without high 24-h blood pressure: the Ohasama study. J Hypertens 2002; 20(11):2183–9.
55. McHill AW, Velasco J, Bodner T, et al. Rapid changes in overnight blood pressure after transitioning to early-morning shiftwork. Sleep 2021. https://doi.org/10.1093/sleep/zsab203.
56. Mason IC, Qian J, Adler GK, et al. Impact of circadian disruption on glucose metabolism: implications for type 2 diabetes. Diabetologia 2020;63(3): 462–72.
57. Arble DM, Bass J, Laposky AD, et al. Circadian timing of food intake contributes to weight gain. Obes (Silver Spring) 2009;17(11):2100–2.
58. Salgado-Delgado R, Angeles-Castellanos M, Saderi N, et al. Food intake during the normal activity phase prevents obesity and circadian desynchrony in a rat model of night work. Endocrinology 2010;151(3):1019–29.
59. Westerterp KR. Diet induced thermogenesis. Nutr Metab (Lond) 2004;1(1):5.
60. Morris CJ, Garcia JI, Myers S, et al. The human circadian system has a dominating role in causing the morning/evening difference in diet-induced thermogenesis. Obesity (Silver Spring) 2015;23(10): 2053–8.
61. McHill AW, Melanson EL, Higgins J, et al. Impact of circadian misalignment on energy metabolism during simulated nightshift work. Proc Natl Acad Sci U S A 2014;111(48):17302–7.
62. Rubio-Sastre P, Scheer FA, Gómez-Abellán P, et al. Acute melatonin administration in humans impairs glucose tolerance in both the morning and evening. Sleep 2014;37(10):1715–9.
63. Buxton OM, Cain SW, O'Connor SP, et al. Adverse metabolic consequences in humans of prolonged sleep restriction combined with circadian disruption. Sci Transl Med 2012;4(129): 129ra43.
64. Qian J, Dalla Man C, Morris CJ, et al. Differential effects of the circadian system and circadian misalignment on insulin sensitivity and insulin secretion in humans. Diabetes Obes Metab 2018;20(10): 2481–5.
65. Mattson MP, Allison DB, Fontana L, et al. Meal frequency and timing in health and disease. Proc Natl Acad Sci U S A 2014;111(47):16647–53.
66. Stumvoll M, Goldstein BJ, van Haeften TW. Type 2 diabetes: principles of pathogenesis and therapy. Lancet 2005;365(9467):1333–46.
67. Wittmann M, Dinich J, Merrow M, et al. Social jetlag: misalignment of biological and social time. Chronobiol Int 2006;23(1–2):497–509.
68. Roenneberg T, Wirz-Justice A, Merrow M. Life between clocks: daily temporal patterns of human chronotypes. J Biol Rhythms 2003;18(1):80–90.
69. Hena M, Garmy P. Social jetlag and its association with screen time and nighttime texting among adolescents in Sweden: a cross-sectional study. Front Neurosci 2020;14:122.
70. Paine SJ, Gander PH, Travier N. The epidemiology of morningness/eveningness: influence of age, gender, ethnicity, and socioeconomic factors in adults (30-49 years). J Biol Rhythms 2006;21(1): 68–76.
71. Suh S, Yang HC, Kim N, et al. Chronotype differences in health behaviors and health-related quality of life: a population-based study among aged and older adults. Behav Sleep Med 2017;15(5):361–76.
72. Merikanto I, Lahti T, Puolijoki H, et al. Associations of chronotype and sleep with cardiovascular diseases and type 2 diabetes. Chronobiol Int 2013;30(4):470–7.
73. Parsons MJ, Moffitt TE, Gregory AM, et al. Social jetlag, obesity and metabolic disorder: investigation in a cohort study. Int J Obes (Lond) 2015;39(5):842–8.
74. Gamboa Madeira S, Reis C, Paiva T, et al. Social jetlag, a novel predictor for high cardiovascular risk in blue-collar workers following permanent atypical work schedules. J Sleep Res 2021;e13380. https://doi.org/10.1111/jsr.13380.
75. Arntz HR, Müller-Nordhorn J, Willich SN. Cold Monday mornings prove dangerous: epidemiology of sudden cardiac death. Curr Opin Crit Care 2001;7(3):139–44.
76. Barnett AG, Dobson AJ. Excess in cardiovascular events on Mondays: a meta-analysis and prospective study. J Epidemiol Community Health 2005; 59(2):109–14.
77. Eckel RH, Depner CM, Perreault L, et al. Morning circadian misalignment during short sleep duration impacts insulin sensitivity. Curr Biol 2015;25(22): 3004–10.
78. Giuntella O, Mazzonna F. Sunset time and the economic effects of social jetlag: evidence from US time zone borders. J Health Econ 2019;65:210–26.
79. Crowley SJ, Wolfson AR, Tarokh L, et al. An update on adolescent sleep: new evidence informing the perfect storm model. J Adolesc 2018;67:55–65.
80. Carskadon MA. Sleep in adolescents: the perfect storm. Pediatr Clin North Am 2011;58(3):637–47.
81. Crowley SJ, Acebo C, Fallone G, et al. Estimating dim light melatonin onset (DLMO) phase in adolescents using summer or school-year sleep/wake schedules. Sleep 2006;29(12):1632–41.
82. Crowley SJ, Cain SW, Burns AC, et al. Increased sensitivity of the circadian system to light in early/mid-puberty. J Clin Endocrinol Metab 2015; 100(11):4067–73.
83. Touitou Y, Touitou D, Reinberg A. Disruption of adolescents' circadian clock: the vicious circle of media

use, exposure to light at night, sleep loss and risk behaviors. J Physiol Paris 2016;110(4 Pt B):467–79.
84. Mathew GM, Li X, Hale L, et al. Sleep duration and social jetlag are independently associated with anxious symptoms in adolescents. Chronobiol Int 2019;36(4):461–9.
85. Mathew GM, Hale L, Chang AM. Social jetlag, eating behaviours and BMI among adolescents in the USA. Br J Nutr 2020;124(9):979–87.
86. Carvalho-Mendes RP, Dunster GP, de la Iglesia HO, et al. Afternoon school start times are associated with a lack of both social jetlag and sleep deprivation in adolescents. J Biol Rhythms 2020;35(4): 377–90.
87. Schweitzer PK, Randazzo AC, Stone K, et al. Laboratory and field studies of naps and caffeine as practical countermeasures for sleep-wake problems associated with night work. Sleep 2006;29(1):39–50.
88. McHill AW, Smith BJ, Wright KP Jr. Effects of caffeine on skin and core temperatures, alertness, and recovery sleep during circadian misalignment. J Biol Rhythms 2014;29(2):131–43.
89. Carrier J, Fernandez-Bolanos M, Robillard R, et al. Effects of caffeine are more marked on daytime recovery sleep than on nocturnal sleep. Neuropsychopharmacology 2007;32(4):964–72.
90. Czeisler CA, Walsh JK, Roth T, et al. Modafinil for excessive sleepiness associated with shift-work sleep disorder. N Engl J Med 2005;353(5):476–86.
91. Broughton RJ, Fleming JA, George CF, et al. Randomized, double-blind, placebo-controlled crossover trial of modafinil in the treatment of excessive daytime sleepiness in narcolepsy. Neurology 1997; 49(2):444–51.
92. Kuan YC, Wu D, Huang KW, et al. Effects of modafinil and armodafinil in patients with obstructive sleep apnea: a meta-analysis of randomized controlled trials. Clin Ther 2016;38(4):874–88.
93. Sharkey KM, Fogg LF, Eastman CI. Effects of melatonin administration on daytime sleep after simulated night shift work. J Sleep Res 2001;10(3): 181–92.
94. Wallace PJ, Haber JJ. Top 10 evidence-based countermeasures for night shift workers. Emerg Med J 2020;37(9):562–4.
95. Harrison EM, Walbeek TJ, Maggio DG, et al. Circadian profile of an emergency medicine department: scheduling practices and their effects on sleep and performance. J Emerg Med 2020;58(1):130–40.
96. Gupta CC, Centofanti S, Dorrian J, et al. Altering meal timing to improve cognitive performance during simulated nightshifts. Chronobiology Int 2019; 36(12):1691–713.
97. Smith MR, Eastman CI. Shift work: health, performance and safety problems, traditional countermeasures, and innovative management strategies to reduce circadian misalignment. Nat Sci Sleep 2012;4:111–32.
98. Eastman CI, Martin SK. How to use light and dark to produce circadian adaptation to night shift work. Ann Med 1999;31(2):87–98.
99. Smith MR, Fogg LF, Eastman CI. Practical interventions to promote circadian adaptation to permanent night shift work: study 4. J Biol Rhythms 2009;24(2): 161–72.

Sleep Deficiency in Pregnancy

Arlin Delgado, MD, Judette M. Louis, MD, MPH*

KEYWORDS

• Pregnancy • Sleep deficiency • Maternal outcomes • Labor outcomes • Sleep health equity

KEY POINTS

- Sleep is critical and necessary for a person to maintain a healthy lifestyle, requiring 7 to 8 hours nightly during adulthood.
- During pregnancy, sleep deficiency may be caused by many physiologic, emotional, and mental health changes.
- Sleep deficiency is associated with an increased risk of adverse maternal outcomes (gestational diabetes, hypertensive disorders, and depression) as well as preterm labor and delivery.
- Socioeconomic factors and social determinants of health are critical factors that must be evaluated further to best address sleep health disparities in these at-risk populations.
- Future research needs to evaluate if sleep deficiency is a causal factor in adverse maternal and neonatal outcomes.

INTRODUCTION

Sleep is considered a critical and necessary aspect of one's daily life for overall health. The National Sleep Foundation recommends that a person sleep approximately 7 to 9 hours per 24 hour during adulthood, ages 26 to 64 years of age.[1] However, in 2014, up to 35% of adults reported short sleep duration, and up to 34% (CI 34.4%–35.2%) of women were affected.[2] Abnormalities in sleep duration, poor sleep quality, and abnormal timing of sleep all contribute to morbidity in the affected individual. Although studies in pregnancy are limited, in the general populations, existing data indicate that these sleep disturbances are associated with mortality risk, impaired metabolism, impaired learning and cognitive functioning, and overall poorer quality of life.[3,4] In the 2018 "Sleep in America Poll," women reported a lower effectiveness, defined as ability to complete daily tasks and responsibilities, when analyzing their sleep health compared with men.[5] This finding is further supported by several studies in which women were found to report higher levels of self-reported sleep deprivation and sleep problems.[6,7]

Despite these concerning statistics, this literature fails to comprehensively address the challenges specific to women. Sleep in women is affected by a multitude of factors—including socioeconomic factors, natural physiologic changes, and demographic characteristics.

One impactful socioeconomic factor is the entrance of women into the work force. As women enter careers, they are now juggling family-related responsibilities and the demands of a workforce that are negatively affecting their sleep hygiene. This was found in a secondary analysis of data from The Sister Study, a prospective cohort study of women aged 35 to 74 years. Cross-sectional and longitudinal sleep data was available for more than 20,000 women. Patient perceived sex-specific and sexual orientation-specific job discrimination was significantly and independently associated with shorter sleep duration and higher odds of having short sleep duration (less than 7 hours/night) at the start of the study. Among those who did not have abnormal sleep, age-specific job

Department of Obstetrics and Gynecology, Morsani College of Medicine, University of South Florida Morsani College of Medicine, 2 Tampa General Circle, Tampa, FL 33606, USA
* Corresponding author.
E-mail address: Jlouis1@usf.edu

Clin Chest Med 43 (2022) 261–272
https://doi.org/10.1016/j.ccm.2022.02.004

discrimination was associated with the new onset of short sleep at time 2 (OR = 1.21, 95% CI: 1.03, 1.43).[8] Considering these competing responsibilities and tasks, women reported they ran out of time to sleep more frequently than men.[9]

Physiologically, natural hormone fluctuations across varying time points in life (from puberty to menstruation and through postmenopausal states) affect sleep differently. This effect is due to established associations between the fluctuations in estrogen and progesterone that are associated with changes in sleep–wake cycles, affecting the quality and quantity of sleep.[10,11]

Sleep Pattern Changes in Pregnancy

During pregnancy, there are different hormonal and physiologic changes that adversely affect a woman's ability to sleep (**Table 1**).[11] Mindell, Cook, and Nikolovski (2015)[12] distributed a survey to more than 2400 pregnant women and found that 76% reported insufficient nighttime sleep, 49% reported significant daytime sleepiness, and 78% required daytime naps. Meanwhile, Hedman and colleagues (2002)[13] surveyed women before, during, and after pregnancy and found self-reported sleep duration increased during the first trimester of pregnancy but subsequently decreased after delivery. The mean sleep duration was 7.8 hours before pregnancy, 8.2 hours in the first trimester ($P < .001$), and 7 hours after delivery ($P < .001$). Objectively, women who were followed using activity tracking devices during pregnancy were found to have a significant inverse association between gestational age and sleep duration (-B = 0.2; $P < .001$).[14] The nuMoM2b Sleep Duration and Continuity Substudy is a prospective study of a subset of the women enrolled in the nuMoM2b parent study. The primary objective of this substudy was to examine the relationship of objectively assessed sleep duration, continuity, and timing, with cardiovascular and metabolic morbidity related to pregnancy. A total of 782 nulliparous women wore a wrist actigraphic monitor and completed a sleep log for 7 consecutive days before 23 weeks of gestation. Approximately one-third (27.9%) of these women had a sleep duration less than 7 hours.[15] A meta-analysis of 5 studies using polysomnography to quantify and define sleep patterns in pregnancy supports the findings. There was an overall significantly reduced total sleep time from the first to the third trimester of pregnancy by 26.8 minutes (pooled WMD, 95% CI = 12.14–41.56).[16] Increases in a woman's wake after sleep onset, and transition from N3 sleep stage and rapid eye movement sleep to more superficial nonrapid eye movement sleep are hypothesized to cause the observed sleep structure changes. These changes then lead to a subjectively perceived less restorative sleep pattern.

These sleep stage transitions, in part, are due to an increase in estrogen production, which also leads to increasing hyperemia and collapsibility of the upper airways, possibly worsening underlying sleep-related disorders.[17] Furthermore, changes in the metabolism of supplements, such as iron and folate, are associated with increasing restless leg syndrome. An increase in water retention increases renal blood flow that leads to urinary frequency, often requiring multiple awakenings per night, especially in the third trimester.[17] Melatonin, a hormone well established in regulation of the circadian rhythm, is also impacted during pregnancy–with an initial increase in the first trimester, a decrease in the middle of pregnancy, and then a final increase in the third trimester associated with the onset of labor. Although no data in humans is established, rat studies suggest the placenta is a source of melatonin and can cross the maternal–fetal interface increasing serum levels.[18] All of these changes can interact to contribute negatively to a woman's ability to sleep.[11]

SLEEP HEALTH DISPARITIES IN PREGNANCY

Sleep health disparities defined as differences in one or more dimensions of sleep health (duration, efficiency, timing, regularity, alertness, and quality) that adversely affect designated disadvantaged populations are prevalent yet understudied. In a multisite survey and chart review of 267 pregnant women by Kalmbach and colleagues (2019),[19] the researchers found a high prevalence of self-reported sleep disturbance. Short sleep duration was reported in 24% of women who were on average 28 weeks of gestation women (±1.20, range 25–37). Women living in poverty (defined as less than $20K annual household income) were 72% more likely to have an increased score (>8) on the Pittsburgh sleep quality index (PSQI), with higher scores indicating worsening sleep. Moreover, although not statistically significant, it was noted that women in poverty reported less sleep compared with women not in poverty (6.31 hours vs 6.66 hours, respectively). Additionally, women living in poverty were more likely to identify as Black race (67.5% vs 23.9%, $P < .001$). Similarly, in a study of 133 women surveyed during each trimester and between 4 and 11 weeks postpartum, using the PSQI, it was found that African American women subjectively had poor sleep.[20] Most recently, Feinstein, and

Table 1
Factors contributing to sleep deficiency in pregnancy

	First Trimester	Second Trimester	Third Trimester
Factors decreasing sleep	Nausea/vomiting Urinary frequency Backache	Fetal movement Heartburn Cramps Tingling in extremities Shortness of breath Night awakening	

colleagues (2020),[21] published findings on the evaluation of 14 years of cross-sectional National Health Interview Survey showing that compared with pregnant White women, pregnant Black women had a higher short sleep prevalence (prevalence ratio for pregnant Black women = 1.35; 95% CI, 1.08–1.6). Article published by Okun and colleagues[22] further supported this in which 170 pregnant women were assessed between 10 and 20 weeks gestation in which it was found women with household income less than $50K per year was associated with poorer sleep quality on the PSQI ($P < .05$) and greater sleep fragmentation ($P < .05$), using PSQI as well as actigraphy, respectively. These findings are supported by the Nulliparous Pregnancy Outcomes Study: monitoring mothers-to-be sleep activity substudy. The Sleep Duration and Continuity substudy included pregnant women (16–21 weeks of gestation) who underwent 7 days of actigraphy. Among the 782 participants, 27.9% had short sleep duration (<7 hours). Increasing age, race-ethnicity (specifically non-Hispanic Black, and Asian), increasing BMI, insurance (specifically commercial), and recent smoking history were significantly associated with shorter sleep duration.[15] Further, in that sample, there were differences in sleep efficiency and fragmentation. Social inequalities do exist, and their presence predisposes these populations to sleep-related adverse health outcomes.

Sleep Deficiency and Risk for Depression, Antepartum, and Postpartum

Depression is considered one of the most common complications of pregnancy. Research shows that quality and quantity of sleep in pregnancy are predictors of depression in the postpartum period.[23–25] Peripartum and postpartum depression affects approximately 10% to 20% of women.[26] The prevalence has been increasing with as evidenced by a doubling in the rate of antidepressant use during pregnancy since 1999.[27,28] Peripartum depression is defined as the onset of a major depressive disorder during pregnancy. Postpartum depression is defined as the onset of a major depressive episode within 4 weeks from delivery; however, some will argue for inclusions of onset up to 12 weeks from delivery (**Table 2**).[29] Episodes of depression are, in turn, linked with many adverse maternal and neonatal outcomes. Maternal outcomes include risk of preterm delivery, lack of infant bonding, increased risk of suicidality, and use of substances and other risky behaviors.[30] Adverse neonatal outcomes including increased risk of small for gestational age, and potentially low birth weight infants,[31] failure to thrive, and difficulties with development in cognitive, behavioral, and emotional domains.[30]

Field (2007) studied sleep quality, defined as the number of nightly sleep disturbances, and found was linked to an increased risk of depression symptoms in the second and third trimesters.[32] In a prospective study, 63 women were followed through the latter stage of pregnancy (defined between 36 weeks gestation and term), and results indicated a history of sleep disruption during this time was associated with the onset of postnatal blues, a transient mood disturbance within the weeks after delivery.[33] Skouteris and colleagues (2008)[23] established sleep quality early in pregnancy would predict levels of depressive symptoms later in pregnancy, after following women starting at 15 to 23 weeks gestation for 3 times at 8-week intervals. This association held even after controlling for already present depressive symptoms. Similarly, in a cross-sectional study of 360 women who completed a PSQI questionnaire and the Edinburgh Postnatal Depression Scale (EPDS), women with poor sleep quality were 3.34 more times higher than women who reported good sleep quality to have high depression scores (odds ratio = 3.34, CI 2.04–5.48, $P < .001$).[34]

However, these studies do not evaluate the impact of sleep duration on a woman and her pregnancy. In a study by Jomeen and Martin (2007),[35] women with depression in pregnancy were more likely to report short sleep duration on

Table 2
Definitions of maternal and pregnancy-related health outcomes

Health Outcomes	Timing of Onset	Diagnostic Criteria
Maternal-Related Health Disorders and Outcomes		
Peripartum depression	Any gestational age	Depressive episode meeting criteria per the DSMV criteria
Postpartum depression	After delivery until 12 wk from delivery	Depressive episode meeting criteria per the DSMV criteria
GDM	Any gestational age	Two or more elevated glucose values during a 3-h 100g glucose tolerance test[a]
Chronic hypertension	<20 wk gestation	Two or more blood pressures with: • SBP[a] > 140 and/or DBP [b] > 90
Gestational hypertension	>20 wk gestation	2 or more blood pressures with: • SBP[b] > 140 and/or DBP[c]>90
Preeclampsia	–	Chronic or gestational hypertension diagnosis and: 24 h protein >300g or Urine protein/creatinine > 0.3
Preeclampsia with severe features	–	Preeclampsia and (at least one of the following): • Thrombocytopenia (platelets <100K) • Elevated liver enzymes twice upper limit of normal • Severe persistent right upper quadrant or epigastric pain • Abnormal renal clearance (creatinine > 1.1 or twice patient baseline) • New onset headache unresponsive to medical management or visual disturbances • Pulmonary edema
Shoulder dystocia	At time of delivery	Vaginal delivery requiring additional maneuvers to deliver a fetus after gentle traction and pulling have failed to deliver the infant shoulder
Neonate and Infant-Related Health Disorders and Outcomes		
Preterm birth	20 wk 0 d–36 wk 6 d gestation	Periviable and viable delivery (via vaginal delivery or cesarean section)
Stillbirth	–	Delivery of dead infant, previously viable
Macrosomia	–	Infant weighing >4000 g at time of delivery

[a] Based off Carpenter and Coustan.
[b] SBP: systolic blood pressure.
[c] DBP: diastolic blood pressure.

the PSQI (PSQI subscale mean scores of 0.32 vs 0.79, $P = .002$) at 14 weeks gestation. In a prospective study by Okun and colleagues (2013)[36] of 160 pregnant women, up to 38% of women met criteria for sleep deficiency. This was defined as deficiency in duration (with 7 hours as threshold), insufficiency (determined by 5 question measure), or insomnia symptoms (positive case based on Insomnia Sleep Quality scoring criteria) in at least 1 time point during their early gestation (either between 10 and 12, 14 and 16, or 18 and 20 weeks gestation). At 10 to 12 weeks gestation, 14 to 16 weeks gestation, and 18 to 20 weeks gestation, the prevalence of reported short sleep duration decreased from approximately 10% to 5%. Women who were sleep deficient across all 3 study time points reported more perceived stress when comparing the Perceived Stress Scale (PSS) scores between the sleep-deficient and nonsleep-deficient groups ($F_{2,157} = 5.53$; $P < .01$), as well as an increase in depressive symptoms calculated from the Inventory of Depressive Symptomatology scale (IDS; $F_{2,157} = 3.85$; $P = .02$). Wrist actigraphs with a sleep deficiency defined as less than 6 hours supported these qualitative findings—regardless of which gestational age time point (either between 10 and 12, 14 and 16, or 18 and 20 weeks gestation), a woman's score for depressive symptomology and pregnancy-related distress (using PSS and IDS, respectively) did not differ among those sleep deficient or not ($F_{2,157} = 1.71$; $P = .18$ and $F_{2,157} = 2.86$; $P = .06$, respectively). A woman's perceived stress level was significantly related to sleep deficiency ($F_{2,157} = 5.31$, $P < .01$; **Table 3**).

The association between sleep deficiency and depression is challenging to delineate as it is uncertain which factors impact or leads to the other first. The studies suggesting an association between sleep quality and quantity with depression are often based on self-reported data with minimal objective data and are often cross-sectional, precluding the establishment of causation. In addition, the association between sleep quality, quantity, and depression is confounded and impacted by socioeconomics, age, education, occupation, and familial responsibilities and expectations among women.[27,37,38] Future literature should seek to establish causation between sleep deficiency and depression as the adverse neonatal and maternal outcomes associated with depression are economically and emotionally costly.

Sleep Deficiency and Risk for Gestational Diabetes

Gestational diabetes (GDM) in pregnancy is defined as carbohydrate intolerance that develops during pregnancy. It is one of the most common medical complications faced during pregnancy, and it is the cause of up to 86% of all reported diabetes during pregnancy.[39–41] Physiologically, a woman's increase in hormones (estrogen, progesterone, leptin, cortisol, placental lactogen, and growth hormone) promotes a state of insulin resistance and gluconeogenesis. This state can lead to hyperglycemia, and therefore promotes an imbalance of oxidants leading to oxidative stress and increasing inflammatory state in tissues (muscle and/or adipose). Insulin resistance additionally creates neurohormonal imbalances that upregulate satiety and hunger signals, leading to increased caloric intake, which further exacerbates the situation.[42]

Women diagnosed with GDM are at increased risk for adverse maternal and neonatal outcomes. Maternal outcomes include an increased risk for preeclampsia,[43] and development of diabetes long term.[44] The affected neonates are at increased risk for macrosomia, neonatal hypoglycemia, shoulder dystocia, and stillbirth[45,46] (see **Table 2**).

Several studies within the last 12 years have sought to study the association between sleep and the development of GDM. Early work found self-reported sleep less than 7 hours per night was associated with an increased risk for GDM.[47] In another study of more than 1200 women, self-reported sleep duration of less than 4 hours per night was associated with a significantly increased relative risk of GDM compared with those reporting 9 hours per night even after adjusting for age and ethnicity (RR = 5.56, 95% CI 1.31–23.69.[48] However, this study's definition of sleep duration (<4 hours per night) was considered extreme as it only represented 1.6% of the cohort and is not an accepted definition. Recently, several studies[49–51] sought to study these associations among Asian women and once again found associations between sleep deficiency and GDM. Zhou and colleagues (2016)[49] and Cai and colleagues (2017)[51] both found an increased risk of GDM with short sleep duration (less than 7 hours and less than 6 hours nightly, respectively). Conversely, a study by Reutrakul and colleagues (2011)[52] did not find the same association. In a group of 169 women with 26 cases of GDM, the association between GDM and short sleep duration defined as less than 7 hours was not statistically significant (unadjusted OR = 2.4, 95% CI 1.0–5.9, $P = .06$). Additionally, Wang and colleagues (2017)[50] found self-reported sleep duration less than 7 hours was not associated with GDM (aOR = 1.36, 95% CI 0.87–2.14).

These studies were limited by their sample size and limited power to detect an association between sleep duration and GDM. The cohorts were also not generalizable as they tended to be homogenous in race/ethnicity among the patient population and from single-site centers. These concerns were subsequently addressed between two studies recently published within the last

Table 3
Sleep deficiency and depression, antepartum, and postpartum

Study	Study Type	Study Population	Evaluation	Conclusions
Field et al (2007)	Prospective cohort	83 depressed; 170 depressed (divided by formal interview) in second and third trimester	Self-reported scales: CES-D, STAI, STAXI, VITAS, and sleep scale[a]; Urine assays—cortisol and norepinephrine	Depressed women had high depression ($P < .05$), anxiety ($P < .01$), and sleep disturbance scores ($P < .01$) in both trimesters
Wilkie, et al (1992)	Prospective cohort	63 women in third trimester and postnatal period	Self-reported scale: Stein questionnaire; Kendell score	90% reported worse sleep at end of third trimester Poorer sleep quality recorded the increasing emotional distress recorded
Skouteris, et al (2008)	Prospective cohort	273 women followed at 15–23 wk with q8week intervals for 3 follow-ups	Self-reported scale: PSQI[b] and Beck depression inventory	Sleep quality in early pregnancy predicted levels of depressive symptoms later in pregnancy
Iranpour, et al (2016)	Cross-sectional	360 pregnant women	Self-reported scale: PSQI and EPDS[c]	Women with poor sleep quality were more likely to have higher depression score
Jomeen and Martin, 2007	Cross-sectional	148 pregnant women	Self-reported scale: PSQI and EPDS[c]	Women with higher depression scores had shorter sleep duration ($P = .002$)
Okun, et al (2013)	Prospective cohort	160 pregnant at 10–12, 14–16, and 18–20 wk gestation	Self-reported sleep diary Actigraphy	Women who were sleep deficiency across all time points perceived higher stress ($P < .01$) and depressive levels ($P = .02$)

[a] CES-D = Clinical Epidemiologic Studies Depression Scale; STAI = State/trait anxiety index; STAXI = State/trait anger inventory; VITAS = VITAS healthcare corporation.
[b] PSQI = Pittsburgh sleep questionnaire index.
[c] EPDS = Edinburgh postnatal depression scale.

5 years. In a study across 12 clinical sites with more than 2581 women when exposed to short or long sleep durations were compared with GDM regardless of obesity, no association was found, but when compared among nonobese women, sleep duration in the second trimester only was associated with GDM after adjustment for multiple confounding factors (prepregnancy BMI, family history, age, ethnicity, gestational age, parity, and marital status).[53] Finally, a study by Facco and colleagues (2017)[54] objectively assessed sleep parameters and found exposure to less than 7 hours of sleep per night during pregnancy was associated with an increased odds of GDM compared with longer sleep, adjusting for other confounding factors (like BMI) with a 2-fold increased risk.

Overall, the literature suggests a clear association between sleep deficiency and GDM. However, it is unclear whether that association is limited to populations that would otherwise be at low risk for GDM. Future work should establish if there is causation and the implementation of protective factors to reduce the risk of GDM.

Sleep Deficiency and Risk for Hypertensive Disorders

Hypertensive disorders in pregnancy include chronic hypertension, gestational hypertension, and preeclampsia. Chronic hypertension and gestational hypertension, as well as preeclampsia, are disorders defined based on elevated blood pressure values and laboratory abnormalities[55] (see **Table 2**). These disorders have been previously associated with adverse maternal outcomes,[56] including myocardial infarct, acute respiratory distress, renal failure, coagulopathy, and adverse fetal outcomes,[57] including oligohydramnios, intrauterine growth restriction, and preterm delivery. One earlier study by Edwards and colleagues (2000)[58] found women with these disorders may have underlying altered sleep patterns. The authors studied sleep architecture using a polysomnogram in 25 preeclamptic patients and compared them to 17 primigravida women to find that preeclamptic patients had an increased percentage of time spent in slow-wave sleep ($P < .001$), as well as a decrease in rapid eye movement; however, these patients were simultaneously on clonidine—an antihypertensive medication known to alter sleep architecture.

Very few studies have examined the association between sleep quantity or quality and hypertension. Williams and colleagues (2010)[59] completed a prospective cohort study of 1272 healthy pregnant women. Medical records were extracted to find blood pressure values and sleep deficiency assessed using self-reported sleep duration. Women with short sleep (defined as less than 5 hours) had an increased likelihood of pregnancy-induced hypertension and development of preeclampsia (OR 9.52, 95% CI 1.82–49.4). In a case series of 9 women with preeclampsia and 8 women with normal term pregnancy, sleep quality was evaluated using recorded nocturnal body movement activity with a static charge-sensitive bed and found women with preeclampsia had a significantly increased total frequency of body movements.[60] However, both groups self-reported similar subjective sleep complaints, and this study did not define sleep duration as a complaint. Furthermore, although essential demographic characteristics were collected in these studies, no further analysis was performed to risk stratify women (**Table 5**).

Table 4
Sleep deficiency and preterm birth

Study	Study Type	N (Preterm/ Full Term)	Comparison Made	Relative Risk (95% CI)	Adjusted Odds Ratio (95% CI)
Michell, et al 2011	Prospective cohort	131/960	<5 h vs 6–7 h vs >8 h	1.7 (1.1–2.8)[a] 0.9 (0.6–1.4) 1.0	
Kajeepeta, 2014	Case-control	479/480	<6 h vs 7–8 h vs ≥9 h		**1.53 (1.08–2.17)**[b] 1 (referent) 1.5 (1.04–2.16)
Okun, et al (2012)	Prospective cohort	26/186	<7 h vs >9 h		0.86 (0.29–0.2.59) 1.19 (0.38–3.75)

Bold indicates ratio was significant, at $P < .05$.
[a] Adjusted for maternal age, education, prepregnancy BMI, and smoking status.
[b] Adjusted for maternal age, prepregnancy weight, unplanned pregnancy, no vitamin use and sleep duration, as well as vital exhaustion.

Table 5
Sleep deficiency and hypertensive disorders

Study	Study Type	Population	Evaluation Methods	Conclusions
Ekholm, et al (1992)	Cross-sectional	9 preeclamptic, 8 nonpreeclamptic	Nocturnal body movement activity	Preeclamptic women had increased body movement frequency
Edwards, et al (2000)	Cross-sectional	25 preeclamptic, 17 nonpreeclamptic	Polysomnogram	Preeclamptic patients with increased time spent in slow-wave sleep, and less rapid eye movement sleep
Williams, et al (2010)	Prospective cohort	1272 pregnant followed through pregnancy	Self-reported sleep duration Chart extraction	Sleep duration <5 h associated with increased likelihood of pregnancy-induced hypertension and preeclampsia development

Sleep Deficiency and Risk of Preterm Birth

Preterm birth is defined as birth between 20 weeks 0 days and 36 weeks 6 days gestation and is a leading cause of perinatal morbidity and mortality in the United States (see **Table 2**).[61] It affects approximately 10% of all pregnancies[62] and accounts for up to 50% of long-term disability (neurodevelopmental or physical) among children.[63] Analysis of health-care costs shows these disabilities cost billions annually within the first 6 months alone.[64]

The pathophysiological link between sleep deficiency and preterm birth has been a topic of interest for researchers worldwide. It has been long thought inflammatory cytokines play a role in the initiation of labor. Okun and colleagues (2007)[65] subsequently studied 19 women in late pregnancy (defined at 36 weeks gestation) and found that those who self-reported poorer sleep quality as measured by the PSQI had higher serum interleukin 6, a known proinflammatory cytokine.

In a study by Micheli and colleagues (2011),[66] sleep patterns of Greek women were analyzed. It was found that women who self-reported less than 5 hours of sleep nightly during the third trimester were at high risk for preterm birth (relative risk 1.7, CI 1.1–2.8) even after controlling for maternal age, education, smoking exposure, and prepregnancy BMI. However, when the types of preterm birth were evaluated, medically indicated preterm birth, defined as maternal or fetal complications necessitating earlier delivery (RR 2.4, CI 1.0–6.4), was associated with sleep deprivation but not spontaneous preterm birth (RR 1.6, CI 0.8–2.9). This association was supported by a case-control study of 479 Peruvian women who had a preterm birth compared with 480 women with a full-term delivery at the same hospital.[67] In this study, it was found that short sleep duration (defined as $\leq$6 hours) when compared with women who slept 7 to 8 hours was significantly associated with preterm birth. This association persisted after accounting for potential confounders such as maternal age, weight, use of vitamins, and planned pregnancy status (adjusted odds ratio [aOR] = 1.56; 95% CI 1.11–2.19). In 2021, Okun, Obetz, and Feliciano[68] used sleep diaries, as well as actigraphy (an objective measure), to assess sleep for three 2-week periods in early gestation (between 10 and 20 weeks) in addition to laboratory testing for fasting levels of interleukin 6 (ILK-6), interferon gamma (IFN y), and tumor necrosis factor alpha (TNF-α). During weeks 10, 14, and 18, it was found that ILK-6, IFN y, and TNF-α did not vary significantly (IL-6: 0.27 vs 0.25 vs 0.37; F_{2170} = 1.85; IFN y: 1. 6 vs 1. 66 vs 1.66, F_{2168} = 0.17; IFN-y: 6.98 vs 10.22 vs 5.37, F_{2164} = 0.75) and were not predictive of neonatal birth weight or gestational age. However, analysis showed diary assessed total sleep time and actigraphy assessed sleep latency were negatively associated with gestational age (β = −0.21, $t = -2.11$, $P < .05$) and β = −0.26, $t = -1.95$, $P = .05$, respectively).

Conversely, Okun et.al (2012)[69] found no significant difference in preterm birth among a cohort of 217 women who self-reported less than 7 hours of sleep in unadjusted and adjusted models ($P = 0.77$ and $P = .88$, respectively). Preterm birth was found among women that reported an increased amount of time in bed; however, when adjusted for the presence of major depressive disorder, selective serotonin receptor use, employment, age, and history of preterm birth, this no longer was significant ($P = .15$). This study was limited by its small sample size. It was not powered to answer the question regarding whether sleep deficiency is an independent risk factor in addition to knowing the used self-reported sleep analysis is subject to recall bias (see **Table 4**). More sleep studies gathering objective clinical data are required to further address and delineate the relationship between sleep deficiency and preterm birth.

Sleep Deficiency and Labor Outcomes

Not only does sleep deficiency affect maternal health and pregnancy outcomes, but limited data also indicates a link to a patient's perception and experience during labor and delivery. Studies have shown a link between sleep deficiency and a patient's labor course and duration of labor. In a cohort of 131 healthy primiparous women, 48-hour actigraphy and subjective sleep questionnaires were used to assess the association among fatigue, sleep disturbance, and duration, as well as the mode of delivery.[70] Women were categorized into 3 categories: average of 6 hours or less per night (<6 hours), average of 6 to 6.9 hours per night (6–6.9 hours), or greater than average of 7 hours per night (7+ hours). It was found women who reported an average of 6 hours of sleep or less during the last month of pregnancy had a statistically longer duration of labor (<6 hours: average 29 hours vs 6–6.9 hours: average 20 hours vs 7+ hours: average 17.7 hours, $P < .05$). These women also had a higher rate of cesarean birth (<6 hours: 37% vs 7+ hours:11%, $P < .05$). Similarly, in a study of 88 women who completed the PSQI three times per week during their last 3 weeks of prenatal care as well as at the initial postpartum visit, it was found that women who described poor sleep quality defined by higher PSQI scores were found to have shorter sleep duration (average 6.45 ± 2.07 hours) and were 20% more likely to have a cesarean section and longer duration of labor.[71] A study by Beebe and Lee (2007)[72] assessed a woman's sleep patterns in the 5 days before labor and noted in 35 nulliparous women that those with worst reported sleep, especially the evening before hospitalization, had increased perception of pain with spontaneous labor onset. These women were enrolled at greater than 38 weeks gestation (to avoid preterm delivery in the sample) and recruited in childbirth classes. Sleep was recorded via wrist actigraphy monitors. The total amount of sleep decreased in the last 5 nights of pregnancy progressively from on average 452 minutes ± 58 (approximately 7.5 hours) to an average of 274 minutes ± 145 (approximately 4.5 hours); this change was significant between 2 nights before delivery and the night of delivery ($t = -4.94$, $P < .001$). The women's scores on fatigue in early labor had a moderate correlation with a woman's total sleep time the night before birth (r's = −0.39), yet not statistically significant given the small sample size. Although these studies suggest an association, they do not establish causation of whether the sleep duration was the cause of longer labor or if other emotional and physical stressors (not examined) are the cause of these perceptions.

SUMMARY

In conclusion, sleep deficiency is a common problem faced among our population, especially among pregnant women. Sleep deprivation during pregnancy may be due to multiple physiologic, emotional, and physical factors. The existing literature supports an association between sleep deficiency and an increased risk for pregnancy-related complications, including GDM and hypertensive disorders in pregnancy. Moreover, a woman's mental health may be placed at risk secondary to peripartum depression. However, major gaps in knowledge remain. Future clinical research should focus on establishing causation as well as exploring effective interventions to mitigate and reduce the occurrence of adverse maternal and neonatal outcomes with sleep deficiency.

CLINICS CARE POINTS

- Sleep Deficiency affects up to one third of women throughout their life, and pregnancy related changes may lead to onset of sleep deficiency.
- Women should be screened and evaluated early in pregnancy for predisposing risk factors, such as low socioeconomic status, and provided resources when possible.

- Causation of pregnancy related complications (gestational diabetes, depression, hypertensive disorders) in patients with sleep deficiency has not been evaluated in research.

DISCLOSURE

The authors have no conflicting interests to report.

REFERENCES

1. Nation Sleep Foundation. National sleep foundation recommends new sleep times. National Sleep Foundation; 2019. Available at: https://www.sleepfoundation.org/press-release/national-sleep-foundation-recommends-new-sleep-times. Accessed February 1, 2021.
2. Center for Disease Control and Prevention. Cdc - data and statistics - sleep and sleep disorders. Sleep 2017;1. Available at: https://www.cdc.gov/sleep/data_statistics.html. Accessed February 1, 2021.
3. Rod NH, Vahtera J, Westerlund H, et al. Sleep disturbances and cause-specific mortality: results from the GAZEL cohort study. Am J Epidemiol 2011;173(3):300–9.
4. Choi JW, Song JS, Lee YJ, et al. Increased mortality in relation to insomnia and obstructive sleep apnea in Korean patients studied with nocturnal polysomnography. J Clin Sleep Med 2017;13(1):49–56.
5. National Sleep Foundation. Sleep & effectiveness are linked, but few plan their sleep 2018. Available at: https://sleepfoundation.org/sites/default/files/Sleep in America 2018_prioritizing sleep.pdf. Accessed February 14, 2021.
6. Lindberg E, Janson C, Gislason T, et al. Sleep disturbances in a young adult population: can gender differences be explained by differences in psychological status? Sleep 1997;20(6):381–7.
7. Arber S, Bote M, Meadows R. Gender and socio-economic patterning of self-reported sleep problems in Britain. Soc Sci Med 2009;68(2):281–9.
8. Lee S, Chang AM, Buxton OM, et al. Various types of perceived job discrimination and sleep health among working women: findings from the sister study. Am J Epidemiol 2020;189(10):1143–53.
9. National sleep foundation. Summary of findings 2005. (March 2005). Retrieved from: https://www.sleepfoundation.org/wp-content/uploads/2018/10/2005_summary_of_findings.pdf
10. Pengo MF, Won CH, Bourjeily G. Sleep in women across the life span. Chest 2018;154(1):196–206.
11. Reichner CA. Insomnia and sleep deficiency in pregnancy. Obstet Med 2015;8(4):168–71.
12. Mindell JA, Cook RA, Nikolovski J. Sleep patterns and sleep disturbances across pregnancy. Sleep Med 2015;16(4):483–8.
13. Hedman C, Pohjasvaara T, Tolonen U, et al. Effects of pregnancy on mothers' sleep. Sleep Med 2002;3(1):37–42.
14. Kominiarek MA, Yeh C, Balmert LC, et al. Sleep duration during pregnancy using an activity tracking device. AJP Rep 2020;10(3):E309–14.
15. Reid KJ, Facco FL, Grobman WA, et al. Sleep during pregnancy: the nuMoM2b pregnancy and sleep duration and continuity study. Sleep 2017;40(5):zsx045.
16. Garbazza C, Hackethal S, Riccardi S, et al. Polysomnographic features of pregnancy: a systematic review. Sleep Med Rev 2020;50.
17. Santiago JR, Nolledo MS, Kinzler W, et al. Sleep and sleep disorders in pregnancy. Ann Intern Med 2001;134(5):396–408.
18. McCarthy R, Jungheim ES, Fay JC, et al. Riding the rhythm of melatonin through pregnancy to deliver on time. Front Endocrinol (Lausanne) 2019;10:616.
19. Kalmbach DA, Cheng P, Sangha R, et al. Insomnia, short sleep, and snoring in mid-to-late pregnancy: disparities related to poverty, race, and obesity. Nat Sci Sleep 2019;11:301–15.
20. Christian LM, Carroll JE, Porter K, et al. Sleep quality across pregnancy and postpartum: effects of parity and race. Sleep Heal 2019;5(4):327–34.
21. Feinstein L, McWhorter KL, Gaston SA, et al. Racial/ethnic disparities in sleep duration and sleep disturbances among pregnant and non-pregnant women in the United States. J Sleep Res 2020;29(5):e13000.
22. Okun ML, Tolge M, Hall M. Low socioeconomic status negatively affects sleep in pregnant women. J Obstet Gynecol Neonatal Nurs 2014;43(2):160–7.
23. Skouteris H, Germano C, Wertheim EH, et al. Sleep quality and depression during pregnancy: a prospective study. J Sleep Res 2008;17(2):217–20.
24. Bei B, Milgrom J, Ericksen J, et al. Subjective perception of sleep, but not its objective quality, is associated with immediate postpartum mood disturbances in healthy women. Sleep 2010;33(4):531–8.
25. Dørheim SK, Bjorvatn B, Eberhard-Gran M. Can insomnia in pregnancy predict postpartum depression? A longitudinal, population-based study. PLoS One 2014;9(4):e94674.
26. Kettunen P, Koistinen E, Hintikka J. Is postpartum depression a homogenous disorder: time of onset, severity, symptoms and hopelessness in relation to the course of depression. BMC Pregnancy Childbirth 2014;14(1):402.
27. Gale S, Harlow BL. Postpartum mood disorders: a review of clinical and epidemiological factors. J Psychosom Obstet Gynecol 2003;24(4):257–66.

28. Yonkers K, Wisner KL, Stewart DE, et al. Management of depression during pregnancy. Obstet Gynecol 2014;114(3). https://doi.org/10.1002/pnp.113.
29. Langan RC, Goodbred AJ. Identification and management of peripartum depression. Vol 93. 2016. Available at: http://www.wpspublish.com/. Accessed May 18, 2021.
30. Bonari L, Pinto N, Ahn E, Einarson A, Steiner M, Koren G. Perinatal risks of untreated depression during pregnancy. Canadian journal of psychiatry 2004; 49(11):726–35.
31. Szegda K, Markenson G, Bertone-Johnson ER, et al. Depression during pregnancy: a risk factor for adverse neonatal outcomes? A critical review of the literature. J Matern Fetal Neonatal Med 2014; 27(9):960–7.
32. Field T, Diego M, Hernandez-Reif M, et al. Sleep disturbances in depressed pregnant women and their newborns. Infant Behav Dev 2007;30(1):127–33.
33. Wilkie G, Shapiro CM. Sleep deprivation and the postnatal blues. J Psychosom Res 1992;36(4): 309–16.
34. Iranpour S, Kheirabadi GR, Esmaillzadeh A, et al. Association between sleep quality and postpartum depression. J Res Med Sci 2016;21(8):110.
35. Jomeen J, Martin C. Assessment and relationship of sleep quality to depression in early pregnancy. J Reprod Infant Psychol 2007;25(1):87–99.
36. Okun ML, Kline CE, Roberts JM, et al. Prevalence of sleep deficiency in early gestation and its associations with stress and depressive symptoms. J Women's Health (Larchmt) 2013;22(12):1028–37.
37. Lusskin SI, Pundiak TM, Habib SM. Perinatal depression: hiding in plain sight. Can J Psychiatry 2007;52(8):479–88.
38. Beck CT. Predictors of postpartum depression: an update. Nurs Res 2001;50(5):275–85.
39. Correa A, Bardenheier B, Elixhauser A, et al. Trends in prevalence of diabetes among delivery hospitalizations, United States, 1993–2009. Matern Child Health J 2015;19(3):635–42.
40. Coustan DR. Gestational diabetes mellitus. Clin Chem 2013;59(9):1310–21.
41. American Diabetes Association. American diabetes standards of medical care in diabetes. Diabetes Care 2016;39(Supplement 1):S1–106.
42. Plows JF, Stanley JL, Baker PN, et al. Molecular sciences the pathophysiology of gestational diabetes mellitus. doi:10.3390/ijms19113342
43. Yogev Y, Xenakis EMJ, Langer O. The association between preeclampsia and the severity of gestational diabetes: the impact of glycemic control. Am J Obstet Gynecol 2004;191(5):1655–60.
44. England LJ, Dietz PM, Njoroge T, et al. Preventing type 2 diabetes: public health implications for women with a history of gestational diabetes mellitus. Am J Obstet Gynecol 2009;200(4):365.e1–8.
45. Rosenstein MG, Cheng YW, Snowden JM, et al. The risk of stillbirth and infant death stratified by gestational age in women with gestational diabetes. American journal of obstetrics and gynecology, 206. Mosby Inc.; 2012. p. 309.e1–7.
46. O'sullivan JB. Body weight and subsequent diabetes mellitus. JAMA 1982;248(8):949–52.
47. Facco FL, Grobman WA, Kramer J, et al. Self-reported short sleep duration and frequent snoring in pregnancy: impact on glucose metabolism. Am J Obstet Gynecol 2010;203(2):142.e1–5.
48. Qiu C, Enquobahrie D, Frederick IO, et al. Glucose intolerance and gestational diabetes risk in relation to sleep duration and snoring during pregnancy: a pilot study. BMC Womens Health 2010;10:17.
49. Zhou FM, Yang LQ, Zhao RP, et al. Effect of sleep in early pregnancy on gestational diabetes; a prospective study. J Sichuan Univ (Medical Sci Ed 2016; 47(6):964–8. Available at: https://pubmed.ncbi.nlm.nih.gov/28598132/. Accessed January 20, 2021.
50. Wang H, Leng J, Li W, et al. Sleep duration and quality, and risk of gestational diabetes mellitus in pregnant Chinese women. Diabet Med 2017;34(1): 44–50.
51. Cai S, Tan S, Gluckman PD, et al. Sleep quality and nocturnal sleep duration in pregnancy and risk of gestational diabetes mellitus. Sleep 2017;40(2). https://doi.org/10.1093/sleep/zsw058.
52. Reutrakul S, Zaidi N, Wroblewski K, et al. Sleep disturbances and their relationship to glucose tolerance in pregnancy. Diabetes Care 2011;34(11): 2454–7.
53. Rawal S, Hinkle SN, Zhu Y, et al. A longitudinal study of sleep duration in pregnancy and subsequent risk of gestational diabetes: findings from a prospective, multiracial cohort. American journal of obstetrics and gynecology, 216. Mosby Inc.; 2017. p. 399. e1–8.
54. Facco FL, Grobman WA, Reid KJ, et al. Objectively measured short sleep duration and later sleep midpoint in pregnancy are associated with a higher risk of gestational diabetes. Am J Obstet Gynecol 2017;217(4):447.e1–13.
55. Roccella EJ. Report of the national high blood pressure education program working group on high blood pressure in pregnancy. Am J Obstet Gynecol 2000;183(1):s1–22.
56. Steegers EAP, Von Dadelszen P, Duvekot JJ, et al. Pre-eclampsia. In: The lancet, 376. Elsevier B.V.; 2010. p. 631–44.
57. Bokslag A, Van Weissenbruch M, Mol BW, et al. Preeclampsia; short and long-term consequences for mother and neonate. 2016. doi:10.1016/j.earlhumdev.2016.09.007
58. Edwards N, Blyton DM, Kesby GJ, et al. Preeclampsia is associated with marked alterations in sleep architecture. Sleep 2000;23(5):619–25.

59. Williams MA, Miller RS, Qiu C, et al. Associations of early pregnancy sleep duration with trimester-specific blood pressures and hypertensive disorders in pregnancy. Sleep 2010;33(10):1363–71.
60. Ekholm EMK, Polo O, Rauhala ER, et al. Sleep quality in preeclampsia. Am J Obstet Gynecol 1992;167(5):1262–6.
61. Byrne B, Morrison JJ. Preterm birth. Clin Evid (Online) 2003;10:1700–15. Available at: https://www.who.int/news-room/fact-sheets/detail/preterm-birth. Accessed June 1, 2021.
62. Martin JA, Brady MPH, Hamilton E, et al. National vital statistics reports, Volume 66, Number 1, January 5, 2017. Vol 66. 2015. Available at: http://www.cdc.gov/nchs/data_access/Vitalstatsonline.htm. Accessed February 27, 2021.
63. Wood NS, Marlow N, Costeloe K, et al. Neurologic and developmental disability after extremely preterm birth. N Engl J Med 2000;343(6):378–84.
64. Beam AL, Fried I, Palmer N, et al. Estimates of healthcare spending for preterm and low-birthweight infants in a commercially insured population: 2008â€"2016. J Perinatol 2020;40:1091–9.
65. Okun ML, Hall M, Coussons-Read ME. Sleep disturbances increase interleukin-6 production during pregnancy: implications for pregnancy complications. Reprod Sci 2007;14(6):560–7.
66. Micheli K, Komninos I, Bagkeris E, et al. Sleep patterns in late pregnancy and risk of preterm birth and fetal growth restriction. Epidemiology 2011;22(5):738–44.
67. Kajeepeta S, Sanchez SE, Gelaye B, et al. Sleep duration, vital exhaustion, and odds of spontaneous preterm birth: a case-control study. BMC Pregnancy Childbirth 2014;14(1):337.
68. Okun ML, Obetz V, Feliciano L. Sleep disturbance in early pregnancy, but not inflammatory cytokines, may increase risk for adverse pregnancy outcomes. Int J Behav Med 2021;28(1):48–63.
69. Okun ML, Luther JF, Wisniewski SR, et al. Disturbed sleep, a novel risk factor for preterm birth? J Women's Heal 2012;21(1):54–60.
70. Lee KA, Gay CL. Sleep in late pregnancy predicts length of labor and type of delivery. Am J Obstet Gynecol 2004;191(6):2041–6.
71. Naghi I, Keypour F, Ahari SB, et al. Sleep disturbance in late pregnancy and type and duration of labour. J Obstet Gynaecol 2011;31(6):489–91.
72. Beebe KR, Lee KA. Sleep disturbance in late pregnancy and early labor. J Perinat Neonatal Nurs 2007;21(2):103–8.

Sleep Deficiency in the Elderly

Jane Alexandra Pappas, MM[a,1], Brienne Miner, MD, MHS[b,*]

KEYWORDS

• Sleep • Aging • Sleep deficiency • Circadian rhythm • Sleep quality • Sleep duration • Cognition • Physical function

KEY POINTS

- With normal aging, there are changes to sleep architecture and circadian rhythmicity that contribute to sleep deficiency through their impact on sleep duration, quality, and timing.
- Causes of sleep deficiency in older age are multifactorial, including medical and psychiatric diseases, medication and substance use, social isolation, loneliness, loss of physical function, caregiving, and bereavement.
- Sleep deficiency has been associated in older adults with increased mortality, cognitive impairment, depression, and impaired physical function.
- Nonpharmacologic interventions are available for the treatment of older adults with sleep deficiency and are preferred to pharmacologic interventions due to the risk profile of the latter.

INTRODUCTION

Sleep deficiency, characterized by impairments in daytime function that arise due to insufficient sleep duration, poor sleep quality, and/or sleep that is out-of-sync with the body's natural clock,[1–3] presents a unique challenge in the elderly. Aging itself exerts cellular alterations that predispose older adults to sleep changes, which may be associated with an increased risk of disease and mortality, while the increasing prevalence of chronic health conditions also contributes to an acceleration of these effects and to sleep deficiency in particular.[4] Moreover, the unique changes to lifestyle, routine, experience, and daily stimulation or lack thereof that tend to accompany aging and, in the western context, retirement, also can contribute to sleep deficiency.[5] Therefore, in considering sleep deficiency, we need to be aware of the impact of normal changes in sleep physiology that result from aging itself—and which occur in both healthy and unhealthy older adults—and of age-related changes to sleep, resulting from the health-related and psychosocial/behavioral factors typical of aging.[4]

In this article, we describe the syndrome of sleep deficiency in older adults, often defined as aged 65 years and older. First, we describe normative changes to sleep physiology, which may not be pathologic but nonetheless predispose older adults to sleep deficiency via changes in sleep duration, quality, and/or timing. Second, we discuss health-related and psychosocial/behavioral factors that precipitate sleep deficiency in this age group. Third, we review the consequences of sleep deficiency in older adults, focusing specifically on important age-related outcomes, including mortality, cognition, depression, and physical function. Finally, we review treatments for sleep deficiency in older persons, focusing especially on nonpharmacologic interventions, which are much preferred in this age group due to the potential for adverse effects of pharmacologic interventions.

[a] San Juan Bautista School of Medicine, Salida 21 Carr. 172 Urb. Turabo Gardens, Caguas 00726, Puerto Rico; [b] Section of Geriatrics, Yale University School of Medicine, 333 Cedar Street, New Haven, CT 06520, USA

[1] Present address: PO Box 429, Ludlow, VT 05149.

* Corresponding author.

E-mail address: brienne.miner@yale.edu

Clin Chest Med 43 (2022) 273–286
https://doi.org/10.1016/j.ccm.2022.02.005
0272-5231/22/

Normative Changes to Sleep Architecture and Circadian Rhythm in Aging

Sleep duration and quality

Aging-related physiologic changes to sleep architecture are well established (**Table 1**). It has been shown that sleep duration decreases with age,[6,7] which may be at odds with a recommended sleep duration of 7 to 8 hours in older adults.[8] This recommendation is supported by evidence that older adults sleeping for 7 to 8 hours overnight have better mental and physical health, cognition, and quality of life compared with older adults with shorter or longer sleep durations.[8] Thus, the recommended sleep duration is not reduced in older adults, even though the ability to get the recommended amount of sleep may be decreased because of normal changes in sleep architecture.[9] Further support for the recommended 7 to 8 hours of sleep is the robust association of both shorter (6 hours or less) and longer (greater than 9 hours) sleep durations with adverse health consequences, including cardiovascular, metabolic, immunologic, and cognitive outcomes, as well as mortality.[10] Because of differences across studies in how short and long sleep durations are defined, the National Sleep Foundation recommendations acknowledge that a sleep duration anywhere from 6 to 9 hours may be appropriate.[8]

Changes in sleep architecture across the life span are well demonstrated by two large meta-analyses.[6,7] Older adults spend more time in non-rapid eye movement (NREM) stages N1 and N2, and less time in N3 (slow wave sleep) and rapid eye movement (REM) sleep,[6,7] and also experience shorter and fewer NREM–REM sleep cycles.[11] Sleep efficiency (the ratio of time spent asleep while in bed) seems to be particularly impacted by aging, as it continues to decrease as a function of age past 90 years.[6] The observed quantitative change in arousal frequency from young adulthood (18–34 years) to older age (65–79 years) is dramatic, doubling from 9.6 to 18.8 events per hour.[7] However, an increased arousal frequency does not seem to affect the ability of healthy older adults to fall back to sleep.[5] Other age-dependent changes in sleep parameters seem to stabilize by the age of 60. For example, there is an age-related increase in sleep latency and in wake after sleep onset (WASO) only up to the age of 60.[6]

There are also significant qualitative changes to the microarchitecture of REM, N2, and N3. Older adults exhibit shorter REM latency and reduced REM activity and density.[12] There are also marked changes in sleep spindles with age, including a reduction in sleep spindle and K-complex density and a decrease in spindle duration and amplitude.[13] In older adults, sleep spindle frequency diminishes progressively over the course of a night's sleep.[14] These changes have profound implications. Sleep spindles, a defining feature of N2, have been associated with neuronal plasticity and memory consolidation.[15] Studies show a positive correlation between increases in spindle density and episodic learning, hippocampal encoding, and recall ability.[15] Moreover, sleep spindles may not only affect memory and learning due to sleep but also seem to have an effect on the ability of a sleeper to remain asleep. Awakenings from sleep secondary to external auditory stimuli are significantly reduced when they occur during sleep spindles. In this way, spindles seem to be protective of sleep continuity.[13]

With regard to N3, a marked reduction in delta wave amplitude and density has been observed, possibly because of cortical neuron loss.[12] These age-related changes are more pronounced across the frontal lobe.[12] Slow wave activity impairment is dramatic in older adults, who exhibit 75% to 80% less slow wave activity over the prefrontal cortex during the first NREM sleep cycles as compared with younger adults.[11]

Structural changes in the brain secondary to aging may have an important role in the decline of sleep duration and increase in sleep fragmentation in older people.[16] With aging, a small group of cells in the hypothalamic preoptic area, responsible for sleep initiation and maintenance via expression of the inhibitory neuropeptide galanin, diminish in number. The severity of this loss, observed postmortem, correlates with previous sleep fragmentation, whereas a greater change is seen in those with Alzheimer disease (AD).[11] Up to 50% of the neurons in this aforementioned region of the brain, referred to as the "sleep switch," are lost during the course of the normal aging process. It has been proposed that this network of cells lose the ability to fire simultaneously, thereby impairing the brain's transition from a wakeful state to sleep.[3]

Circadian rhythmicity

Changes to the circadian system seen in aging populations (see **Table 1**) significantly affect the overall pattern of the sleep–wake cycle. Perhaps, the most recognized change to circadian patterns is the tendency for a phase advance, resulting in an earlier time for the sleep period.[17] Many rhythms controlled by the circadian system reflect this advance, including melatonin and core body temperature rhythms. The timing of melatonin release has been reported to move to an earlier time with age.[17] Similarly, core body temperature

Table 1
Age-related changes to sleep physiology

Architecture	Circadian Rhythm
• Decreases in: o total sleep time o sleep efficiency o slow wave sleep o REM sleep • Increases in: o WASO o arousals from sleep o sleep latency	• Phase advance is common • Decreased rhythm amplitude • Decrease in ability to phase shift

peaks earlier in the day in the elderly and, in turn, declines earlier. Alertness increases as body temperature increases, whereas there is increased sleepiness with lower body temperatures. This pattern tracks neatly with the increased daytime napping and earlier sleep onset often seen in older adults, which occur as the core body temperature decreases.[4]

A decrease in the amplitude of the circadian rhythm in older adults has also been reported. For example, there is a diminished range of temperatures experienced in the older population.[18] The most substantial discrepancy between the ages spans the "sleep propensity zone," which occurs between 4:00 AM and 7:00 AM Younger adults achieve a more precipitous decline in body temperature during this time, which will act as a cue to maintain sleepiness. Older adults, however, have less of a reduction in their body temperature, a signal of a less potent circadian stimulus to maintain sleep. As a result, they may experience a greater number of awakenings during the night or awaken earlier in the morning than younger adults.[19] Similarly, a reduction in the amplitude of melatonin and other hormone rhythms has also been reported.[17] Importantly, most studies have documented an overall decrease in the secretion of melatonin with aging, although some suggest there may be no change in healthy elderly. This decrease in production is largely reflected in lower nocturnal melatonin levels.[20]

Aging has also been associated with alteration in the circadian rhythm of cortisol, which may have implications for sleep. In particular, a marked elevation of cortisol levels has been associated with aging and linked to decreased N3 sleep and increased nighttime arousals.[21] A recent cross-sectional study found an association between sleep disruption on actigraphy and elevated daytime cortisol levels.[22]

Older adults also experience a reduction in the ability to phase shift and to adapt to a new sleep time.[23] Evidence suggest that this vulnerability may be related to both changes intrinsic to the signaling of the circadian timing system itself as well as disruption of entrainment mechanisms.[24] An example of disruption in entrainment is visual impairment, which leads to impaired entrainment by light, the primary circadian entrainment cue. Those with conditions affecting vision, such as macular degeneration and cataracts, are 30% to 60% more likely to suffer from sleep deficiency.[5]

Napping

Napping is prevalent in aging populations, ranging from 25% to 46% in landmark studies of persons aged 65 years and older.[25,26] Napping has been associated with adverse outcomes, including cardiovascular disease, dementia, depression, diabetes, falls, impaired quality of life, and mortality.[27] However, other studies have suggested potential benefits for napping with respect to reduced cardiovascular risk and improved cognitive performance and well-being.[28,29] In particular, a recent study found that subjects who napped one to two times per week had lower risk of incident cardiovascular events, whereas no association was found with incidence of cardiovascular disease for more frequent napping or for daily nap duration (ie, durations <1 hour vs ≥1 hour as compared with no napping).[29] This study shows the importance of accounting for nap frequency when assessing the effect of naps on cardiovascular health. Similarly, a study among persons aged 75 to 94 years found that daytime naps were protective for mortality if nighttime sleep durations were short (<7 hours), but increased mortality risk if nighttime sleep durations were long (>9 hours).[30] Whether napping is helpful or harmful probably has to do with the nap characteristics (ie, frequency, duration) and total overnight sleep duration. Other characteristics, including nap timing and whether napping is habitual or intentional may also be important.[27,29,31]

Risk Factors for Sleep Deficiency in Older Adults

Comorbidities

Aging is commonly associated with multiple factors that can affect sleep, ranging from an increasing prevalence of health-related factors (eg, chronic medical and psychiatric conditions, including primary sleep disorders) and psychosocial/behavioral factors. With an increasing number of health problems, the likelihood of sleep disturbance increases,[32] in part, because these health problems are associated with symptoms (eg, pain, dyspnea) and/or medication effects that may disrupt sleep.[5] Notably, 75% of adults aged

65 years and older suffer, at a minimum, from at least two chronic health conditions.[33] Chronic pain is one of the most common conditions to cause disturbed sleep in older and has been associated with greater sleep latency and reduced sleep efficiency. Osteoarthritis is a major underlying cause of chronic pain. Other medical comorbidities associated with sleep deficiency are cancer, heart disease, stroke, respiratory, and neurologic diseases.[33,34]

Specific sleep disorders are important to consider as risk factors for sleep deficiency, as nearly all of them increase in prevalence with age. Among older adults, restless legs syndrome and periodic limb movements during sleep are present in 12% and 45%, respectively, 29% have insomnia, and 24% have obstructive sleep apnea (OSA).[35] OSA requires special mention, as its presentation may differ in older adults. With aging, structural changes to the airway (eg, loss of tissue elasticity and muscle wasting, fat deposits in the pharyngeal walls) are a more significant contributor than obesity to OSA, and older adults with OSA are more likely to present with nocturia and daytime sleepiness than snoring and witnessed apneas.[35]

Circadian rhythm disorders, while rare overall, increase in prevalence with age and may contribute to sleep deficiency. Advanced sleep–wake phase disorder (ASWPD) is an advance to an earlier time of the major sleep period. As opposed to an advanced sleep phase, ASWPD additionally includes a complaint of difficulty staying awake until a desired bedtime and/or an inability to remain asleep until the desired wake time as a result of the advanced sleep phase.[36] Sleepiness in the early evening may impede participation in valued activities.[37] The prevalence of ASWPD in the general population is unknown but may be present in 1% of individuals aged 40 to 64 years.[36] Irregular sleep–wake rhythm disorder (ISWRD) causes multiple irregular sleep and wake episodes throughout a 24-hour period due to the absence of a well-defined circadian sleep–wake cycle.[36] Individuals may have insomnia symptoms during the scheduled sleep period and/or daytime sleepiness during periods in which wake is desired. Those affected by ISWRD are usually institutionalized older adults with dementia or those with moderate-to-severe cognitive defects.[38,39] The overall prevalence of this disorder is unknown, but its prevalence increases with age, neurologic disease, mental disability, and dementia.[40]

Medication and substance use

With greater incidence of medical conditions comes greater use of medications in older adults, which can have profound implications for sleep. In a survey of Medicare beneficiaries, 46% experienced "polypharmacy," defined as taking five or more medications.[41] Sedating drugs (eg, antihistamines, anticholinergics, antiepileptics, opiates) may cause depressed respiration and daytime drowsiness, whereas activating drugs (eg, stimulants, certain antidepressants, corticosteroids) may negatively affect the ability to initiate or maintain sleep.[5] Still other drugs may cause sleep-disruptive symptoms (eg, diuretics, hypoglycemic agents).[5] Moreover, drugs affecting the central nervous system can reduce slow wave and REM sleep and exacerbate sleep disorders.[4] Nonprescription drugs are equally significant; diphenhydramine or pseudoephedrine is commonly used medications that may disturb sleep–wake patterns.[5]

Substance use, particularly caffeine, nicotine, and alcohol, may also negatively affect sleep. The stimulating effects of caffeine can increase sleep latency and arousals, leading to shorter sleep durations.[42] Smoking has been correlated with difficulty initiating sleep, maintaining sleep, and waking up, as well as sleep durations of less than 6 hours per night, with nicotine serving as the potential mediator of this effect.[34] Alcohol can worsen sleep disordered breathing by relaxing pharyngeal muscles and has been shown to promote sleep disturbance and arousals, leading to reduced sleep durations.[42]

Nocturia

Nocturia, resulting from multifactorial causes, is another major contributor to impairments in sleep duration and quality in older adults. Older adults naturally produce less antidiuretic hormone and have less bladder capacity.[43] Men also commonly suffer from benign prostatic hyperplasia, which may cause urgency, whereas postmenopausal women may suffer from a lack of the protective effects of estrogen on nocturia.[44,45] However, a crucially important cause, which should not be overlooked, is the role of OSA. Hypoxemia, resulting from collapse of the airway, causes diaphragmatic contractions that lead to pressure changes in the thorax. When this leads to cardiac venous distension that impacts normal flow, the heart receives an incorrect signal of fluid overload and atrial natriuretic peptide is excreted, causing increased urine production.[45] Anyone experiencing nocturia at least three times nightly should be referred for polysomnography, as this is suggestive of OSA.[44]

Psychosocial/behavioral factors

A constellation of psychosocial and behavioral factors, exerting effects through multiple pathways, may predispose to or precipitate sleep deficiency in older adults. Particularly relevant are the effects of social isolation, loneliness, loss of physical function, caregiving, and bereavement, which may contribute to sleep deficiency via effects on sleep hygiene, exposure to zeitgebers (cues from the environment [eg, light, exercise, meals, social activity] that entrain circadian rhythms, promoting normal sleep–wake habits),[46] and/or increased risk of psychiatric comorbidity. Social isolation (having few social relationships or infrequent social contact) and loneliness (a subjective feeling of being isolated) are prevalent in older populations.[47,48] Because of retirement and living alone, nearly one-third of older adults may be socially isolated.[49] Isolation and loneliness can affect sleep through effects on sleep hygiene, promoting behaviors that are counter to the promotion of healthy sleep, such as napping and irregular bedtimes. In addition, isolation and loneliness may be associated with decreased exposure to zeitgebers.[46] A prospective cohort study of persons aged 60 years and older found that a poor social network led to a greater risk of both short sleep (<6 hours) and poor sleep quality.[50] A 2020 study found an intriguing relationship between social support and the impact of rumination (intrusive thoughts) on sleep quality. Specifically, perceived support from a spouse, but not from family or friends, while not reducing rumination, did appear to reduce its harmful impact on sleep quality. Researchers speculated that spousal support may be more relevant to sleep because of access to such support at bedtime.[51] A variety of studies have linked both social isolation and loneliness with poorer sleep quality, whereas close relationships have been shown to improve self-reported (Pittsburgh sleep quality index) and objective (actigraphy) measures of sleep quality.[50]

Loss of physical function is also common among older adults and may decrease physical activity and exposure to zeitgebers.[52] Older adults with decreased physical function (defined as difficulty walking one-half mile without help and/or difficulty walking a flight of stairs without help) are more likely to report symptoms of sleep deficiency.[32] Up to 20% of all caregivers in the United States are 65 years of age or older[53] and may be subject to tremendous physical, emotional, and financial strains, including middle-of-the-night sleep disruptions due to the needs of the care recipient.[4] Avoidant coping styles, which are characterized by attempts to suppress, rather than accept, unwanted or intrusive thoughts (eg, use of distraction or denial), have been linked to poor sleep efficiency in caregivers for persons with dementia.[54] Bereavement, or suffering from the loss of a loved one to death,[55] may be experienced by as many as 70% of older adults.[56] This condition may contribute to sleep deficiency through worsening health and functional impairment,[57] increased risk for mood disorders,[55] as well as increasing loneliness and social isolation.[57]

Consequences of Sleep Deficiency in Older Adults

Mortality

Robust evidence links measures of sleep deficiency, including sleep duration, quality, and timing, with mortality. A well-known U-shaped association has been described for the relationship of sleep duration with mortality. Both short and long self-reported sleep have been associated with mortality.[10,58,59,60] Similar results have been demonstrated for actigraphy-measured sleep duration and mortality.[10] It should be noted that these associations are derived mainly from cross-sectional studies, precluding causal inference. The relationship between short or long sleep duration and mortality is likely driven more by the underlying comorbidity causing alterations in sleep duration than by sleep duration per se.[10]

The relationship between poor sleep quality and mortality may vary depending on the method used to define the former. A recently published meta-analysis found that subjective poor sleep quality was not associated with the increased risk of death. This meta-analysis included studies with a wide range of sleep quality measures (eg, disturbed or restless sleep, subjective poor sleep quality, subjective sleep problems, sleep difficulties, difficulty maintaining sleep).[60] When using objective measures of sleep quality, investigators from the osteoporotic fractures in men (MrOS) sleep study found objective sleep quality/sleep continuity as measured by actigraphy minutes a WASO to be one of the strongest predictors of mortality.[61] This relationship was maintained even after controlling for a host of serious diseases. Only age, cognition, and history of cardiovascular disease had a greater impact on mortality than sleep continuity.

The effect of sleep timing on mortality has been evaluated by studies that examine the rhythmicity, stability and/or regularity of the sleep period from day to day. In the aforementioned study from the MrOS sleep cohort, older men with less robust rest-activity rhythms had higher all-cause and cardiovascular-related mortality rates.[62] Similar findings were shown in the study of osteoporotic fractures (SOF) among older women, where weaker circadian activity rhythms were associated with higher mortality risk. In a separate analysis of the MrOS cohort, lower rhythmicity, as represented by the pseudo-F statistical from actigraphy, was one of the strongest sleep characteristics to predict mortality. In fact, lower rhythmicity ranked higher in importance than sleep continuity in predicting mortality.[61] Other studies examining the prospective association between fragmented circadian activity rhythms (as measured by actigraphy) and mortality found that older adults with less stable activity rhythms had a 20% increase in all-cause mortality.[63] Thus, whatever the pattern of bedtime or wake time was, the "interday stability" (a measure of the similarity of the sleep–wake rhythm across several days) was protective, whereas "intraday variability," which measured the frequency of variation between rest and activity during a 24-hour period, imposed a significantly higher mortality risk.[63]

Cognition

As with mortality, robust evidence links measures of sleep duration, quality, and timing, with cognition. Both shorter and longer sleep durations have been associated with cognitive impairment. A recent analysis of 7959 participants in the Whitehall II study, who were followed for 25 years to assess incident dementia, found an increased risk for dementia among participants with short (≤6 hours) compared with normal (7 hours) sleep duration, even after adjusting for sociodemographic, behavioral, cardiometabolic, and mental health factors.[64] Similarly, in a prospective analysis from the Nurses' Health study, shorter and longer sleep durations in both midlife and old age were associated with worse cognition later in life.[65] Several large surveys of older adults found that both short and long sleep duration were associated with poorer cognitive function in areas such as verbal fluency and recall, but that long sleep duration was more deleterious.[66]

Several studies have also compared the effects of experimental sleep deprivation on older adults as compared with younger adults, finding that older adults exhibit greater decrements in tasks such as vigilance, reaction times, addition, and object use.[66] Acute sleep deprivation has also been shown to increase accumulation of β-amyloid in the hippocampus, suggesting a link between insufficient sleep duration and AD.[67]

Various markers of poor sleep quality have been associated with adverse cognitive outcomes. In the MrOS study, reduced sleep efficiency, greater nighttime wakefulness, and poor self-reported sleep quality were associated with subsequent cognitive decline in community-dwelling older men.[68] In the study of the National Social Life, Health, and Aging Project, a nationally representative cohort of older US adults, actigraphic sleep disruption measures (eg, WASO, fragmentation) were associated with a 5-year cognitive decline. WASO had the strongest association with cognitive decline, whereas self-reported sleep-disruption measures showed little association with cognitive function.[69]

With respect to sleep timing, analyses of actigraphy data from the MrOS cohort found that parameters of disrupted rest-activity rhythms (eg, lower amplitude, pseudo F-statistic [overall circadian rhythmicity], phase-advanced acrophase [time of peak activity level]) were associated with cognitive decline.[70] Similarly, in the SOF, older women with decreased circadian activity rhythm amplitude and robustness had increased odds of developing mild cognitive impairment (ie, memory loss with maintenance of the ability to independently perform most activities of daily living) and dementia.[71] In contrast to the findings for mortality mentioned above, there was no relationship between other parameters representing rest-activity rhythm disruption (eg, intradaily variability, interdaily stability) and dementia risk in the SOF cohort.[72]

When discussing the relationship between sleep deficiency and cognition/dementia, it is important to acknowledge their bidirectional relationship. Although sleep deficiency can affect cognition, so too can dementia itself produce changes in sleep. Persons with AD experience neurodegeneration and structural changes to the brain that may contribute to sleep deficiency. For example, persons with AD have fewer posterior NREM fast spindles compared with healthy older adults, and the severity of the discrepancy is predictive of the degree of memory impairment.[73] Neurofibrillary tangles in the preoptic area of the hypothalamus are also correlated with the degree of fragmented sleep. Amyloid β accumulation is associated with reduced REM sleep in both healthy adults and those with AD. Tau-associated neurofibrillary tangles within the medial-temporal lobe are a hallmark of AD, and tau levels in cerebrospinal fluid have been associated with diminished slow wave sleep in persons diagnosed with AD. Tau deposition in other areas of the brain has been found in cognitively normal older adults, which has led to interest as to whether these abnormalities could lead to sleep changes predictive of the onset of neurodegenerative disease. If so, the potential exists for patterns of sleep disturbance to be used as a diagnostic tool.[11]

Interestingly, OSA also appears to have a bidirectional relationship with dementia. Patients with OSA have an 85% increased risk of developing mild cognitive impairment, whereas AD patients are more prone to develop OSA. AD is believed to damage neurons responsible for upper airway tone.[74] OSA patients have been found to develop more AD biomarkers, including amyloid β plaques or tau proteins, than those without the condition.[75]

Depression

Many studies demonstrate a connection between impairments in sleep duration, quality, and/or timing and mental health. Although the relationship between sleep and mental health has been studied widely, most studies focus on depression, and no meta-analyses of the relationship between psychiatric disease (eg, depression, anxiety, or other disorders) have been performed. Short self-reported sleep duration (most often defined at ≤6 hours) has been associated in cross-sectional and longitudinal studies with depressive symptoms and diagnosis.[76] Some studies also support an increased risk for depression with long sleep duration (ie, longer than 8–9 hours).[76] A study of Parkinson disease (PD) patients found that self-reported short sleep duration was highly correlated with depression severity, an effect that while significant in controls, was even greater in PD sufferers. The effect may be more pronounced in PD patients as a consequence of dopaminergic dysfunction that would inhibit such patients' ability to increase dopamine production following sleep loss.[77]

The link between poor sleep quality and depression is well established and has additional implications for older adults due to the interconnectedness of sleep deficiency, depression, and cognitive impairment.[74,78] The IMPACT study of older adults revealed that 44% of patients with persistent insomnia symptoms continue to suffer with depression 6 months later, although that was true for only 16% of participants not suffering insomnia symptoms.[79] Moreover, in assessing depression risk, sleep disturbance has been shown to have a 2.6 higher odds ratio than prior depression or disability.[80] Depression is a particular concern in older adults as a risk factor for cognitive impairment, with a recent study demonstrating that reported difficulty in initiating sleep entirely mediated the harmful effects of depression on cognitive impairment.[78]

Parameters of disrupted rest-activity rhythms have also been linked with depression. In the SOF cohort of older women, depressive symptoms were associated with greater desynchronization of circadian activity rhythms, manifested by decreased amplitude, rhythm robustness, and mesor.[81] Similarly, a study from the Rotterdam cohort found that depressive symptoms were related to less stable and more fragmented rest-activity rhythms.[82] Finally, a recent study in older adults looked at the sleep regularity index from actigraphy, which captures rapid changes in sleep timing by calculating the percent probability of a person being asleep at any two time points 24 hours apart.[83] In this study, sleep irregularity was associated with an increased risk of depression.

Physical function

Sleep duration, quality, and timing have been linked to impairments in physical function among older adults. An analysis of 6020 adults aged 65 and older participating in the National Health and Nutrition Examination Survey between the years of 2007 to 2016 looked at the effect of sleep duration on "functional limitations" (ie, reporting at least some difficulty in performing a basic task of daily living). Those achieving 7 to 8 hours of sleep per weeknight had a reduced likelihood of functional limitations, whereas the extremes of inappropriate sleep duration increased the odds of reporting functional limitations. Reporting greater than 9 hours of sleep had the most profound impact, demonstrating a nearly threefold greater odds of functional limitations.[84] Elderly women sleeping less than 5 hours per night had 1.5 times the odds of having two or more falls in the next year when compared with older women who slept the recommended 7 to 8 hours.[85] Self-reported long sleep duration was also associated with an increased incidence of falls.[86]

With respect to poor sleep quality, a study of 215 older adults found that poor sleep quality (greater than 5 on PSQI) conferred two times the odds of physical disability, defined as difficulty in performing activities necessary for living. This relationship remained even after controlling for known risk factors.[87] Actigraphy-measured parameters of sleep fragmentation have also been linked to fall risk in a study of older men. Sleep efficiency less than 70% increased the odds of falling by 36%.[86] In older women, greater WASO and lower sleep efficiency increased the risk for functional or physical decline.[88]

Evidence in the domain of sleep timing and its relationship to physical function comes again from the MrOS cohort, where later acrophase was associated with an increase in risk of falls, but not fractures.[89] Additional support comes from a cross-sectional study of heart failure patients, which evaluated circadian rhythm robustness by calculating circadian quotient.[90] The circadian quotient provides a normalized amplitude compared with mesor (individual average activity level), accounting for daytime and nighttime activities and allowing comparison between participants with different activity levels. The results demonstrated that persons with higher circadian quotients (ie, more robust rhythms) had better functional performance, as assessed by a 6-minute walk test and the medical outcomes study short form physical function scale.[91]

Treatment of Sleep Deficiency in Older Adults

Nonpharmacologic interventions

Common pharmacologic treatments for sleep deficiency may be associated with increased risk of adverse outcomes and/or be potentially inappropriate for use in the elderly.[92,93]

Because of the loss of lean muscle mass and increase in body fat, the drug elimination half-life in the elderly is increased. Medications that effect the central nervous system, such as benzodiazepines (BZDs), nonbenzodiazepine receptor-agonists (BZRAs), and some antidepressants, are known to increase the risk of falls, hospitalizations, and even death, as well as disrupt sleep architecture.[4,92] BZDs have well documented harms in the elderly including dizziness, daytime drowsiness, cognitive impairment, and delirium.[94] Furthermore, BZDs are associated with falls, hip fractures, and car accidents. Moreover, their benefits are minimal, tolerance develops with repeated use, and rebound insomnia can occur after just 1 or 2 weeks of taking them. Although some BZRAs can be used short term at low doses in the elderly with fewer side effects, in general, their benefits may not justify their risks. Therefore, the 2019 American Geriatrics Society Beers Criteria strongly advises against the use of both BZDs and BZRAs.[93] Moreover, behavioral interventions have demonstrated benefits without the adverse effects of pharmacologic interventions.

Light exposure Although some studies have not found a change in melatonin secretion with age, a study of elderly with insomnia symptoms in Japan found that it is possible to increase melatonin levels via exposure to light. Among a group of older Japanese, those with insomnia symptoms who were also significantly deficient in environmental light exposure were exposed to 4 hours of midday bright light for a period of 2 weeks. Not only were they able to increase their levels to those seen in a control group of young adults without circadian phase shifting but there also was a parallel in the magnitude of increase in melatonin secretion and improvements in sleep disturbance.[95] Bright light therapy is also useful specifically for disorders of sleep timing.[96] In these situations, bright light may be used to bring about more consolidated sleep (as with ISWRD) or to delay the major sleep period (as with ASWPD).[97]

Physical and social activities Physical and social activities have been linked to improved biomarkers of sleep, including a more robust lowering of body temperature and a greater proportion of N3.[98] The relationship between sleep and physical activities is bidirectional; therefore, while poorer quality and less sleep predict less physical activity, physical activity also has been shown to promote better sleep.[99] Aerobically fit people aged 60 years and older have shorter sleep onset latency, less WASO, and greater sleep efficiency.[100] Several studies have found powerful benefits to sleep from exercise. Moderate intensity exercise has been shown to improve objective sleep quality and 3 months of aerobic training was shown to reduce fragmentation of the rest-activity rhythm in postmenopausal women.[100] A randomized controlled trial of aquatic exercise among older adults with mild sleep disturbance found significant improvements in sleep onset latency and sleep efficiency for persons in the intervention when compared with the control group.[43] One simple mechanism by which exercise is proposed to promote sleep is that it will deplete glycogen stores, thereby provoking an increase in adenosine, which triggers sleep.[101] This may be particularly important in older adults because of the observed loss of adenosine A1 receptors in older brains, a reduction that remains notable even after accounting for reduced brain cells and volume. This may render the elderly brain less sensitive to extracellular adenosine, requiring more to achieve adequate homeostatic sleep drive.[11]

Two more recent studies demonstrated a synergistic reduction in the risk of insomnia symptoms from the combination of social and physical activities. The first, which examined data from 7162 community-dwelling older adults, and which controlled for health status, found that participants who reported having engaged in walking in the last month were 30% less likely to report insomnia symptoms, those that participated in an organized activity other than religious services in the last month were 22% less likely, and those who participated in both organized social events and walking were 40% less likely to experience insomnia symptomatology.[102] A follow-up prospective study that tracked participants 65 years and older for 3 years found that lowest risk for insomnia symptoms was found in those who engaged in organized social activity as well as vigorous exercise (vs walking alone).[103]

Behavioral treatment for insomnia Cognitive behavioral treatment of insomnia (CBT-I) is highly efficacious in the short-term and long-term.[104] Moreover, a 2019 study demonstrated that the therapy had multiple benefits, significantly reducing depression, maladaptive thinking, and hyperarousal in postmenopausal women, a population with increased risk of depression. The effect was measurable immediately following treatment as well as at 6 months.[105] Given the compounding and mediating relationships of insomnia, depression, and cognitive decline, this therapy is attractive when feasible. However, its implementation imposes a burden from the standpoint of availability, cost, and time; it requires 6 to 8 individual treatment sessions with a trained clinician.[104] A brief behavioral intervention (BBTI), by contrast, may be carried out by any allied health professional and may require fewer sessions.[106] Rather than using a cognitive behavioral approach, BBTI teaches participants about sleep hygiene and circadian mechanisms, explaining the "why" behind the 4 behaviors emphasized: reducing time in bed, getting up at the same time each day, not going to bed unless sleepy, and not staying in bed unless asleep. BBTI was demonstrated to be an effective, simple, and long-lasting nonpharmacologic intervention for the treatment of insomnia in older adults.[106]

Sleep restriction therapy is a key component of CBT-I and BBTI, but is also effective on its own as treatment. In particular, studies have demonstrated that it helps reduce sleep latency, WASO, and sleep efficiency.[94] In this technique, patients are instructed to be in bed attempting to sleep for a duration determined by calculating their average sleep duration during the course of a 2-week sleep diary. As sleep efficiency improves, patients will gradually increase their time in bed.[96]

Music therapy A recent meta-analysis that evaluated the effect of music on sleep quality in older adults found that older persons who listened to music had significantly better quality sleep than those who did not.[107] Music therapy lasting greater than 4 weeks was most effective and "sedative" (slow tempo [60–80 beats per minute], soft volume, and smooth melody) music was more beneficial than "rhythmic" music (fast tempo, loud volume, and rhythmic patterns). Music is believed to improve sleep by reducing anxiety as a result of modulating the sympathetic nervous system response and reducing the release of cortisol.[107]

Pharmacologic treatments

As noted above pharmacologic treatments for sleep deficiency in older adults have been associated with many adverse outcomes and should only be considered as a last resort when other interventions have failed. When behavioral changes are neither feasible nor sufficient to treat sleep deficiency, pharmacologic treatments, particularly with ramelteon, suvorexant, or doxepin, may be considered. Ramelteon activates melatonin MT1 and MT2 receptors in the suprachiasmatic nucleus of the hypothalamus, decreasing the alerting signal and promoting sleep. It is preferred over benzodiazepines as it causes less sedation and has a better safety profile. It exhibits a higher binding affinity and longer half-life than exogenous melatonin, which may account for its increased hypnotic effects.[92,108]

Suvorexant is as an orexin antagonist, blocking the wakefulness effects of orexin neurons by selectively inhibiting the binding of neuropeptides orexin A and B to OX1 and OX2 receptors. It has been shown to decrease sleep latency and increase mean sleep duration by 39 minutes, compared with 16 minutes with placebo. Its major side effect is daytime somnolence, but it has neither been shown to impair memory or balance the day after its use, nor has it been associated with withdrawal or rebound of symptoms on discontinuation.[92,109]

Doxepin at low doses ($\leq$6 mg) represents another pharmacologic option for persons with difficulty maintaining sleep.92 Although technically in the tricyclic antidepressant class, at doses less than 10 mg, this drug has mainly antihistaminergic effects. It is US Food and Drug Administration approved for the treatment of insomnia and appropriate per the Beers criteria when used at doses of 3 to 6 mg.93 Caution is required when persons are taking other medications metabolized by the Cytochrome P450 enzyme pathways (eg, proton pump inhibitors, cimetidine, amiodarone, bupropion, paroxetine) as concurrent use may lead to increased systemic concentrations of doxepin.[92]

Limitations of Current Knowledge

Major challenges in the study of sleep deficiency in older adults are the multifactorial nature of underlying causes and the lack of aging-specific tools for the assessment of sleep deficiency. Many of the traditional questionnaires commonly used to evaluate sleep complaints were developed in younger populations and tend to focus on one sleep complaint (eg, insomnia or daytime sleepiness),[110–112] rather than taking a more comprehensive approach. Such an approach is needed in older adults, who may experience several sleep-related symptoms and multiple concurrent causes for sleep disruption.[5] In addition, atypical presentations of sleep disorders (eg, nocturia from OSA)[35] and specific situational factors (eg, greater flexibility in sleep–wake schedules, different expectations about health)[113] may decrease the sensitivity of traditional questionnaires to detect underlying sleep–wake disturbances.[113,114] However, objective, laboratory-based methods (eg, polysomnography, serial measurement of melatonin levels) are burdensome and often not practical.[115] Thus, there is a need to develop age-appropriate self-reported and objective sleep assessment tools and/or biomarkers of sleep deficiency for effective evaluation of sleep disturbances in older adults. Such tools would also allow for rigorous and reproducible monitoring of sleep-promoting interventions.

SUMMARY

The older adult simultaneously confronts multiple risk factors for sleep deficiency and suffers a great health burden and reduced quality of life consequent to its effects. Predisposing and precipitating factors are diverse and interconnected. These include aging-related alterations in sleep physiology, which predispose older adults to changes in sleep duration, quality, and timing. Although not necessarily specific to older adults, aging is associated with an increasing prevalence of diverse precipitants for sleep deficiency, including increasing rates of medical and psychiatric comorbidities, medication and substance use, and psychosocial/behavioral factors. Sleep deficiency in older adults leads to many adverse health outcomes, particularly with respect to mortality, cognition, depression, and physical function. In view of the disabling impact of sleep deficiency in the elderly, especially with respect to outcomes that impact the ability of older adults to live independently for as long as possible with good quality of life, it is incumbent on health-care providers to aggressively treat sleep deficiency and its root causes. Nonpharmacologic approaches, including light exposure, physical and social activities, BBTI, and music therapy, should be considered as first-line treatment due to their efficacy and safety profiles as compared with many of the traditional pharmacologic treatments. Additional research is needed to develop aging-specific self-reported and objective sleep measures and to identify biomarkers diagnostic of sleep deficiency.

CLINICS CARE POINTS

- Sleep deficiency is commonly experienced by older adults. I should not be assumed to be due to normal aging, especially given its associations with many adverse outcomes in this population
- The etiology of sleep deficiency is usually multifactorial and multiple predisposing and precipitating risk factors should be considered in the diagnostic work-up.
- Pharmacologic therapies for sleep deficiency may have many adverse side effects, especially among older adults. Therefore, nonpharmacologic interventions should be the mainstay of therapy.

ACKNOWLEDGMENTS

Dr Miner is supported by the Claude D. Pepper Older Americans Independence Center at Yale School of Medicine (P30AG021342), the American Academy of Sleep Medicine Foundation, a foundation of the American Academy of Sleep Medicine, and the National Institute on Aging (R03AG073991 and K76AG074905).

DISCLOSURE

The authors have nothing to disclose.

REFERENCES

1. National Institutes of Health Sleep Disorders Research Plan. 2011.
2. Joho S, Oda Y, Ushijima R, et al. Effect of adaptive servoventilation on muscle sympathetic nerve activity in patients with chronic heart failure and central sleep apnea. J Card Fail 2012;18:769–75.
3. Czeisler CA. Impact of sleepiness and sleep deficiency on public health–utility of biomarkers. J Clin Sleep Med 2011;7:S6–8.
4. Vaz Fragoso CA, Gill TM. Sleep complaints in community-living older persons: a multifactorial geriatric syndrome. J Am Geriatr Soc 2007;55:1853–66.
5. Miner B, Kryger MH. Sleep in the aging population. Sleep Med Clin 2017;12:31–8.
6. Ohayon MM, Carskadon MA, Guilleminault C, et al. Meta-analysis of quantitative sleep parameters from childhood to old age in healthy individuals: developing normative sleep values across the human lifespan. Sleep 2004;27:1255–73.
7. Boulos MI, Jairam T, Kendzerska T, et al. Normal polysomnography parameters in healthy adults: a systematic review and meta-analysis. Lancet Respir Med 2019;7:533–43.
8. Hirshkowitz M, Whiton K, Albert SM, et al. National Sleep Foundation's sleep time duration recommendations: methodology and results summary. Sleep Health 2015;1:40–3.
9. Avidan AY. Normal sleep in humans. In: Kryger Meir HAAY, Berry Richard B, editors. Atlas of

clinical sleep medicine. 2nd edition. Philadelphia (PA): Saunders; 2014. p. 65–97.
10. Watson NF, Badr MS, Belenky G, et al. Joint consensus statement of the American Academy of Sleep Medicine and Sleep Research Society on the recommended amount of sleep for a healthy adult: methodology and discussion. J Clin Sleep Med 2015;11:931–52.
11. Mander BA, Winer JR, Walker MP. Sleep and human aging. Neuron 2017;94:19–36.
12. Hornung OP, Danker-Hopfe H, Heuser I. Age-related changes in sleep and memory: commonalities and interrelationships. Exp Gerontol 2005;40:279–85.
13. Crowley K. The effects of normal aging on sleep spindle and K-complex production. Clin Neurophysiol 2002;113:1615–22.
14. De Gennaro L, Ferrara M. Sleep spindles: an overview. Sleep Med Rev 2003;7:423–40.
15. Alger SE, Chambers AM, Cunningham T, et al. The role of sleep in human declarative memory consolidation. Curr Top Behav Neurosci 2015;25:269–306.
16. Lim AS, Kowgier M, Yu L, et al. Sleep fragmentation and the risk of incident alzheimer's disease and cognitive decline in older persons. Sleep 2013;36:1027–32.
17. Duffy JF, Zitting KM, Chinoy ED. Aging and circadian rhythms. Sleep Med Clin 2015;10:423–34.
18. Vaz Fragoso CA, Gill TM. Sleep complaints in community-living older persons: a multifactorial geriatric syndrome. J Am Geriatr Soc 2007;55:1853–66.
19. Monk TH. Sleep and circadian rhythms. Exp Gerontol 1991;26:233–43.
20. Touitou Y. Human aging and melatonin. Clinical relevance. Exp Gerontol 2001;36:1083–100.
21. Li J, Vitiello MV, Gooneratne NS. Sleep in normal aging. Sleep Med Clin 2018;13:1–11.
22. Morgan E, Schumm LP, McClintock M, et al. Sleep characteristics and daytime cortisol levels in older adults. Sleep 2017;40.
23. Monk TH. Aging human circadian rhythms: conventional wisdom may not always be right. J Biol Rhythms 2005;20:366–74.
24. Carrier J, Monk TH, Buysse DJ, et al. Amplitude reduction of the circadian temperature and sleep rhythms in the elderly. Chronobiol Int 1996;13:373–86.
25. Foley DJ, Monjan AA, Brown SL, et al. Sleep complaints among elderly persons: an epidemiologic study of three communities. Sleep 1995;18:425–32.
26. National Sleep Foundation Sleep in America Poll. National sleep foundation. 2003. Available at: https://sleepfoundation.org/sites/default/files/2003SleepPollExecSumm.pdf. Accessed December 19, 2019.
27. Miner B, Lucey B. Normal aging. In: Kryger MH, editor. Principles and practice of sleep medicine. 7th edition. Philadelphia (PA): Elsevier; 2021. p. 27–34.
28. Milner CE, Cote KA. Benefits of napping in healthy adults: impact of nap length, time of day, age, and experience with napping. J Sleep Res 2009;18:272–81.
29. Hausler N, Haba-Rubio J, Heinzer R, et al. Association of napping with incident cardiovascular events in a prospective cohort study. Heart (British Cardiac Society) 2019;105:1793–8.
30. Cohen-Mansfield J, Perach R. Sleep duration, nap habits, and mortality in older persons. Sleep 2012;35:1003–9.
31. Milner CE, Cote KA. Benefits of napping in healthy adults: impact of nap length, time of day, age, and experience with napping. J Sleep Res 2009;18:272–81.
32. Sleep in America poll. 2003. Available at: https://sleepfoundation.org/sites/default/files/2003SleepPollExecSumm.pdf. Accessed July 13, 2016.
33. Onen SH, Onen F. Chronic medical conditions and sleep in the older adult. Sleep Med Clin 2018;13:71–9.
34. Ohayon MM. Epidemiology of insomnia: what we know and what we still need to learn. Sleep Med Rev 2002;6:97–111.
35. Bloom HG, Ahmed I, Alessi CA, et al. Evidence-based recommendations for the assessment and management of sleep disorders in older persons. J Am Geriatr Soc 2009;57:761–89.
36. American Academy of Sleep Medicine. International classification of sleep disorders: diagnostic and coding manual. 3rd edition Darien (IL).2014.
37. Gulyani S, Salas RE, Gamaldo CE. Sleep medicine pharmacotherapeutics overview: today, tomorrow, and the future (Part 1: insomnia and circadian rhythm disorders). Chest 2012;142:1659–68.
38. Morgenthaler TI, Lee-Chiong T, Alessi C, et al. Practice parameters for the clinical evaluation and treatment of circadian rhythm sleep disorders. An American Academy of Sleep Medicine report. Sleep 2007;30:1445–59.
39. Pillar G, Shahar E, Peled N, et al. Melatonin improves sleep-wake patterns in psychomotor retarded children. Pediatr Neurol 2000;23:225–8.
40. Amara AW, Maddox MH. Epidemiology of sleep medicine. In: Kryger MH, Roth T, Dement WC, editors. Principles and practice of sleep medicine. Philadelphia (PA): Elsevier; 2017. p. 627–37.
41. Safran DG, Neuman P, Schoen C, et al. Prescription drug coverage and seniors: findings from a 2003 national survey. Health Aff (Millwood) 2005;(Suppl Web Exclusives). W5-152-W5-66.
42. Barczi SR, Teodorescu MC. Psychiatric and medical comorbidities and effects of medications in

older adults. In: Kryger MH, Roth T, Dement WC, editors. Principles and practices of sleep medicine. 5th edition. Philadelphia (PA): Elsevier; 2011. p. 1524–35.
43. Dzierzewski JM, Griffin SC, Ravyts S, et al. Psychological interventions for late-life insomnia: current and emerging science. Curr Sleep Med Rep 2018;4:268–77.
44. Vaughan CP, Bliwise DL. Sleep and nocturia in older adults. Sleep Med Clin 2018;13:107–16.
45. Umlauf MG, Chasens ER, Greevy RA, et al. Obstructive sleep apnea, nocturia and polyuria in older adults. Sleep 2004;27:139–44.
46. Gabehart RJ, Van Dongen, Hans PA. Circadian rhythms in sleepiness, alertness, and performance. In: Kryger Meir HRT, Dement William C, editors. Principles and practice of sleep medicine. 5th edition. Philadelphia (PA): Elsevier; 2011. p. 445–55.
47. Pooler JA, Hartline-Grafton H, DeBor M, et al. Food insecurity: a key social determinant of health for older adults. J Am Geriatr Soc 2019;67:421–4.
48. Perissinotto C, Holt-Lunstad J, Periyakoil VS, et al. A practical approach to assessing and mitigating loneliness and isolation in older Adults. J Am Geriatr Soc 2019;67:657–62.
49. West LA, Cole S, Goodkind D, et al. 65+ in the United States: 2010. Washington (DC): United States Census Bureau; 2014.
50. Leon-Gonzalez R, Rodriguez-Artalejo F, Ortola R, et al. Social network and risk of poor sleep outcomes in older adults: results from a Spanish Prospective Cohort Study. Nat Sci Sleep 2021;13:399–409.
51. Marini CM, Wilson SJ, Nah S, et al. Rumination and sleep quality among older adults: examining the role of social support. Journals Gerontol Ser B 2021;76(10):1948–59.
52. Older Americans 2012: key indicators of well-being. Available at: http://www.agingstats.gov/main_site/data/2012_documents/docs/entirechartbook.pdf. Accessed June 26, 2016.
53. Caregiving in the US. 2015. Available at: http://www.aarp.org/content/dam/aarp/ppi/2015/caregiving-in-the-united-states-2015-report-revised.pdf. Accessed July 13, 2016.
54. Taylor BJ, Irish LA, Martire LM, et al. Avoidant coping and poor sleep efficiency in dementia caregivers. Psychosomatic Med 2015;77:1050–7.
55. Shear MK. Clinical practice. Complicated grief. N Engl J Med 2015;372:153–60.
56. Williams BR, Sawyer Baker P, Allman RM, et al. Bereavement among African American and White older adults. J Aging Health 2007;19:313–33.
57. Shear MK, Ghesquiere A, Glickman K. Bereavement and complicated grief. Curr Psychiatry Rep 2013;15:406.
58. Aurora RN, Kim JS, Crainiceanu C, et al. Habitual sleep duration and all-cause mortality in a general community sample. Sleep 2016;39:1903–9.
59. Gallicchio L, Kalesan B. Sleep duration and mortality: a systematic review and meta-analysis. J Sleep Res 2009;18:148–58.
60. Kwok CS, Kontopantelis E, Kuligowski G, et al. Self-reported sleep duration and quality and cardiovascular disease and mortality: a dose-response meta-analysis. J Am Heart Assoc 2018;7:e008552.
61. Wallace ML, Yu L, Buysse DJ, et al. Multidimensional sleep health domains in older men and women: an actigraphy factor Analysis. Sleep 2021;44(2):zsaa181.
62. Paudel ML, Taylor BC, Ancoli-Israel S, et al. Rest/activity rhythms and mortality rates in older men: MrOS Sleep Study. Chronobiol Int 2010;27:363–77.
63. Zuurbier LA, Luik AI, Hofman A, et al. Fragmentation and stability of circadian activity rhythms predict mortality: the Rotterdam study. Am J Epidemiol 2015;181:54–63.
64. Sabia S, Fayosse A, Dumurgier J, et al. Association of sleep duration in middle and old age with incidence of dementia. Nat Commun 2021;12:2289.
65. Devore EE, Grodstein F, Duffy JF, et al. Sleep duration in midlife and later life in relation to cognition. J Am Geriatr Soc 2014;62:1073–81.
66. Dzierzewski JM, Dautovich N, Ravyts S. Sleep and cognition in older adults. Sleep Med Clin 2018;13:93–106.
67. Shokri-Kojori E, Wang G-J, Wiers CE, et al. β-Amyloid accumulation in the human brain after one night of sleep deprivation. Proc Natl Acad Sci 2018;115:4483–8.
68. Blackwell T, Yaffe K, Laffan A, et al. Associations of objectively and subjectively measured sleep quality with subsequent cognitive decline in older community-dwelling men: the MrOS sleep study. Sleep 2014;37:655–63.
69. McSorley VE, Bin YS, Lauderdale DS. Associations of sleep characteristics with cognitive function and decline among older adults. Am J Epidemiol 2019;188:1066–75.
70. Rogers-Soeder TS, Blackwell T, Yaffe K, et al. Rest-activity rhythms and cognitive decline in older men: the osteoporotic fractures in men sleep study. J Am Geriatr Soc 2018;66:2136–43.
71. Tranah GJ, Blackwell T, Stone KL, et al. Circadian activity rhythms and risk of incident dementia and mild cognitive impairment in older women. Ann Neurol 2011;70:722–32.
72. Posner AB, Tranah GJ, Blackwell T, et al. Predicting incident dementia and mild cognitive impairment in older women with nonparametric analysis of circadian activity rhythms in the Study of Osteoporotic Fractures. Sleep 2021;44(10):zsab119.

73. Gorgoni M, Lauri G, Truglia I, et al. Parietal fast sleep spindle density decrease in Alzheimer's disease and amnesic mild cognitive impairment. Neural Plast 2016;2016:8376108.
74. Gooneratne NS, Vitiello MV. Sleep in older adults: normative changes, sleep disorders, and treatment options. Clin Geriatr Med 2014;30:591–627.
75. Baril A-A, Carrier J, Lafrenière A, et al. Biomarkers of dementia in obstructive sleep apnea. Sleep Med Rev 2018;42:139–48.
76. Consensus Conference P, Watson NF, Badr MS, et al. Joint consensus statement of the American Academy of sleep medicine and sleep research Society on the recommended amount of sleep for a healthy adult: methodology and discussion. Sleep 2015;38:1161–83.
77. Kay DB, Tanner JJ, Bowers D. Sleep disturbances and depression severity in patients with Parkinson's disease. Brain Behav 2018;8:e00967.
78. Wu CR, Chen PY, Hsieh SH, et al. Sleep mediates the relationship between depression and cognitive impairment in older men. Am J Mens Health 2019; 13:1–10, 1557988319825765.
79. Pigeon WR, Hegel M, Unützer J, et al. Is insomnia a perpetuating factor for late-life depression in the IMPACT cohort? Sleep 2008;31:481–8.
80. Cole MG, Nandini D. Risk factors for depression among elderly community subjects: a systematic review and meta-analysis. Am J Psychiatry 2003; 160:1147–56.
81. Maglione JE, Ancoli-Israel S, Peters KW, et al. Depressive symptoms and circadian activity rhythm disturbances in community-dwelling older women. Am J Geriatr Psychiatry 2014;22:349–61.
82. Luik AI, Zuurbier LA, Hofman A, et al. Stability and fragmentation of the activity rhythm across the sleep-wake cycle: the importance of age, lifestyle, and mental health. Chronobiol Int 2013;30:1223–30.
83. Lunsford-Avery JR, Engelhard MM, Navar AM, et al. Validation of the sleep regularity index in older adults and associations with cardiometabolic risk. Sci Rep 2018;8:14158.
84. Vincent BM, Johnson N, Tomkinson GR, et al. Sleeping time is associated with functional limitations in a national sample of older Americans. Aging Clin Exp Res 2021;33:175–82.
85. Stone KL, Ancoli-Israel S, Blackwell T, et al. Actigraphy-measured sleep characteristics and risk of falls in older women. Arch Intern Med 2008;168: 1768–75.
86. Stone KL, Blackwell TL, Ancoli-Israel S, et al. Sleep disturbances and risk of falls in older community-dwelling men: the outcomes of sleep disorders in older men (MrOS sleep) study. J Am Geriatr Soc 2014;62:299–305.
87. Chien MY, Chen HC. Poor sleep quality is independently associated with physical disability in older adults. J Clin Sleep Med 2015;11:225–32.
88. Spira AP, Covinsky K, Rebok GW, et al. Poor sleep quality and functional decline in older women. J Am Geriatr Soc 2012;60:1092–8.
89. Rogers TS, Blackwell TL, Lane NE, et al. Rest-activity patterns and falls and fractures in older men. Osteoporos Int 2017;28:1313–22.
90. Jeon S, Conley S, Redeker NS. Rest-activity rhythms, daytime symptoms, and functional performance among people with heart failure. Chronobiol Int 2020;37:1223–34.
91. Conley S, Knies A, Batten J, et al. Agreement between actigraphic and polysomnographic measures of sleep in adults with and without chronic conditions: a systematic review and meta-analysis. Sleep Med Rev 2019;46:151–60.
92. Schroeck JL, Ford J, Conway EL, et al. Review of safety and efficacy of sleep medicines in older adults. Clin Ther 2016;38:2340–72.
93. American Geriatrics Society 2019 Updated AGS Beers Criteria® for potentially inappropriate medication use in older adults. J Am Geriatr Soc 2019; 67:674–94.
94. Flaxer JM, Heyer A, Francois D. Evidenced-based review and evaluation of clinical significance: nonpharmacological and pharmacological treatment of insomnia in the elderly. Am J Geriatr Psychiatry 2021;29:585–603.
95. Mishima K, Okawa M, Shimizu T, et al. Diminished melatonin secretion in the elderly caused by insufficient environmental illumination1. J Clin Endocrinol Metab 2001;86:129–34.
96. Suzuki K, Miyamoto M, Hirata K. Sleep disorders in the elderly: diagnosis and management. J Gen Fam Med 2017;18:61–71.
97. Miner B, Jiwa N, Koo B. Treatment of RLS/PLMD, hypersomnolence, circadian disorders, and parasomnias. In: Savard JOM, editor. Handbook of sleep disorders in medical conditions. Massachusettes (MA): Academic Press; 2019. p. 77–95.
98. Endeshaw YW, Yoo W. Association between social and physical activities and insomnia symptoms among community-dwelling older adults. J Aging Health 2016;28:1073–89.
99. Varrasse M, Li J, Gooneratne N. Exercise and sleep in community-dwelling older adults. Curr Sleep Med Rep 2015;1:232–40.
100. Benloucif S, Orbeta L, Ortiz R, et al. Morning or evening activity improves neuropsychological performance and subjective sleep quality in older adults. Sleep 2004;27:1542–51.
101. Scharf MT, Naidoo N, Zimmerman JE, et al. The energy hypothesis of sleep revisited. Prog Neurobiol 2008;86:264–80.

102. Endeshaw Y. Clinical characteristics of obstructive sleep apnea in community-dwelling older adults. J Am Geriatr Soc 2006;54:1740–4.
103. Endeshaw YW, Yoo W. Organized social activity, physical exercise, and the risk of insomnia symptoms among community-dwelling older adults. J Aging Health 2019;31:989–1001.
104. Koffel E, Bramoweth AD, Ulmer CS. Increasing access to and utilization of cognitive behavioral therapy for insomnia (CBT-I): a narrative review. J Gen Intern Med 2018;33:955–62.
105. Kalmbach DA, Cheng P, Arnedt JT, et al. Treating insomnia improves depression, maladaptive thinking, and hyperarousal in postmenopausal women: comparing cognitive-behavioral therapy for insomnia (CBTI), sleep restriction therapy, and sleep hygiene education. Sleep Med 2019;55:124–34.
106. Buysse DJ, Germain A, Moul DE, et al. Efficacy of brief behavioral treatment for chronic insomnia in older adults. Arch Intern Med 2011;171:887–95.
107. Chen C-T, Tung H-H, Fang C-J, et al. Effect of music therapy on improving sleep quality in older adults: a systematic review and meta-analysis. J Am Geriatr Soc 2021;69:1925–32.
108. Neubauer DN. A review of ramelteon in the treatment of sleep disorders. Neuropsychiatr Dis Treat 2008;4:69–79.
109. Rhyne DN, Anderson SL. Suvorexant in insomnia: efficacy, safety and place in therapy. Ther Adv Drug Saf 2015;6:189–95.
110. Johns MW. A new method for measuring daytime sleepiness: the epworth sleepiness scale. Sleep 1991;14:540–5.
111. Onen F, Moreau T, Gooneratne NS, et al. Limits of the epworth sleepiness scale in older adults. Sleep Breath 2013;17:343–50.
112. Bastien CH, Vallieres A, Morin CM. Validation of the insomnia severity index as an outcome measure for insomnia research. Sleep Med 2001;2:297–307.
113. Miner B, Gill TM, Yaggi HK, et al. The epidemiology of patient-reported hypersomnia in persons with advanced age. J Am Geriatr Soc 2019;67:2545–52.
114. Miner B, Gill TM, Yaggi HK, et al. Insomnia in community-living persons with advanced age. J Am Geriatr Soc 2018;66:1592–7.
115. Yalamanchali S, Farajian V, Hamilton C, et al. Diagnosis of obstructive sleep apnea by peripheral arterial tonometry: meta-analysis. JAMA Otolaryngology–Head Neck Surg 2013;139:1343–50.

Adding Insult to Injury

Sleep Deficiency in Hospitalized Patients

Wissam Mansour, MD[a], Melissa Knauert, MD, PhD[b,*]

KEYWORDS

• Sleep deficiency • Circadian • Environment • Sound • Light • Critical illness • Acute illness

KEY POINTS

- Sleep deficiency, including short sleep, poor quality sleep, and abnormally timed sleep, is common in hospitalized patients.
- Key factors contributing to the risk and severity of sleep deficiency include preexisting sleep and other disorders, illness severity, the hospital environment, and treatment-related effects.
- Sleep deficiency results in deleterious health effects impacting various organ systems.
- Sleep and circadian markers are difficult to study in the hospital setting.
- Nonpharmacologic treatments are currently guideline recommended; pharmacologic treatments are under investigation, but their use is limited by established harms.

INTRODUCTION

Sleep is vital for human health and has a critical role in brain function, and regulation of the immune, metabolic, hormonal, and cardiovascular systems.[1,2] Accordingly, sleep disruption results in a wide range of adverse health effects, impacting mood, cognition, metabolism, cardiovascular disease, seizures, immune response, and overall mortality.[3–9] Hospitalized patients experience short sleep, poor sleep quality, insomnia, and marked circadian rhythm misalignment.[10–12] The impact of this on hospital outcomes is difficult to measure, given its variation with illness severity and paucity of feasible objective tests. Regardless, current evidence supports that sleep disruption among hospitalized patients is a risk factor for "post-hospital syndrome," an entity defined by a transient period of increased vulnerability after discharge.[13] Limited studies also suggest associations between poor sleep and in-hospital mortality in intensive care unit (ICU) patients.[14]

This article will provide a review of sleep deficiency in the hospital setting. We will provide an overview of the negative health effects of sleep deficiency, discuss predisposing medical risk factors for poor hospital sleep. We will also discuss environmental and treatment-related factors that contribute to poor sleep. We will review the literature regarding sleep assessment tools for hospitalized patients, and, finally, discuss hospital-based sleep promotion interventions.

SLEEP DISTURBANCES IN HOSPITALIZED PATIENTS

Hospitalized patients frequently suffer from all aspects of sleep deficiency: poor sleep quality, restricted total sleep time, and circadian rhythm misalignment.[11,15,16] Such sleep disturbances appear to be more pronounced with severe illness and during the immediate postoperative period.[17–19] They also appear to persist beyond

[a] Department of Internal Medicine, Division of Pulmonary, Allergy and Critical Care Medicine, Duke University School of Medicine, 1821 Hillandale Road, Suite 25A, Durham, NC 27705, USA; [b] Department of Internal Medicine, Section of Pulmonary, Critical Care, and Sleep Medicine, Yale University School of Medicine, 300 Cedar Street, PO Box 208057, New Haven, CT 06520-8057, USA
* Corresponding author.
E-mail address: Melissa.Knauert@yale.edu

Clin Chest Med 43 (2022) 287–303
https://doi.org/10.1016/j.ccm.2022.02.009

the acute illness and following hospital discharge.[20,21]

Poor Sleep Quality

Poor sleep quality is commonly reported by hospitalized patients in various inpatient settings. Results from questionnaire studies assessing sleep in patients admitted to the regular ward noted patients reporting more frequent nighttime awakenings, sleeping difficulties, and less satisfaction with sleep quality compared with home sleep.[11,22] These findings appear to be worse for critically ill patients admitted to the ICU. In fact, surveys of ICU patients showed self-reporting of sleep disturbance reaching 100% in certain studies.[23,24] Further objective characterization of sleep in the ICU utilizing polysomnography (PSG) revealed frequent arousals, poor nocturnal sleep efficiency, and altered sleep architecture with increased N1 and N2 stages and reduced or absent N3 and REM stages.[23,25,26]

Short Sleep Duration

Sleep quantity can also be impacted by acute illness and hospitalization. Observational data from surveys estimating total sleep time in the hospital ward compared with the home environment of nearly 1500 patients showed that the hospital sleep time was reduced by 83 minutes.[11] Data from wrist activity monitors assessing sleep duration in the hospital wards revealed similar reductions in sleep time when compared to home sleep duration.[27] Studies from the ICU did not necessarily show a similar reduction in sleep quantity over a 24-h period but did note abnormal sleep-wake cycles and nonconsolidated sleep with a significant portion of sleep occurring during the day.[19,26]

Circadian Rhythm Misalignment

The disarrangement of circadian cues (ie, zeitgebers) such as light, sleep-wake, physical activity, meals, and social interactions is the likely driving factor for circadian rhythm misalignment in the hospital. In addition, systemic inflammation and exposure to medications disrupt circadian rhythmicity through alteration of melatonin secretion and clock gene expression.[16] Studies generally demonstrate that critically ill patients have a disorganized circadian rhythmicity.[28–30] However, one study of nonseptic ICU patients (N = 40) showed maintenance of diurnal variation of cortisol and melatonin.[31] Data comparing septic to nonseptic ICU patients showed loss of normal periodicity of melatonin levels and reduced expression of peripheral circadian genes in the septic group only.[32,33] The heterogeneity of study results suggest that circadian rhythm dysregulation is not ubiquitous in critical illness but rather influenced by illness type and severity, degree of encephalopathy, and exposure to certain medications.[30]

ENVIRONMENTAL FACTORS AFFECTING SLEEP

Environmental factors are major contributors to sleep disturbances in hospitalized patients. Numerous studies have evaluated the impact of sound levels, noncircadian light exposure, and patient care interactions on sleep quality in the hospital setting. This section will review available data for environmental disturbances.

Sound Levels

Excessive sound (ie, noise) has been reported at various locations within the hospital. The World Health Organization recommends that overnight equivalent sound pressure level (Leq) for continuous background noise should not exceed 30 A-weighted decibels (dBA). Individual sound events, which may correlate more with the probability of being awakened, should not exceed 45 dBA.[34] A study evaluating the change in hospital noise levels over the years between 1960 and 2005 showed an increase in average nighttime noise from 42 dBA to 60 dBA.[35] A recently published review of 33 studies from different countries demonstrated a hospital daytime Leq range of 37 to 88 dBA and nighttime Leq range of 38 to 68 dBA.[36] ICU-based investigations demonstrated similar sound levels with an overnight minimum average Leq of 50 dBA and peaks greater than 85 dBA occurring 16 times per hour (>85 dBA is equivalent to standing 10 m from heavy traffic).[37,38] Mapping of noise sources in the ICU demonstrated that the majority of loud sounds originate from ventilators, medical alarms, and talking.[39]

The impact of noise in the hospital setting on sleep quality has been evaluated mostly in critically ill patients. An observational study of 64 ICU patients demonstrated that increased background noise correlated with subjective worsening of sleep quality.[40] Small sample polysomnographic studies in critically ill patients showed that sound elevations contributed to 20% of arousals from sleep.[41] Exposing healthy volunteers to simulated ICU noise resulted in poorer sleep quality, increased arousals, and decreased REM sleep.[42,43] Arousal response curves varied by sound level, sound type, and sleep stage.[44] These findings suggest that the influence of sound on sleep is more complex than being predicted by average sound level only.

Noncircadian Light

Circadian rhythms are essential elements in the regulation of sleep timing and indirectly sleep quality. Light-dark patterns are the most important circadian cues (ie, zeitgebers) for circadian entrainment, and light impact depends on intensity, duration, and spectra, as well as light history.[45,46] Studies in the ICU consistently showed a low mean daytime light intensity exposure with an average below 100 to 150 lux compared with normal living environments (sunny day: >50,000 lux; office: 500 lux).[29,47–49] A study comparing the sleep environment between ICU and non-ICU wards demonstrated a similar pattern of dim daytime light in both settings.[50] Nighttime hospital light levels appear appropriately low on average; however, there remain periods of elevated light lasting an average of 1.75 hours per night.[51] Improving insufficient daytime light exposure may be a feasible and rewarding strategy. Studies have shown that daytime bright light interventions can improve sleep quality in the elderly,[52,53] cardiology,[54] and postoperative patients,[55] but not in hospitalized decompensated cirrhosis patients.[56] A combination of morning bright light and nighttime use of short-wavelength filter glasses for medical patients resulted in improved daytime sleepiness, mood, and a decrease in nighttime awakenings.[57] Further work has suggested a role for daytime bright light interventions in reducing delirium in critically ill,[58,59] postoperative patients,[55] and mortality postmyocardial infarction.[60] Conversely, other studies did not show an impact of light therapy on ICU outcomes.[61,62] The differences in outcomes may be secondary to variations in study protocols regarding the timing, spectra, and intensity of light exposure.[46]

Nonphotic Cues

Nonphotic circadian cues (ie, nonlight zeitgebers) also have an important influence on circadian phase entertainment.[45] These nonphotic cues include sleep-wake timing, meal schedules, and physical activity, which are likely to be altered in the hospitalized patients and particularly the critically ill. Meal schedule and nutrition delivery in the ICU is most frequently delivered via continuous 24-h drips despite limited evidence for this practice.[63] Continuous feeding conflicts both with normal gastrointestinal function and with peripheral circadian clocks of the digestive system likely resulting in internal circadian desynchronization, poor sleep, and poor glucose tolerance.[64] A time-restricted daytime feeding regimen may be a proposed solution to help realign the biological rhythm of hospitalized patients.[64] Similarly, hospital mobility programs may promote sleep and circadian alignment via circadian and other pathways; however, this has not been investigated to date.

Patient Care Interactions

Nocturnal care activities rank as a major source of sleep disruption in hospitalized patients; these care activities can wake patients but are also accompanied by pain, anxiety, sound, and light. In a survey study, 20% of hospitalized ward patients reported being awakened by hospital staff.[11] ICU survivors considered sleep disruption from human interventions and diagnostic testing to be as disruptive as environmental noise[24]; studies indicate that nocturnal patient care activities occurred around 4 to 8 times per hour and correlated with 7% of total arousals and awakenings.[41,65] Data from nighttime patient interaction for 200 ICU patients estimated that 14% of nocturnal interactions were not time critical.[66] Expert guidelines currently recommend rescheduling and clustering nocturnal care interactions as part of sleep promotion protocols.[67,68]

MEDICAL CONDITIONS PREDISPOSING TO POOR HOSPITAL SLEEP

Preexisting sleep disorders and certain comorbidities may increase patients' risk for poor sleep in the hospital (**Table 1**). The following section will focus on preexisting conditions with available research evaluating its association with sleep disturbances in the hospital.

Preexisting Sleep Disorders

Preexisting sleep disorders are closely linked to hospital sleep deficiency. Insomnia is one of the most common sleep disorders, and observational studies demonstrate that patients with preexisting insomnia are likely to experience an exacerbation during and after hospitalization.[21,69] Sleep-disordered breathing (SDB) is common, underdiagnosed, and often goes untreated during hospital admissions.[70–73] A retrospective study evaluating the use of positive airway pressure (PAP) therapy in patients with a history of SDB during their hospital stay showed that it was only provided to 5% of patients.[74] In addition, acute sleep deprivation can worsen obstruction in SDB, which in turn will result in worse sleep disruption forming a vicious cycle for hospitalized patients with SDB.[75] Unsurprisingly, SDB is associated with

Table 1
Common medical conditions predisposing to poor hospital sleep

Condition	Sleep Problem	Treatment Options
Obstructive Sleep Apnea	Fragmented sleep, snoring, hypoxemia	Positional therapy, obtain home positive airway pressure settings, minimize use of respiratory depressants
Restless Leg Syndrome	Prolonged sleep latency, periodic limb movements of sleep	Encourage ambulation, continue home RLS medications, avoid unnecessary blood draws, avoid medications that worsen RLS
Chronic Obstructive Pulmonary Disease	Hypoxemia, sleep-related worsening of hypoventilation, dyspnea, obstructive sleep apnea	Treatment of hypoxemia and increased work of breathing, noninvasive ventilation for hypercapnic respiratory failure, head of bed elevation, avoid respiratory depressants
Congestive Heart Failure	Orthopnea, nocturnal diuresis, central sleep apnea	Favor daytime diuresis, optimize cardiac therapy, positive airway pressure for respiratory distress
Stroke	Reduced sleep efficiency, increased daytime sleep, increased risk of sleep apnea	Head of bed elevation, aspiration precautions, continuous positive airway pressure, early rehabilitation programs
Chronic Kidney Disease	Restless leg syndrome, periodic limb movements of sleep	Encourage ambulation, avoid excessive blood draws, correct uremia and electrolyte abnormalities
Gastroesophageal reflux disease	Arousals	Head of bed elevation, avoid meals 4 h before sleep onset

increased risk of complications and poor hospital outcomes in medical and surgical patients.[76,77]

Restless legs syndrome (RLS) is a sensorimotor neurologic disorder that impacts patients' ability to initiate and maintain sleep; RLS is associated with multiple comorbidities that are prevalent in the hospitalized population.[78] Several factors can contribute to the worsening or unmasking of RLS during a hospital stay including immobility, sleep deprivation, blood loss, and possible cessation of RLS medications. Medications that are commonly added in the hospital setting such as antipsychotics, dopamine antagonist antiemetics, and antihistamines can also exacerbate RLS.[79]

Preexisting Medical Disorders

Several common medical disorders are associated with poor sleep including chronic obstructive pulmonary disease (COPD),[80] heart failure,[81] stroke,[82] chronic kidney disease,[83] and gastroesophageal reflux.[84] Patients with COPD are particularly affected with a high prevalence of insomnia, SDB, and RLS.[85] This overlap and association with sleep disorders may explain the vulnerability of patients hospitalized with COPD to sleep disturbances. A cohort study evaluating sleep in medical wards patients using questionnaires and actigraphy found that patients with a history of COPD had a reduced in-hospital sleep quality and quantity compared with those without COPD.[80]

Another patient population of particular concern is patients with cerebrovascular accidents (CVA). The prevalence of sleep disorders in patients after CVA is estimated to be greater than 50%.[86] The rate of obstructive sleep apnea (OSA) after stroke has been found to be as high as 70%.[87] This is likely secondary to positional sleep apnea, upper airway tone changes, and untreated OSA preceding the stroke.[86] Small trials have demonstrated a trend toward improvement in stroke severity and recovery in patients receiving early PAP therapy.[88,89] Stroke patients are also at risk for developing central sleep apnea (CSA). This is thought to be an uncommon consequence that tends to resolve with time.[90] In addition to sleep disturbances from SDB, patients admitted with stroke have a higher subjective reporting of prolonged sleep latency and more daytime napping.[82]

PATIENT FACTORS AFFECTING SLEEP

Illness Severity and Sepsis

Illness severity and acuity has been shown to correlate with the frequency of patient care interactions limiting the availability of rest periods.[65] An observational study of 100 patients showed a significant correlation between disease severity evaluated by Acute Physiologic Assessment and Chronic Health Evaluation II (APACHE II) score and perceived poor sleep quality in the ICU.[91] Increased illness severity is also likely associated with increased pain, anxiety, and delirium that may impact sleep.

The effect of sepsis on sleep has been well documented in the literature but the pathogenesis of this association remains poorly understood. Septic patients have been noted to have alterations in the electroencephalography (EEG) signal showing low-voltage mixed frequency waves with variable theta and delta, referred to as "sepsis-associated encephalopathy."[92] REM sleep was reduced in association with increased N1 and N2 stages.[93] Sepsis also appears to result in a loss of normal circadian rhythm independent of ICU environmental changes. In a study comparing septic to nonseptic ICU patients, sepsis appeared to result in alteration of melatonin secretion and suppression of circadian genes expression.[32] Sleep alterations in sepsis, particularly reduction in REM sleep, may be an appropriate response to stress given the sympathetic-parasympathetic imbalance and increased susceptibility to breathing abnormalities experienced in REM.[94]

Pain

A bidirectional relationship appears to exist between poor sleep and pain. Prevalence rates of insomnia in patients with chronic pain range between 50% and 70%.[95] On the other hand, several prospective studies reported that poor sleep increases the risk for new-onset cases of chronic pain and worsens existing headaches and musculoskeletal pain.[96] Pain increases cortical arousals resulting in sleep fragmentation. The mechanism for the hyperalgesic effect of sleep deprivation and disruption remains under investigation. Sleep deprivation can result in inhibition of opioid synthesis and reduced affinity to opioid receptors.[97] In a study including hospitalized burn patients, a temporal relationship between sleep and pain was noted such that poor night sleep was followed by more painful days.[98] These data support the hypothesis that hospitalized patients with acute or chronic pain are at higher risk for sleep disturbances.

Postoperative Recovery

Postsurgical patients report pain to be the most common cause of sleep disruption during recovery.[99,100] In the postoperative period, patients have absent or markedly depressed REM sleep along with increases in stages N1 and N2, regardless of whether general or regional anesthesia was provided.[101,102] Factors playing a role in REM suppression postoperatively include increases in catecholamine and cortisol levels, in addition to the receipt of opioids.[17] REM rebound phenomenon, described as an increase in REM duration and density, has been reported in postabdominal surgery patients occurring between postoperative days 3 and 6.[101] This may precipitate a period of vulnerability with patients being at higher risk for REM-related respiratory and cardiovascular instability.[103]

Mechanical Ventilation

Poor sleep quality has been reported in critically ill patients requiring mechanical ventilation. Sleep disturbances in this population are caused by a mismatch between patient demand and ventilator supply (patient-ventilator asynchrony), central apneas due to overventilation with consequent hyperpnea, and increased respiratory effort secondary to improper settings or air leaks.[104] Small sample studies have investigated the impact of ventilator mode on sleep. The work of Parthasarathy and colleagues[104] and Toublanc and colleagues[105] demonstrated that assist control ventilation resulted in better sleep quality when compared with pressure support ventilation. In contrast, a study by Cabello and colleagues[106] showed no impact of ventilator modes on sleep quality when pressure support was adjusted to achieve low tidal volumes. These findings suggest that correcting patient-ventilator mismatch, rather than using specific ventilator modes results in improved sleep quality.

Medications

Several medications prescribed to hospitalized patients result in sleep disruption, and alteration of sleep architecture, in addition to associated dangers of increased falls and carryover prescribing (**Table 2**).[107] Commonly used off-label sleep-promoting medications such as antihistamines, antipsychotics, and benzodiazepines actually inhibit deep sleep stages and increase the risk of

Table 2
Effects of commonly used medications on sleep

Medication	Mode of Action	Effects on Sleep
Sedatives-Hypnotics		
Benzodiazepines	GABAA R modulator	↑TST, ↓WASO, ↑N2, ↓N3, ↓REM, ↓SOL
Propofol	GABAA R potentiator	↑TST, ↓REM
Dexmedetomidine	α2 Agonist	↓N3, ↓REM Role in maintaining sleep day-night cycle
Analgesics		
Opioids	μ opioid R agonist	↓TST, ↑WASO, ↓N3, ↓REM, ↑CSA
NSAID	Prostaglandin synthesis inhibition	↓TST, ↑WASO
Antipsychotics		
Haloperidol	D2 antagonism	↑TST, ↑N3, ↓REM, ↓SOL, ↑PLMS
Quetiapine	5-HT2A, D2 antagonism	↑TST, ↓SOL, ↓REM, ↑PLMS
Antidepressants		
Selective serotonin reuptake inhibitor	5-HT reuptake inhibition	↓TST, ↓REM, ↑SOL, ↑PLMS
Trazodone	5-HT2A antagonism; 5-HT reuptake inhibition; α 1, H 1 antagonism	↑TST, ↑N3, ↓REM, ↓SOL
Tricyclic antidepressants	5-HT > NE reuptake inhibition; 5-HT 2 antagonism	↑TST, ↓REM, ↑PLMS
Cardiovascular		
Lipophilic β-blocker	CNS β-blockade	↑WASO, ↓ REM, ↑ nightmares
Norepinephrine Epinephrine	α and β R agonist	↓ REM, ↓ N3
Phenylephrine	α1 R agonist	↓ REM, ↓ N3
Other Medications		
Antihistamine	H1 antagonism	↓ REM, ↓ SOL
Corticosteroids	Unclear, ↓ melatonin	↑WASO, ↓ REM, ↓ N3

Abbreviations: ↓, decrease; ↑, increase; 5HT, serotonin; D, dopamine; H, histamine; NSAID, nonsteroidal anti-inflammatory drug; REM, rapid eye movement; SOL, sleep onset latency; TST, total sleep time; WASO, wake after sleep onset.

Data from PK S., AC R. Chapter 45 - Drugs that Disturb Sleep and Wakefulness. In: Kryger M, Roth T, Dement WC, eds. Principles and Practice of Sleep Medicine (Sixth Edition). Elsevier; 2017:480 to 498.e8 and KA H. Sleep in the ICU: potential mechanisms and clinical implications. *Chest*. 2009 Jul 2009;136(1).

delirium, falls, and daytime cognitive impairment.[108,109] Benzodiazepines have been shown to improve sleep latency and total sleep time, but this should be weighed against disturbances in sleep architecture (decreased N3 and REM) and the increased risk of delirium.[110] Narcotics are known to provoke sleep disruption with increased awakenings and suppression of N3 and REM sleep.[111] These agents also increase the risk of CSA.[111] Propofol and dexmedetomidine have also been shown to result in reduced REM sleep.[112,113] Conversely, propofol may improve sleep efficiency and dexmedetomidine may help preserve the day-night cycle.[113,114]

HEALTH EFFECTS OF SLEEP DISTURBANCES

Sleep disturbances can result in deleterious effects on various body systems.[9] Most available studies involved healthy subjects, with limited research including hospitalized patients. The following section will focus on the impact of short

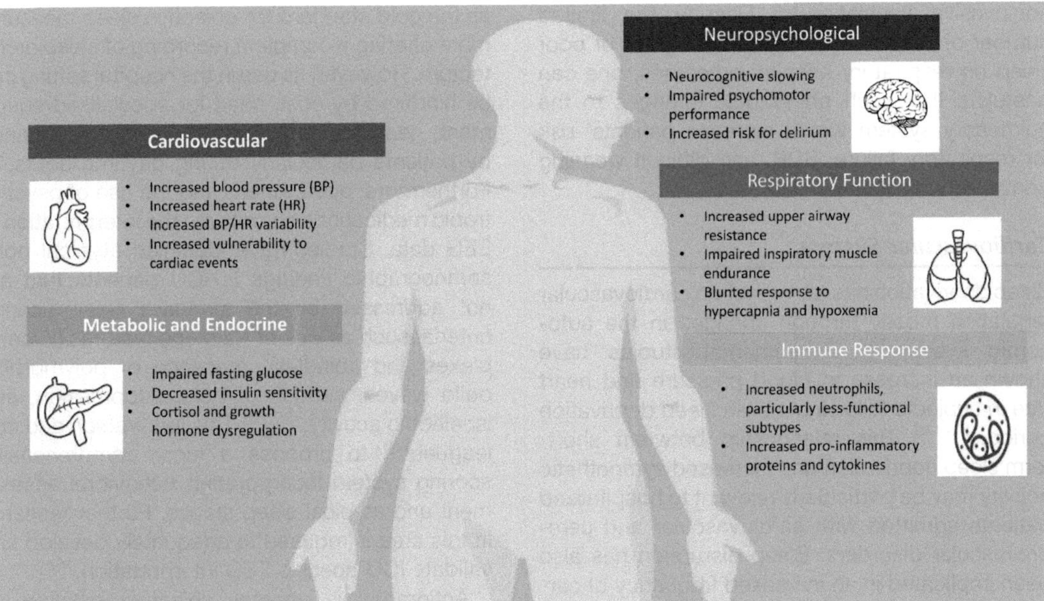

Fig. 1. Potential consequences of sleep deficiency in hospitalized patients.

and long-term sleep disturbances on specific organ systems with extrapolation to the hospitalized population when appropriate (**Fig. 1**).

Immune Response and Inflammation

A bidirectional relationship appears to exist between sleep loss and the immune system.[3] Subacute and chronic sleep deprivation have been shown to reduce the immune response to vaccination, increase the risk for inflammatory disorders, and increase susceptibility to respiratory tract infections.[115–117]

Acute sleep loss has been shown to increase the leukocyte population through increases in neutrophils (innate immunity), while circulating numbers of lymphocytes (adaptive immunity) remain stable.[118,119] Concerningly, a study looking at the subpopulation of neutrophils following one night of sleep deprivation revealed a disproportionate increase of less functional neutrophil subtypes suggesting a less effective proinflammatory state.[120] Studies have also demonstrated an increase in proinflammatory proteins and cytokines following one night of sleep deprivation.[121,122] Though evidence continues to evolve, it appears that sleep disturbances result in an early proinflammatory milieu that may increase hospitalized patients' susceptibility to infectious and inflammatory disorders.

Neuropsychological Effects

Behavioral consequences of sleep deprivation include impaired cognition, psychomotor performance, and mood.[123,124] Delirium has been the subject of multiple studies in critically ill patients given its association with prolonged length of stay, long-term cognitive impairment, functional decline, and increased 1-year mortality.[125,126] The relationship between sleep disturbances and delirium seems plausible as both phenomena share similar clinical and neurophysiologic risk factors.[5] Studies have suggested poor sleep as a modifiable risk factor for delirium in hospitalized patients.[127,128] Sleep promoting interventions in ICU patients seem to be promising at improving delirium-related outcomes; however, evidence is limited by studies heterogeneity and multiple confounders.[129] Research suggests a possible role for exogenous melatonin in delirium prevention for hospitalized patients.[130] Though this finding has not been consistent.[131]

Respiratory Function

Experimental studies have shown that sleep deprivation can have a detrimental impact on the respiratory system by diminishing respiratory response to hypoxemia and hypercapnia, reducing respiratory motor output, increasing upper airway resistance, and impairing inspiratory muscle endurance.[75,132–134] Data from patients with COPD demonstrate a reduction in both forced expiratory volume in 1 second and forced vital capacity following one night of sleep deprivation.[135] In patients with hypercapnic respiratory failure, those with poor sleep and circadian misalignment were found to be at higher risk for late failure of noninvasive ventilation.[136] Despite the limited number of studies evaluating the impact of poor sleep on respiratory hospital outcomes, one can postulate that such physiologic changes to the pulmonary system would increase patients' risk for respiratory failure, SDB, and difficult weaning from mechanical ventilation.

Cardiovascular System

Sleep deprivation has an impact on cardiovascular regulation mostly through changes in the autonomic system.[137] Experimental studies have shown an increase in blood pressure and heart rate in subjects following a 24-h sleep deprivation period.[137–139] This relationship between short-term sleep deprivation and increased sympathetic activity may be particularly relevant to hospitalized patients admitted with cardiovascular and cerebrovascular disorders. Sleep disruption has also been implicated in an increased frequency of cardiac events. Telemetry data from 87 patients demonstrated that the incidence of ventricular ectopy and subsequent cardiac arrest events increased, in correlation with increased sleep disruption from hospital emergency codes overheads.[140] Patients recovering from operative procedures or critical illness may have an increase in REM sleep quantity and phasic events known as "REM rebound." This period may precipitate cardiovascular events in vulnerable patients secondary to blood pressure variations, cardiac arrhythmias, and hypoxemia.[141,142]

Metabolic and Endocrine System

Endocrine functions are influenced by sleep with multiple hormones having a circadian pattern. Loss of periodicity for cortisol and growth hormone has been seen during periods of sleep loss.[143,144] Sleep deprivation alters glucose metabolism with experimental studies demonstrating a reduction in glucose sensitivity in healthy subjects.[145] Data from hospitalized patients showed that shorter sleep duration and worse efficiency determined by actigraphy were associated with greater odds of hyperglycemia.[146] This association might be particularly important in patients with neurologic conditions that could have worse outcomes with hyperglycemia.[147]

ASSESSMENT OF SLEEP IN HOSPITALIZED PATIENTS

Sleep measurement must evaluate sleep duration, quality, and timing. Obtaining such measures in hospitalized patients has been a major challenge for clinicians and investigators.[148] PSG is regarded as the gold standard for objective sleep measurement offering a complete recording of sleep architecture. However, its use in the hospital setting can be hindered by cost, need for specialized equipment, need for trained staff, and poor tolerance by patients particularly during daytime hours.[149] Furthermore, acute illness and the use of psychotropic medications complicate the interpretation of EEG data. Studies have identified atypical polysomnographic findings in ICU patients that are not addressed by the standard sleep scoring criteria, such as lack of N2 stage features (K-complexes and spindles), presence of polymorphic delta waves, periods of burst suppression, and isoelectric activity.[150,151] This led Watson and colleagues[150] to propose a more comprehensive scoring system incorporating behavioral assessment and atypical sleep stages. Further research in this area is required to adequately develop and validate ICU-specific EEG interpretation.[152]

Actigraphy is another objective measure of sleep that offers data on total sleep time, sleep efficiency, and wake after sleep onset.[153] Actigraphy uses accelerometer technology mounted on a wristwatch-like device capable of collecting movement data that is translated by validated algorithms into rest-wake periods.[149] Actigraphy correlates reasonably with PSG in multiple settings and various populations, but may overestimate sleep especially in patients with reduced sleep efficiency.[154] Given its poor ability to differentiate sleep from restful wake, actigraphy may underperform in hospitalized patients. A review of available studies comparing the use of actigraphy in the ICU to other methods of sleep measurement reveals that it tends to report higher sleep quantity and efficiency.[155] Despite these limitations, actigraphy offers a feasible and user-friendly method with a promising role in evaluating sleep changes and trends for the duration of a hospital admission and beyond.[156,157]

Subjective questionnaires are a tempting approach given their feasibility and low cost. Validated sleep questionnaires can be used alone or in conjunction with previously described objective tools. The Richard Campbell Sleep Questionnaire (RCSQ), developed and validated in critically ill patients, is a widely used 5-item visual analog scale measuring the perception of sleep depth, number of awakenings, sleep onset latency, time spent awake, and overall sleep quality.[158] The questionnaire is short and can be applied by novice personnel.[159] In a single ICU group of patients, RCSQ was found to have a moderate correlation with PSG.[158] However, the reliability of self-reported surveys can be impacted by delirium and impaired memory recall. For example, 20%

to 50% of ICU patients were unable to complete the RCSQ in observational studies.[149,160] Although important, use of subjective patient sleep assessment tools may be limited in the hospital population.

INTERVENTIONS TO IMPROVE SLEEP IN HOSPITALIZED PATIENTS

The value of improving sleep in hospitalized patients is increasingly recognized by patients, clinical staff, and hospital administrators. Survey data have demonstrated that most patients and clinicians believe that sleep in the hospital is poor and may adversely affect patient outcomes.[11,161,162] Current expert guidelines for pain, agitation, and delirium prevention in the ICU recommend sleep promotion through a multidisciplinary bundled approach.[67] Despite these recommendations, a large gap remains between our understanding of the problem and implementation of hospital sleep promotion interventions.[162] This section will review current strategies for improving hospital sleep.

Nonpharmacologic Sleep Promotion Protocols

Sleep promotion protocols should follow a multifaceted approach that includes addressing sleep-disrupting medical conditions and medications, limiting external stimuli, promoting relaxation and quiet time, sleep education, controlling pain, and maintaining circadian alignment.[163,164] Researchers have looked at different interventions that variably examined one or more of those elements. Unfortunately, sleep measurement and outcomes varied across different studies, making it difficult to compare the results.[164]

Environmental interventions aimed at noise reduction, light control, and limiting unnecessary nighttime interactions have been commonly used.[164] Noise reduction techniques may include use of earplugs, "white noise" machines, behavioral modifications to improving medical device alarm volume, using remote monitors, and installing acoustic material.[165] Earplugs and sound masking appear to modestly improve patients' subjective perception of sleep.[166–169] Acoustic room adjustments such as using sound-absorbing tiles, resulted in reduced patient pulse amplitude postmyocardial infarction and improved patient experience.[170] Eye masks have been used to block nighttime light stimulation, either alone,[171,172] or in conjunction with earplugs,[173,174] resulting in improved subjective sleep quality for patients; however, eye masks tend to be poorly tolerated by a significant proportion of patients.[175] Behavioral modifications implemented through "quiet time" protocols and clustering of patient care activities showed a successful reduction in perceived noise levels and improved subjective and observed sleep.[176,177] Complementary therapies that promote relaxation such as music, massage, aromatherapy, and acupressure appear to be safe and may achieve minor improvement in sleep.[157,178–180]

In addition to providing patients with the opportunity to sleep, circadian disruption is an important dimension that should be addressed by hospital sleep promotion interventions.[181] Circadian alignment could be promoted via increased exposure to daytime light, encouraging daytime activity, and feeding schedules that mimic daytime meals. Data from interventions with bright light therapy are discussed earlier.

Bundled interventions in medical and surgical ICUs have been associated with a reduction in delirium, even in the absence of a change in subjective sleep scores.[182,183] A pilot study promoting environmental control and limitation of nonurgent bedside care between 00:00 and 04:00 resulted in decreased in-room activity and sound levels.[68] Sleep promoting multimodal initiatives on the general ward have been found to result in modest improvements in subjective and objective sleep measures.[184,185] The low-risk nature of sleep-promoting interventions in the setting of their proven and potential benefits have prompted experts to recommend their implementation before pharmacologic therapy.[152] We acknowledge the need for higher quality evidence from large rigorous studies to encourage hospital-wide interventions that require effort, funding, and resources.

Pharmacotherapy to Treat Sleep Disruption in the Hospital

Prescribing sleep aids to hospitalized patients is a common practice. Single-center studies showed that approximately 20% to 30% of patients admitted to the hospital receive a sleep medication.[186–188] Concerningly, newly prescribed sleep aids were continued for 10% to 30% of patients after discharge.[186,188] Despite the widespread use of pharmacotherapy to treat in-hospital sleep disturbances, there is a paucity of data regarding the safety and efficacy of commonly used agents in this patient population. We will discuss commonly used medications in the following.

Melatonin and melatonin receptor agonists have the potential to support sleep promotion and circadian organization in hospitalized patients; this has led researchers to investigate its application in various settings.[189,190] So far, published small sample trials evaluating the use of exogenous melatonin in the ICU have yielded conflicting results.[156,191,192] Differences in study design, melatonin administration protocol (dose and time), and measured outcomes have made it difficult to compare data and draw conclusions. A systematic review of 4 heterogeneous randomized controlled trials with 151 participants found insufficient evidence to determine the impact of melatonin use on sleep, mortality, and delirium in ICU patients.[193] More recent trials have also had mixed results in improving sleep quality.[194–196]

Trazodone, a serotonin modulator with sedative effect, is commonly used in the hospital setting for the treatment of insomnia.[186] A recent meta-analysis of randomized placebo-controlled trials evaluating trazodone use for the treatment of insomnia showed that trazodone was effective in decreasing the number of early awakenings and improving perceived sleep quality.[197] A small observational study of hospitalized psychiatric patients showed that trazodone resulted in better subjective sleep quality when compared with quetiapine.[198] However, clinicians should note that side effects include daytime somnolence, orthostatic hypotension, QT prolongation, risk of arrhythmias, and increased risk of serotonin syndrome.[199]

Other medications have a very limited role in hospital sleep promotion. First-generation antihistamines such as diphenhydramine and hydroxyzine have limited effectiveness as sleep aids,[200] and potential side effects such as daytime somnolence, delirium, orthostatic hypotension, QT prolongation, and urinary retention render their use in the vulnerable hospitalized population risky and harmful.

Similarly, atypical antipsychotics including quetiapine and olanzapine are being used frequently in the hospital setting for the treatment of insomnia and delirium. Studies in patients with mood and psychotic disorders demonstrated improved sleep among subjects treated with quetiapine; however, there is no evidence supporting its efficacy for the treatment of insomnia in the general population.[201]

Nonbenzodiazepine benzodiazepine receptor agonists such as zolpidem, eszopiclone, and zaleplon are effective sleep aids in the outpatient setting and are commonly prescribed for hospitalized patients.[188] This class of medications is better tolerated than benzodiazepines, but reports of these agents being associated with increased risk of fall, delirium, parasomnias, and cognitive dysfunction have made their use less desirable during acute illness.[202–205]

Benzodiazepines are effective in improving sleep duration but also lead to undesirable reduction of N3 and REM sleep.[110] Their adverse effects, particularly in the hospitalized patient, include daytime somnolence, delirium, cognitive dysfunction, respiratory depression, and increased risk of fall.[110] In hospitalized adults on the internal medicine ward, the use of benzodiazepines was associated with an increased risk of respiratory deterioration, delirium, and falls.[206]

In sum, the decision to pursue pharmacologic therapy for sleep in hospitalized patients should be made with extreme caution. In general, agents with favorable pharmacokinetics (rapid onset of action, short half-life) and minimal drug-drug interactions should be considered at the lowest effective dose and for a limited duration. Scheduled medications should be avoided to reduce risks for tolerance and dependence and other nonpharmacologic sleep interventions should be pursued along with prescribed medication. Newly prescribed sleep aids should be reconciled and preferably discontinued upon hospital discharge.

SUMMARY

Sleep deficiency is pervasive in the hospital setting and has broad implications for patient outcomes. Patient, environmental, illness, and treatment-related factors contribute to the risk and severity of sleep deficiency, but also provide therapeutic targets for sleep promotion. Though evidence is currently limited, there have been modest improvements in hospital sleep and patient outcomes due to environmental control and changes in care patterns. Key next steps in hospital sleep promotion include improvement in sleep measurement techniques and harmonization of study protocols and outcomes to strengthen existing evidence and facilitate data interpretation across studies.

CLINICS CARE POINTS

1. Care providers should be aware that hospitalized patients have poor sleep and avoid scheduling nonurgent care including medications, laboratories, radiologic studies, skincare, and so forth, during the sleep period.
2. Nonpharmacologic sleep promotion bundles that encourage clustering care and avoiding environmental disturbance are recommended by expert guidelines.
3. Eye masks and earplugs should be offered to patients, but not applied by clinical staff unless requested by the patient.

4. Increasing daytime light by turning on room lights and opening window shades during the day is a low-risk way to promote a normal sleep-wake cycle.
5. Extreme caution should be used in prescribing sleep aids to inpatients and care should be taken to assure medications are stopped upon hospital discharge.

DISCLOSURE

Dr. Knauert was supported by the NHLBI (K23 HL138229), and the Fund to Retain Clinical Scientists at Yale sponsored by the Doris Duke Charitable Foundation award #2015216 and the Yale Center for Clinical Investigation.

REFERENCES

1. Carskadon MA, Dement WC. Chapter 2 - normal human sleep: an overview. In: Kryger M, Roth T, Dement WC, editors. Principles and practice of sleep medicine15, 6th edition. Philadelphia: Elsevier; 2017. p. 24.e13.
2. Watson NF, Badr MS, Belenky G, et al. Joint consensus statement of the american academy of sleep medicine and sleep research society on the recommended amount of sleep for a healthy adult: methodology and discussion. Sleep 2015;38(8): 1161–83.
3. Hurtado-Alvarado G, Pavón L, Castillo-García SA, et al. Sleep loss as a factor to induce cellular and molecular inflammatory variations. Clin Dev Immunol 2013;2013:801341.
4. Grandner MA, Sands-Lincoln MR, Pak VM, et al. Sleep duration, cardiovascular disease, and proinflammatory biomarkers. Nat Sci Sleep 2013;5: 93–107.
5. Figueroa-Ramos MI, Arroyo-Novoa CM, Lee KA, et al. Sleep and delirium in ICU patients: a review of mechanisms and manifestations. Intensive Care Med 2009;35(5):781–95.
6. Samsonsen C, Sand T, Bråthen G, et al. The impact of sleep loss on the facilitation of seizures: a prospective case-crossover study. Epilepsy Res 2016;127:260–6.
7. Babson KA, Trainor CD, Feldner MT, et al. A test of the effects of acute sleep deprivation on general and specific self-reported anxiety and depressive symptoms: an experimental extension. J Behav Ther Exp Psychiatry 2010;41(3):297–303.
8. Itani O, Jike M, Watanabe N, et al. Short sleep duration and health outcomes: a systematic review, meta-analysis, and meta-regression. Sleep Med 2017;32:246–56.
9. Medic G, Wille M, Hemels ME. Short- and long-term health consequences of sleep disruption. Nat Sci Sleep 2017;9:151–61.
10. Stewart NH, Arora VM. Sleep in hospitalized older adults. Sleep Med Clin 2018;13(1):127–35.
11. Wesselius HM, van den Ende ES, Alsma J, et al. Quality and quantity of sleep and factors associated with sleep disturbance in hospitalized patients. JAMA Intern Med 2018;178(9):1201–8.
12. Morse AM, Bender E. Sleep in hospitalized patients. Clocks Sleep 2019;1(1):151–65.
13. Krumholz HM. Post-hospital syndrome–an acquired, transient condition of generalized risk. N Engl J Med 2013;368(2):100–2.
14. Knauert MP, Gilmore EJ, Murphy TE, et al. Association between death and loss of stage N2 sleep features among critically Ill patients with delirium. J Crit Care 2018;48:124–9.
15. Manian FA, Manian CJ. Sleep quality in adult hospitalized patients with infection: an observational study. Am J Med Sci 2015;349(1):56–60.
16. Telias I, Wilcox ME. Sleep and circadian rhythm in critical illness. Crit Care 2019;23(1):82.
17. Rampes S, Ma K, Divecha YA, et al. Postoperative sleep disorders and their potential impacts on surgical outcomes. J Biomed Res 2019;34(4): 271–80.
18. Tembo AC, Parker V, Higgins I. The experience of sleep deprivation in intensive care patients: findings from a larger hermeneutic phenomenological study. Intensive Crit Care Nurs 2013;29(6):310–6.
19. Freedman NS, Gazendam J, Levan L, et al. Abnormal sleep/wake cycles and the effect of environmental noise on sleep disruption in the intensive care unit. Am J Respir Crit Care Med 2001;163(2): 451–7.
20. Wilcox ME, Lim AS, Pinto R, et al. Sleep on the ward in intensive care unit survivors: a case series of polysomnography. Intern Med J 2018;48(7): 795–802.
21. Altman MT, Knauert MP, Pisani MA. Sleep disturbance after hospitalization and critical illness: a systematic review. Ann Am Thorac Soc 2017; 14(9):1457–68.
22. Meissner HH, Riemer A, Santiago SM, et al. Failure of physician documentation of sleep complaints in hospitalized patients. West J Med 1998;169(3): 146–9.
23. Elliott R, Rai T, McKinley S. Factors affecting sleep in the critically ill: an observational study. J Crit Care 2014;29(5):859–63.
24. Freedman NS, Kotzer N, Schwab RJ. Patient perception of sleep quality and etiology of sleep disruption in the intensive care unit. Am J Respir Crit Care Med 1999;159(4 Pt 1):1155–62.
25. Elliott R, McKinley S, Cistulli P, et al. Characterisation of sleep in intensive care using 24-hour

polysomnography: an observational study. Crit Care 2013;17(2):R46.
26. Friese RS, Diaz-Arrastia R, McBride D, et al. Quantity and quality of sleep in the surgical intensive care unit: are our patients sleeping? J Trauma 2007;63(6):1210–4.
27. Adachi M, Staisiunas PG, Knutson KL, et al. Perceived control and sleep in hospitalized older adults: a sound hypothesis? J Hosp Med 2013; 8(4):184–90.
28. Gazendam JAC, Van Dongen HPA, Grant DA, et al. Altered circadian rhythmicity in patients in the ICU. Chest 2013;144(2):483–9.
29. Gehlbach BK, Chapotot F, Leproult R, et al. Temporal disorganization of circadian rhythmicity and sleep-wake regulation in mechanically ventilated patients receiving continuous intravenous sedation. Sleep 2012;35(8):1105–14.
30. Maas MB, Lizza BD, Abbott SM, et al. Factors disrupting melatonin secretion rhythms during critical illness. Crit Care Med 2020;48(6):854–61.
31. Riutta A, Ylitalo P, Kaukinen S. Diurnal variation of melatonin and cortisol is maintained in non-septic intensive care patients. Intensive Care Med 2009; 35(10):1720–7.
32. Li CX, Liang DD, Xie GH, et al. Altered melatonin secretion and circadian gene expression with increased proinflammatory cytokine expression in early-stage sepsis patients. Mol Med Rep 2013; 7(4):1117–22.
33. Mundigler G, Delle-Karth G, Koreny M, et al. Impaired circadian rhythm of melatonin secretion in sedated critically ill patients with severe sepsis. Crit Care Med 2002;30(3):536–40.
34. Schwela D. The new World Health Organization guidelines for community noise. Noise Control Eng J 2001;49:193.
35. Busch-Vishniac IJ, West JE, Barnhill C, et al. Noise levels in johns hopkins hospital. J Acoust Soc Am 2005;118(6):3629–45.
36. de Lima Andrade E, da Cunha E Silva DC, de Lima EA, et al. Environmental noise in hospitals: a systematic review. Environ Sci Pollut Res Int 2021;28(16):19629–42.
37. Darbyshire JL, Young JD. An investigation of sound levels on intensive care units with reference to the WHO guidelines. Crit Care 2013;R187.
38. Knauert M, Jeon S, Murphy TE, et al. Comparing average levels and peak occurrence of overnight sound in the medical intensive care unit on A-weighted and C-weighted decibel scales. J Crit Care 2016;36:1–7.
39. Darbyshire JL, Müller-Trapet M, Cheer J, et al. Mapping sources of noise in an intensive care unit. Anaesthesia 2019;74(8):1018–25.
40. Simons KS, Verweij E, Lemmens PMC, et al. Noise in the intensive care unit and its influence on sleep quality: a multicenter observational study in Dutch intensive care units. Crit Care 2018;22(1):250.
41. Gabor JY, Cooper AB, Crombach SA, et al. Contribution of the intensive care unit environment to sleep disruption in mechanically ventilated patients and healthy subjects. Am J Respir Crit Care Med 2003;167(5):708–15.
42. Topf M, Davis JE. Critical care unit noise and rapid eye movement (REM) sleep. Heart Lung 1993; 22(3):252–8.
43. Topf M, Bookman M, Arand D. Effects of critical care unit noise on the subjective quality of sleep. J Adv Nurs 1996;24(3):545–51.
44. Buxton OM, Ellenbogen JM, Wang W, et al. Sleep disruption due to hospital noises: a prospective evaluation. Ann Intern Med 2012;157(3):170–9.
45. Czeisler CA, Buxton OM. Chapter 35 - the human circadian timing system and sleep–wake regulation. In: Kryger MH, Roth T, Dement WC, editors. Principles and practice of sleep medicine. 5th edition. Philadelphia: W.B. Saunders; 2011. p. 402–19.
46. Vetter C, Pattison PM, Houser K, et al. A review of human physiological responses to light: implications for the development of integrative lighting solutions. LEUKOS 2021;1–28.
47. Fan EP, Abbott SM, Reid KJ, et al. Abnormal environmental light exposure in the intensive care environment. J Crit Care 2017;40:11–4.
48. Tan X, van Egmond L, Partinen M, et al. A narrative review of interventions for improving sleep and reducing circadian disruption in medical inpatients. Sleep Med 2019;59:42–50.
49. Bernhofer EI, Higgins PA, Daly BJ, et al. Hospital lighting and its association with sleep, mood and pain in medical inpatients. J Adv Nurs 2014; 70(5):1164–73.
50. Jaiswal SJ, Garcia S, Owens RL. Sound and light levels are similarly disruptive in ICU and non-ICU wards. J Hosp Med 2017;12(10):798–804.
51. Missildine K, Bergstrom N, Meininger J, et al. Sleep in hospitalized elders: a pilot study. Geriatr Nurs 2010;31(4):263–71.
52. Kobayashi R, Fukuda N, Kohsaka M, et al. Effects of bright light at lunchtime on sleep of patients in a geriatric hospital I. Psychiatry Clin Neurosci 2001;55(3):287–9.
53. Fukuda N, Kobayashi R, Kohsaka M, et al. Effects of bright light at lunchtime on sleep in patients in a geriatric hospital II. Psychiatry Clin Neurosci 2001;55(3):291–3.
54. Giménez MC, Geerdinck LM, Versteylen M, et al. Patient room lighting influences on sleep, appraisal and mood in hospitalized people. J Sleep Res 2017;26(2):236–46.
55. Ono H, Taguchi T, Kido Y, et al. The usefulness of bright light therapy for patients after oesophagectomy. Intensive Crit Care Nurs 2011;27(3):158–66.

56. De Rui M, Middleton B, Sticca A, et al. Sleep and circadian rhythms in hospitalized patients with decompensated cirrhosis: effect of light therapy. Neurochem Res 2015;40(2):284–92.
57. Formentin C, Carraro S, Turco M, et al. Effect of morning light glasses and night short-wavelength filter glasses on sleep-wake rhythmicity in medical inpatients. Front Physiol 2020;11.
58. Gehlbach BK, Patel SB, Van Cauter E, et al. The effects of timed light exposure in critically ill patients: a randomized controlled pilot clinical trial. Am J Respir Crit Care Med 2018;198(2):275–8.
59. Smonig R, Magalhaes E, Bouadma L, et al. Impact of natural light exposure on delirium burden in adult patients receiving invasive mechanical ventilation in the ICU: a prospective study. Ann Intensive Care 2019;9(1):120.
60. Beauchemin KM, Hays P. Dying in the dark: sunshine, gender and outcomes in myocardial infarction. J R Soc Med 1998;91(7):352–4.
61. Verceles AC, Liu X, Terrin ML, et al. Ambient light levels and critical care outcomes. J Crit Care 2013;28(1):110.e1-8.
62. Zhang KS, Pelleg T, Hussain S, et al. Prospective randomized controlled pilot study of high-intensity lightbox phototherapy to prevent ICU-acquired delirium incidence. Cureus 2021;13(4):e14246.
63. Stroud M, Duncan H, Nightingale J. Guidelines for enteral feeding in adult hospital patients. Gut 2003; 52(Suppl 7):vii1–12.
64. Sunderram J, Sofou S, Kamisoglu K, et al. Time-restricted feeding and the realignment of biological rhythms: translational opportunities and challenges. J Transl Med 2014;12:79.
65. Tamburri LM, DiBrienza R, Zozula R, et al. Nocturnal care interactions with patients in critical care units. Am J Crit Care 2004;13(2):102–12.
66. Le A, Friese RS, Hsu CH, et al. Sleep disruptions and nocturnal nursing interactions in the intensive care unit. J Surg Res 2012;177(2):310–4.
67. Barr J, Fraser GL, Puntillo K, et al. Clinical practice guidelines for the management of pain, agitation, and delirium in adult patients in the intensive care unit. Crit Care Med 2013;41(1):263–306.
68. Knauert MP, Pisani M, Redeker N, et al. Pilot study: an intensive care unit sleep promotion protocol. BMJ Open Respir Res 2019;6(1):e000411. Accessed 2019.
69. McKinley S, Fien M, Elliott R, et al. Sleep and psychological health during early recovery from critical illness: an observational study. J Psychosom Res 2013;75(6):539–45.
70. Peppard PE, Young T, Barnet JH, et al. Increased prevalence of sleep-disordered breathing in adults. Am J Epidemiol 2013;177(9):1006–14.
71. Sanner BM, Konermann M, Doberauer C, et al. Sleep-Disordered breathing in patients referred for angina evaluation–association with left ventricular dysfunction. Clin Cardiol 2001;24(2):146–50.
72. Schober AK, Neurath MF, Harsch IA. Prevalence of sleep apnoea in diabetic patients. Clin Respir J 2011;5(3):165–72.
73. Motamedi KK, McClary AC, Amedee RG. Obstructive sleep apnea: a growing problem. Ochsner J 2009;9(3):149–53.
74. Spurr K, Morrison DL, Graven MA, et al. Analysis of hospital discharge data to characterize obstructive sleep apnea and its management in adult patients hospitalized in Canada: 2006 to 2007. Can Respir J 2010;17(5):213–8.
75. Leiter JC, Knuth SL, Bartlett D. The effect of sleep deprivation on activity of the genioglossus muscle. Am Rev Respir Dis 1985;132(6):1242–5.
76. Gupta RM, Parvizi J, Hanssen AD, et al. Postoperative complications in patients with obstructive sleep apnea syndrome undergoing hip or knee replacement: a case-control study. Mayo Clin Proc 2001;76(9):897–905.
77. Lindenauer PK, Stefan MS, Johnson KG, et al. Prevalence, treatment, and outcomes associated with OSA among patients hospitalized with pneumonia. Chest 2014;145(5):1032–8.
78. Trenkwalder C, Allen R, Högl B, et al. Comorbidities, treatment, and pathophysiology in restless legs syndrome. Lancet Neurol 2018;17(11): 994–1005.
79. Goldstein C. Management of restless legs syndrome/Willis-Ekbom disease in hospitalized and perioperative patients. Sleep Med Clin 2015; 10(3):303–10.
80. Stewart NH, Walters RW, Mokhlesi B, et al. Sleep in hospitalized patients with chronic obstructive pulmonary disease: an observational study. J Clin Sleep Med 2020;16(10):1693–9.
81. Jorge-Samitier P, Durante A, Gea-Caballero V, et al. Sleep quality in patients with heart failure in the Spanish population: a cross-sectional study. Int J Environ Res Public Health 2020;17(21):7772.
82. Campos TF, Barroso MTM, Silveira ABG, et al. Sleep disturbances complaints in stroke: implications for sleep medicine. Sleep Sci 2021;6(3): 98–102.
83. Maung SC, El Sara A, Chapman C, et al. Sleep disorders and chronic kidney disease. World J Nephrol 2016;5(3):224–32.
84. Fujiwara Y, Arakawa T, Fass R. Gastroesophageal reflux disease and sleep disturbances. J Gastroenterol 2012;47(7):760–9.
85. Budhiraja R, Siddiqi TA, Quan SF. Sleep disorders in chronic obstructive pulmonary disease: etiology, impact, and management. J Clin Sleep Med 2015; 11(3):259–70.
86. Khot SP, Morgenstern LB. Sleep and stroke. Stroke; a J Cereb Circ 2019;50(6):1612–161794.

87. Johnson KG, Johnson DC. Frequency of sleep apnea in stroke and TIA patients: a meta-analysis. J Clin Sleep Med 2010;6(2):131–7.
88. Aaronson JA, Hofman WF, van Bennekom CA, et al. Effects of continuous positive airway pressure on cognitive and functional outcome of stroke patients with obstructive sleep apnea: a randomized controlled trial. J Clin Sleep Med 2016;12(4): 533–41.
89. Khot SP, Davis AP, Crane DA, et al. Effect of continuous positive airway pressure on stroke rehabilitation: a pilot randomized sham-controlled trial. J Clin Sleep Med 2016;12(7):1019–26.
90. Parra O, Arboix A, Bechich S, et al. Time course of sleep-related breathing disorders in first-ever stroke or transient ischemic attack. Am J Respir Crit Care Med 2000;161(2 Pt 1):375–80.
91. Magdy DM, Metwally A, Makhlouf HA. Study of sleep quality among patients admitted to the respiratory intensive care unit. Egypt J Bronchology 2019;13(1):114–9.
92. Maramattom BV. Sepsis associated encephalopathy. Neurol Res 2007;29(7):643–6.
93. Weinhouse GL, Schwab RJ. Sleep in the critically ill patient. Sleep 2006;29(5):707–16.
94. Parthasarathy S, Tobin MJ. Sleep in the intensive care unit. Intensive Care Med 2004;30(2): 197–20698.
95. Barczi SR, Juergens TM. Comorbidities: psychiatric, medical, medications, and substances. Sleep Med Clin 2006;1(2):231–45.
96. Finan PH, Goodin BR, Smith MT. The association of sleep and pain: an update and a path forward. J Pain 2013;14(12):1539–52.
97. Lautenbacher S, Kundermann B, Krieg JC. Sleep deprivation and pain perception. Sleep Med Rev 2006;10(5).
98. Raymond I, Ancoli-Israel S, Choinière M. Sleep disturbances, pain and analgesia in adults hospitalized for burn injuries. Sleep Med 2004;5(6):551–9.
99. Closs SJ. Patients' night-time pain, analgesic provision and sleep after surgery. Int J Nurs Stud 1992; 29(4):381–92.
100. Dolan R, Huh J, Tiwari N, et al. A prospective analysis of sleep deprivation and disturbance in surgical patients. Ann Med Surg (Lond) 2016;6:1–5.
101. Rosenberg-Adamsen S, Skarbye M, Wildschiødtz G, et al. Sleep after laparoscopic cholecystectomy. Br J Anaesth 1996;77(5):572–5.
102. Dette F, Cassel W, Urban F, et al. Occurrence of rapid eye movement sleep deprivation after surgery under regional anesthesia. Anesth Analg 2013;116(4):939–43.
103. Vasu TS, Grewal R, Doghramji K. Obstructive sleep apnea syndrome and perioperative complications: a systematic review of the literature. J Clin Sleep Med 2012;8(2):199–207.
104. Parthasarathy S, Tobin MJ. Effect of ventilator mode on sleep quality in critically ill patients. Am J Respir Crit Care Med 2002;166(11):1423–9.
105. Toublanc B, Rose D, Glérant JC, et al. Assist-control ventilation vs. low levels of pressure support ventilation on sleep quality in intubated ICU patients. Intensive Care Med 2007;33(7):1148–54.
106. Cabello B, Thille AW, Drouot X, et al. Sleep quality in mechanically ventilated patients: comparison of three ventilatory modes. Crit Care Med 2008; 36(6):1749–55.
107. Witcraft EJ, Gonzales JP, Seung H, et al. Continuation of opioid therapy at transitions of care in critically ill patients. J Intensive Care Med 2020;36(8): 879–84, 885066620933798.
108. Schweitzer PK, Randazzo AC. Chapter 45 - drugs that disturb sleep and wakefulness. In: Kryger M, Roth T, Dement WC, editors. Principles and practice of sleep medicine. 6th edition. Elsevier; 2017. p. 480–98.e488.
109. Bourne RS, Mills GH. Sleep disruption in critically ill patients–pharmacological considerations. Anaesthesia 2004;59(4):374–84.
110. Holbrook AM, Crowther R, Lotter A, et al. Meta-analysis of benzodiazepine use in the treatment of insomnia. CMAJ 2000;162(2):225–33.
111. Wang D, Teichtahl H. Opioids, sleep architecture and sleep-disordered breathing. Sleep Med Rev 2007;11(1):35–46.
112. Kondili E, Alexopoulou C, Xirouchaki N, et al. Effects of propofol on sleep quality in mechanically ventilated critically ill patients: a physiological study. Intensive Care Med 2012;38(10):1640–6.
113. Oto J, Yamamoto K, Koike S, et al. Sleep quality of mechanically ventilated patients sedated with dexmedetomidine. Intensive Care Med 2012;38(12): 1982–9.
114. Jean R, Shah P, Yudelevich E, et al. Effects of deep sedation on sleep in critically ill medical patients on mechanical ventilation. J Sleep Res 2020;29(3): e12894.
115. Qazi T, Farraye FA. Sleep and inflammatory bowel disease: an important bi-directional relationship. Inflamm Bowel Dis 2019;25(5):843–52.
116. Spiegel K, Sheridan JF, Van Cauter E. Effect of sleep deprivation on response to immunization. JAMA 2002;288(12):1471–2.
117. Patel SR, Malhotra A, Gao X, et al. A prospective study of sleep duration and pneumonia risk in women. Sleep 2012;35(1):97–101.
118. Kerkhofs M, Boudjeltia KZ, Stenuit P, et al. Sleep restriction increases blood neutrophils, total cholesterol and low density lipoprotein cholesterol in postmenopausal women: a preliminary study. Maturitas 2007;56(2):212–5.
119. Ruiz FS, Andersen ML, Martins RC, et al. Immune alterations after selective rapid eye movement or

total sleep deprivation in healthy male volunteers. Innate Immu 2012;18(1):44–54.
120. Christoffersson G, Vågesjö E, Pettersson US, et al. Acute sleep deprivation in healthy young men: impact on population diversity and function of circulating neutrophils. Brain Behav Immun 2014; 41:162–72.
121. Shearer WT, Reuben JM, Mullington JM, et al. Soluble TNF-alpha receptor 1 and IL-6 plasma levels in humans subjected to the sleep deprivation model of spaceflight. J Allergy Clin Immunol 2001;107(1):165–70.
122. Irwin MR, Wang M, Campomayor CO, et al. Sleep deprivation and activation of morning levels of cellular and genomic markers of inflammation. Arch Intern Med 2006;166(16):1756–62.
123. Pilcher JJ, Huffcutt AI. Effects of sleep deprivation on performance: a meta-analysis. Sleep 1996; 19(4):318–26.
124. Durmer JS, Dinges DF. Neurocognitive consequences of sleep deprivation. Semin Neurol 2005;25(1).
125. Thomason JW, Shintani A, Peterson JF, et al. Intensive care unit delirium is an independent predictor of longer hospital stay: a prospective analysis of 261 non-ventilated patients. Crit Care 2005;9(4): R375–81.
126. Pisani MA, Kong SY, Kasl SV, et al. Days of delirium are associated with 1-year mortality in an older intensive care unit population. Am J Respir Crit Care Med 2009;180(11):1092–7.
127. Sveinsson IS. Postoperative psychosis after heart surgery. J Thorac Cardiovasc Surg 1975;70(4): 717–26.
128. Helton MC, Gordon SH, Nunnery SL. The correlation between sleep deprivation and the intensive care unit syndrome. Heart Lung 1980;9(3):464–8.
129. Flannery AH, Oyler DR, Weinhouse GL. The impact of interventions to improve sleep on delirium in the ICU: a systematic review and research framework. Crit Care Med 2016;44(12):2231–40.
130. Foster J, Burry LD, Thabane L, et al. Melatonin and melatonin agonists to prevent and treat delirium in critical illness: a systematic review protocol. Syst Rev 2016;5(1):199.
131. Asleson DR, Chiu AW. Melatonin for delirium prevention in acute medically ill, and perioperative geriatric patients. Aging Med (Milton) 2020;3(2):132–7.
132. Rault C, Sangaré A, Diaz V, et al. Impact of sleep deprivation on respiratory motor output and endurance. A physiological study. Am J Respir Crit Care Med 2020;201(8):976–83.
133. Chen HI, Tang YR. Sleep loss impairs inspiratory muscle endurance. Am Rev Respir Dis 1989; 140(4):907–9.
134. White DP, Douglas NJ, Pickett CK, et al. Sleep deprivation and the control of ventilation. Am Rev Respir Dis 1983;128(6):984–6.
135. Phillips BA, Cooper KR, Burke TV. The effect of sleep loss on breathing in chronic obstructive pulmonary disease. Chest 1987;91(1):29–32.
136. Roche Campo F, Drouot X, Thille AW, et al. Poor sleep quality is associated with late noninvasive ventilation failure in patients with acute hypercapnic respiratory failure. Crit Care Med 2010;38(2): 477–85.
137. Ogawa Y, Kanbayashi T, Saito Y, et al. Total sleep deprivation elevates blood pressure through arterial baroreflex resetting: a study with microneurographic technique. Sleep 2003;26(8):986–9.
138. Lusardi P, Zoppi A, Preti P, et al. Effects of insufficient sleep on blood pressure in hypertensive patients: a 24-h study. Am J Hypertens 1999;12(1 Pt 1):63–8.
139. Tochikubo O, Ikeda A, Miyajima E, et al. Effects of insufficient sleep on blood pressure monitored by a new multibiomedical recorder. Hypertens 1996; 27(6).
140. Miner SE, Pahal D, Nichols L, et al. Sleep disruption is associated with increased ventricular ectopy and cardiac arrest in hospitalized adults. Sleep 2016; 39(4):927–35.
141. Rosenberg J, Wildschiødtz G, Pedersen MH, et al. Late postoperative nocturnal episodic hypoxaemia and associated sleep pattern. Br J Anaesth 1994; 72(2):145–50.
142. Gabor JY, Cooper AB, Hanly PJ. Sleep disruption in the intensive care unit. Curr Opin Crit Care 2001; 7(1):21–7.
143. Schüssler P, Uhr M, Ising M, et al. Nocturnal ghrelin, ACTH, GH and cortisol secretion after sleep deprivation in humans. Psychoneuroendocrinology 2006;31(8):915–23.
144. Brandenberger G, Gronfier C, Chapotot F, et al. Effect of sleep deprivation on overall 24 h growth-hormone secretion. Lancet 2000;356(9239):1408.
145. Sharma S, Kavuru M. Sleep and metabolism: an overview. Int J Endocrinol 2010;2010:270832.
146. DePietro RH, Knutson KL, Spampinato L, et al. Association between inpatient sleep loss and hyperglycemia of hospitalization. Diabetes Care 2017; 40(2):188–93.
147. Chang VA, Owens RL, LaBuzetta JN. Impact of sleep deprivation in the neurological intensive care unit: a narrative review. Neurocrit Care 2020; 32(2):596–608.
148. Watson PL. Measuring sleep in critically ill patients: beware the pitfalls. Crit Care 2007;11(4):159.
149. Bourne RS, Minelli C, Mills GH, et al. Clinical review: sleep measurement in critical care patients: research and clinical implications. Crit Care 2007; 11(4):226.
150. Watson PL, Pandharipande P, Gehlbach BK, et al. Atypical sleep in ventilated patients: empirical electroencephalography findings and the path

toward revised ICU sleep scoring criteria. Crit Care Med 2013;41(8):1958–67.
151. Drouot X, Roche-Campo F, Thille AW, et al. A new classification for sleep analysis in critically ill patients. Sleep Med 2012;13(1):7–14.
152. Farshidpanah S, Pisani MA, Ely EW, et al. Chapter 135 - sleep in the critically ill patient. In: Kryger M, Roth T, Dement WC, editors. Principles and practice of sleep medicine. 6th edition. Elsevier; 2017. p. 1329–40.e1325.
153. Marino M, Li Y, Rueschman MN, et al. Measuring sleep: accuracy, sensitivity, and specificity of wrist actigraphy compared to polysomnography. Sleep 2013;36(11):1747–55.
154. Van de Water AT, Holmes A, Hurley DA. Objective measurements of sleep for non-laboratory settings as alternatives to polysomnography–a systematic review. J Sleep Res 2011;20(1 Pt 2):183–200.
155. Schwab KE, Ronish B, Needham DM, et al. Actigraphy to evaluate sleep in the intensive care unit. A systematic review. Ann Am Thorac Soc 2018; 15(9):1075–82.
156. Bourne RS, Mills GH, Minelli C. Melatonin therapy to improve nocturnal sleep in critically ill patients: encouraging results from a small randomised controlled trial. Crit Care 2008;12(2):R52.
157. Chen JH, Chao YH, Lu SF, et al. The effectiveness of valerian acupressure on the sleep of ICU patients: a randomized clinical trial. Int J Nurs Stud 2012;49(8):913–20.
158. Richards KC, O'Sullivan PS, Phillips RL. Measurement of sleep in critically ill patients. J Nurs Meas 2000;8(2):131–44.
159. Shahid A, Wilkinson K, Marcu S, et al. Richards-campbell sleep questionnaire (RCSQ). In: Shahid A, Wilkinson K, Marcu S, et al, editors. STOP, THAT and one hundred other sleep scales. New York, NY: Springer New York; 2012. p. 299–302.
160. Frisk U, Nordstrom G. Patients' sleep in an intensive care unit–patients' and nurses' perception. Intensive Crit Care Nurs 2003;19(6):342–9.
161. Grossman MN, Anderson SL, Worku A, et al. Awakenings? Patient and hospital staff perceptions of nighttime disruptions and their effect on patient sleep. J Clin Sleep Med 2017;13(2):301–6.
162. Kamdar BB, Knauert MP, Jones SF, et al. Perceptions and practices regarding sleep in the intensive care unit. A survey of 1,223 critical care providers. Ann Am Thorac Soc 2016;13(8):1370–7.
163. DuBose JR, Hadi K. Improving inpatient environments to support patient sleep. Int J Qual Health Care 2016;28(5):540–53.
164. Hu RF, Jiang XY, Chen J, et al. Non-pharmacological interventions for sleep promotion in the intensive care unit. Cochrane Database Syst Rev 2015;2015(10):CD008808.
165. Xie H, Kang J, Mills GH. Clinical review: the impact of noise on patients' sleep and the effectiveness of noise reduction strategies in intensive care units. Crit Care 2009;13(2):208.
166. Scotto CJ, McClusky C, Spillan S, et al. Earplugs improve patients' subjective experience of sleep in critical care. Nurs Crit Care 2009;14(4):180–4.
167. Van Rompaey B, Elseviers MM, Van Drom W, et al. The effect of earplugs during the night on the onset of delirium and sleep perception: a randomized controlled trial in intensive care patients. Crit Care 2012;16(3):R73.
168. Almberg AK, Mitchell N, Tonna JE. Observations of acoustic interruptions versus ambient sound levels with perceived sleep quality during critical illness. Crit Care Explor 2021;3(2):e0342.
169. Williamson JW. The effects of ocean sounds on sleep after coronary artery bypass graft surgery. Am J Crit Care 1992;1(1):91–7.
170. Hagerman I, Rasmanis G, Blomkvist V, et al. Influence of intensive coronary care acoustics on the quality of care and physiological state of patients. Int J Cardiol 2005;98(2):267–70.
171. Daneshmandi M, Neiseh F, SadeghiShermeh M, et al. Effect of eye mask on sleep quality in patients with acute coronary syndrome. J Caring Sci 2012; 1(3):135–43.
172. Mahran GS, Leach MJ, Abbas MS, et al. Effect of eye masks on pain and sleep quality in patients undergoing cardiac surgery: a randomized controlled trial. Crit Care Nurse 2020;40(1):27–35.
173. Jones C, Dawson D. Eye masks and earplugs improve patient's perception of sleep. Nurs Crit Care 2012;17(5):247–54.
174. Sweity S, Finlay A, Lees C, et al. SleepSure: a pilot randomized-controlled trial to assess the effects of eye masks and earplugs on the quality of sleep for patients in hospital. Clin Rehabil 2019;33(2): 253–61.
175. Fang CS, Wang HH, Wang RH, et al. Effect of earplugs and eye masks on the sleep quality of intensive care unit patients: a systematic review and meta-analysis. J Adv Nurs 2021.
176. Olson DM, Borel CO, Laskowitz DT, et al. Quiet time: a nursing intervention to promote sleep in neurocritical care units. Am J Crit Care 2001; 10(2):74–8.
177. Gardner G, Collins C, Osborne S, et al. Creating a therapeutic environment: a non-randomised controlled trial of a quiet time intervention for patients in acute care. Int J Nurs Stud 2009;46(6): 778–86.
178. Zimmerman L, Nieveen J, Barnason S, et al. The effects of music interventions on postoperative pain and sleep in coronary artery bypass graft (CABG) patients. Sch Inq Nurs Pract 1996;10(2):153–70 [discussion: 171-154].

179. Richards KC. Effect of a back massage and relaxation intervention on sleep in critically ill patients. Am J Crit Care 1998;7(4):288–99.
180. Karadag E, Samancioglu S, Ozden D, et al. Effects of aromatherapy on sleep quality and anxiety of patients. Nurs Crit Care 2017;22(2):105–12.
181. Knauert MP, Kamdar BB, Sleep in the ICUTF. Reply: sleep in the intensive care unit is a priority. Ann Am Thorac Soc 2016;13(10):1868–9.
182. Kamdar BB, King LM, Collop NA, et al. The effect of a quality improvement intervention on perceived sleep quality and cognition in a medical ICU. Crit Care Med 2013;41(3):800–9.
183. Tonna JE, Dalton A, Presson AP, et al. The effect of a quality improvement intervention on sleep and delirium in critically ill patients in a surgical ICU. Chest 2021;160(3):899–908.
184. Gathecha E, Rios R, Buenaver LF, et al. Pilot study aiming to support sleep quality and duration during hospitalizations. J Hosp Med 2016;11(7):467–72.
185. Herscher M, Mikhaylov D, Barazani S, et al. A sleep hygiene intervention to improve sleep quality for hospitalized patients. Jt Comm J Qual Patient Saf 2021;47(6):343–6.
186. Gillis CM, Poyant JO, Degrado JR, et al. Inpatient pharmacological sleep aid utilization is common at a tertiary medical center. J Hosp Med 2014; 9(10):652–7.
187. Frighetto L, Marra C, Bandali S, et al. An assessment of quality of sleep and the use of drugs with sedating properties in hospitalized adult patients. Health Qual Life Outcomes 2004;2:17.
188. Pek EA, Remfry A, Pendrith C, et al. High Prevalence of inappropriate benzodiazepine and sedative hypnotic prescriptions among hospitalized older adults. J Hosp Med 2017;12(5):310–6.
189. Reiter RJ, Tan DX, Fuentes-Broto L. Melatonin: a multitasking molecule. Prog Brain Res 2010;181: 127–51.
190. Claustrat B, Leston J. Melatonin: physiological effects in humans. Neurochirurgie 2015;61(2–3): 77–84.
191. Ibrahim MG, Bellomo R, Hart GK, et al. A double-blind placebo-controlled randomised pilot study of nocturnal melatonin in tracheostomised patients. Crit Care Resusc 2006;8(3):187–91.
192. Mistraletti G, Umbrello M, Sabbatini G, et al. Melatonin reduces the need for sedation in ICU patients: a randomized controlled trial. Minerva Anestesiol 2015;81(12):1298–310.
193. Lewis SR, Pritchard MW, Schofield-Robinson OJ, et al. Melatonin for the promotion of sleep in adults in the intensive care unit. Cochrane database Syst Rev 2018;5(5):CD012455.
194. Gandolfi JV, Di Bernardo APA, Chanes DAV, et al. The Effects of melatonin supplementation on sleep quality and assessment of the serum melatonin in ICU patients: a randomized controlled trial. Crit Care Med 2020;48(12):e1286–93.
195. Bellapart J, Appadurai V, Lassig-Smith M, et al. Effect of exogenous melatonin administration in critically ill patients on delirium and sleep: a randomized controlled trial. Crit Care Res Pract 2020;2020:3951828.
196. Jaiswal SJ, McCarthy TJ, Wineinger NE, et al. Melatonin and sleep in preventing hospitalized delirium: a randomized clinical trial. Am J Med 2018;131(9):1110–1117 e1114.
197. Yi XY, Ni SF, Ghadami MR, et al. Trazodone for the treatment of insomnia: a meta-analysis of randomized placebo-controlled trials. Sleep Med 2018; 45:25–32.
198. Doroudgar S, Chou TI, Yu J, et al. Evaluation of trazodone and quetiapine for insomnia: an observational study in psychiatric inpatients. Prim Care Companion CNS Disord 2013;15(6). PCC. 13m01558.
199. Shin JJ, Saadabadi A. Trazodone. In: StatPearls. Treasure Island FL: © 2021, StatPearls Publishing LLC.; 2021.
200. Vande Griend JP, Anderson SL. Histamine-1 receptor antagonism for treatment of insomnia. J Am Pharm Assoc (2003) 2012;52(6):e210–9.
201. Modesto-Lowe V, Harabasz AK, Walker SA. Quetiapine for primary insomnia: consider the risks. Cleve Clin J Med 2021;88(5):286–94.
202. Mahoney JE, Webb MJ, Gray SL. Zolpidem prescribing and adverse drug reactions in hospitalized general medicine patients at a Veterans Affairs hospital. Am J Geriatr Pharmacother 2004; 2(1):66–74.
203. Kolla BP, Lovely JK, Mansukhani MP, et al. Zolpidem is independently associated with increased risk of inpatient falls. J Hosp Med 2013;8(1):1–6.
204. Torii H, Ando M, Tomita H, et al. Association of hypnotic drug use with fall incidents in hospitalized elderly patients: a case-crossover study. Biol Pharm Bull 2020;43(6):925–31.
205. Richards K, Rowlands A. The impact of zolpidem on the mental status of hospitalized patients older than age 50. Medsurg Nurs 2013;22(3):188–91, 187.
206. Lavon O, Bojol S. Safety of brotizolam in hospitalized patients. Eur J Clin Pharmacol 2018;74(7): 939–43.

Effects of Sleep Deficiency on Risk, Course, and Treatment of Psychopathology

Molly E. Atwood, PhD*

KEYWORDS

• Sleep deficiency • Sleep disturbance • Depression • Anxiety • Posttraumatic stress disorder • Bipolar disorder

KEY POINTS

- Historically, sleep deficiency has been conceptualized as a symptom or consequence of psychiatric disorders.
- However, recent evidence suggests that sleep deficiency is now better conceptualized as a comorbid problem and might also be an underlying risk factor for developing a psychiatric disorder.
- Assessment and treatment of sleep deficiency are important in the care of patients with psychiatric disorders.

INTRODUCTION

Sleep is a fundamental process vital for physical and mental health. Sleep deficiency occurs when there is a deficit in the quantity or quality of sleep versus what is needed for optimal health and well-being. Sleep deficiency can result from sleep deprivation, insufficient sleep duration, sleeping at the wrong time of day relative to one's internal sleep-wake rhythm, and/or a sleep disorder, such as insomnia, that fragments sleep and reduces sleep quality.[1] Epidemiologic data indicate that approximately 20% to 30% of the population complain of general sleep deficiency.[2] Moreover, around 6% to 10% of individuals meet diagnostic criteria for insomnia disorder,[3] and as many as one in 3 adults report experiencing at least one nighttime insomnia symptom.[4–6]

The assessment of sleep deficiency is accomplished through one of the 2 ways: subjective assessment via clinical interview, self-report questionnaires, and/or prospective sleep diaries, and objective assessment via polysomnography or wrist actigraphy. The most commonly measured sleep parameters are total sleep time, sleep onset latency (or the amount of time it takes to fall asleep), wakefulness after sleep onset (or the amount of time awake in the middle of the night after initiating sleep), and sleep efficiency (or the percentage of time spent in bed asleep). Polysomnography is also able to capture information about sleep architecture, including the amount of time spent in various sleep stages. This includes both nonrapid eye movement sleep (NREM) sleep and rapid eye movement (REM) sleep. NREM sleep is further subcategorized into stages 1 (light sleep), 2, and 3 (slow-wave or deep sleep;[7]).

Sleep deficiency is highly comorbid with many, if not most, psychiatric disorders. Indeed, many psychiatric disorders have sleep deficiency listed as a diagnostic criterion, including major depressive disorder (MDD), bipolar disorder (BD), generalized anxiety disorder (GAD), and posttraumatic stress disorder (PTSD;[3]). Moreover, many other disorders have sleep deficiency as a part of their clinical presentation. For example, individuals with panic disorder (PD), social anxiety disorder (SAD), obsessive-compulsive disorder (OCD),

Department of Psychiatry and Behavioral Sciences, Johns Hopkins University School of Medicine, 5510 Nathan Shock Drive, Suite 100 Baltimore, MD 21224-6823, USA
* Department of Psychiatry and Behavioral Sciences, Johns Hopkins University School of Medicine, 5510 Nathan Shock Drive, Suite 100 Baltimore, MD 21224-6823, USA
E-mail address: matwood4@jhmi.edu

Clin Chest Med 43 (2022) 305–318
https://doi.org/10.1016/j.ccm.2022.02.010

alcohol use disorder, and schizophrenia often report disturbed sleep.[8]

In contrast to the longstanding view that sleep deficiency is a consequence or epiphenomenon of psychiatric disorders, converging evidence from several lines of research suggest that the relationship between sleep and psychiatric disorders is bi-directional. For example, sleep deficiency has been shown to predict the subsequent onset of several psychiatric disorders (eg,[9–11]). Further, treatment of the psychiatric disorder often does not fully resolve sleep symptoms (eg,[12–15]), and sleep-focused interventions have been shown to have a positive impact on psychiatric conditions even if the psychiatric disorder is not directly targeted.[16–19] Thus, sleep deficiency is now better conceptualized as a comorbid, rather than secondary, problem in individuals with mental health difficulties and might also be an underlying risk factor for developing a psychiatric disorder.

This article examines the nature of the relationship between sleep deficiency and psychopathology. Several excellent reviews have previously been published on this topic[20,21]; this article offers an update of recent evidence, focusing on commonly seen psychiatric conditions in clinical practice, including unipolar and bipolar depression, anxiety disorders, and PTSD. We focus on the nonspecific problem of sleep deficiency, with an emphasis on insomnia and insomnia symptoms, the most prevalent and researched sleep disorder. Epidemiologic studies are summarized to characterize the extent of comorbidity between sleep deficiency and psychiatric disorders. Longitudinal studies examining sleep deficiency as a risk factor for the development of psychopathology are also discussed. Finally, the impact on sleep of psychological interventions for mental health disorders, as well as the effects of treating sleep on comorbid psychopathology is reviewed.

Effects of Sleep on Risk for Psychopathology and Illness Course

Unipolar depression

Depression is one of the most prevalent mental health disorders. In the United States, approximately 20% of the population will report symptoms that meet the criteria for a depressive disorder in their lifetime.[22] Of those with depression, the majority report co-occurring sleep difficulties, including insomnia (85%) and hypersomnia (48%; ie, extended nocturnal sleep and excessive daytime sleepiness).[23] Furthermore, one study found that individuals with insomnia were 9.82 times more likely than those without insomnia to have clinically significant depression.[24]

There is considerable evidence for objective sleep disturbances in individuals with unipolar depression as compared with healthy controls. Indeed, individuals with depression show increased time to sleep onset and wakefulness after sleep onset, as well as decreased sleep efficiency.[25] Polysomnographic measures of sleep have also shown disturbances in sleep architecture including reduced slow-wave sleep, decreased REM latency, and increased REM density and duration.[25] A few studies to date have compared objective hypersomnia between those with and without depression using polysomnography and multiple sleep latency test (MSLT;[26–29]). All reported no difference. However, individuals with depression tend to spend a greater amount of time in bed, which can contribute to reduced sleep efficiency and increased sleep fragmentation.[30]

In addition to evidence documenting structural abnormalities in sleep during depressive episodes, a plethora of longitudinal studies has shown that insomnia increases the risk of a subsequent depressive episode. These studies have been subject to several meta-analyses.[31–34] For example, Li and colleagues[33] meta-analyzed 34 prospective cohort studies including more than 150,000 participants with an average follow-up period of approximately 5 years. They found that participants with insomnia had a more than the 2-fold increased risk of developing depression over time (pooled risk ratio [RR] = 2.27). Comparable findings were obtained in a more recent meta-analysis of 10 prospective studies also with an average follow-up of 5 years (odds ratio [OR] = 2.83;[34]). In one of the most rigorous longitudinal studies on this topic to date, Buysse and colleagues[9] assessed insomnia and depression in a community sample of 591 adults at 6 time points over the course of 20 years. Diagnoses of insomnia and depression were confirmed by semi-structured clinical interviews. The authors found that between 17% and 50% of participants with insomnia lasting 2 or more weeks at any given assessment time point developed major depressive episodes or MDD at the subsequent assessment time point. Furthermore, insomnia was a stronger predictor of subsequent depression than depression was of subsequent insomnia.[9]

General sleep disturbance likewise is associated with the risk of depression. For example, in a meta-analysis of 23 prospective studies that recruited older adults, those who self-reported sleep disturbances (ie, poor sleep quality and/or insomnia symptoms) at baseline had a greater risk of developing depression 12 to 24 months later than those without sleep disturbances (RR = 1.92;[32]). In addition, those with persistent as opposed to acute sleep disturbances at baseline were at even greater risk (RR = 3.90) and were more likely to experience recurrence of depression (RR = 7.70). A recent prospective study also found that insomnia was associated with persistence of depression over a 6-month period.[10]

Bipolar depression

BD is a chronic and severe mental illness characterized by shifts in mood (between [hypo]mania and depression) and activity (increased goal-directed activity and inactivity).[3] In patients with BD, periods of mania are characterized by reduced need for sleep, whereas during episodes of depression, insomnia and hypersomnia are common.[3] Harvey[35] notes that across studies of patients during a manic episode, around 69% to 99% exhibit a reduced need for sleep. During a depressive episode, one study found that 100% of patients experience insomnia, while rates of hypersomnia (23% to 78%) are somewhat lower.[35] Even in the interepisode period, individuals with BD report sleep disturbance,[36,37] which seems to be related to worse illness course and outcome.[38] In one study, around 55% of euthymic patients with BD met diagnostic criteria for insomnia and around 70% indicated some sleep disturbance.[39] Around 25% report interepisode hypersomnia.[40]

In addition to disturbances in sleep duration and continuity, a sizable proportion of individuals with BD exhibit circadian abnormalities.[41] For example, one study found that approximately 30% of individuals with BD have a delayed sleep–wake phase disorder,[42] indicating a delay in sleep/wake times of at least 2 h from what is socially desired. This can contribute to sleep problems when one tries to sleep at a time that is out of sync with their internal rhythm (either by choice or due to life circumstances). In addition, individuals with BD tend to have unstable 24-hr sleep/wake and activity/rest cycles,[43] which is both a contributor to and consequence of circadian dysregulation.

Evidence from polysomnographic studies show that sleep architecture during periods of mania is characterized by shortened REM latency and increased REM density.[44] During the depressed state, those with BD also show shortened REM latency and increased REM density, as well as more fragmented sleep and longer latency to slow-wave sleep as compared with healthy controls.[44] This suggests that sleep disturbances in mania and depression result, at least in part, from similar processes. As compared with patients with unipolar depression, individuals with BD show longer sleep onset latency, greater fragmentation of REM sleep (especially in BD I), and greater REM density during the depressed state.[44] Two meta-analyses have also shown that, as determined by actigraphy monitoring, interepisode sleep of individuals with BD is characterized by increased sleep onset latency and wakefulness after sleep onset, and poor sleep efficiency.[36,45] Interestingly, longer sleep duration and more time spent in bed are also characteristic of interepisode individuals as compared with controls,[36] with time in bed (which, in excess of total sleep time, reduces sleep efficiency) being more strongly related to measures of hypersomnia than total sleep time.[40] Other than a higher percentage of stage 1 sleep, one meta-analysis found no significant between-group differences in sleep architecture between interepisode individuals and healthy controls.[36]

Most of the individuals with BD identify sleep disturbance as an important prodromal symptom of manic episode onset.[46,47] Several case reports and experimental studies corroborate that sleep deprivation is associated with the onset of (hypo)mania in some patients. For example, Colombo and colleagues[48] exposed 206 patients with BD in a depressive episode to just one night of total sleep deprivation, followed by a recovery night or a recovery night plus medications (lithium, pindolol, fluoxetine, or amineptine). Results showed that around 5% of patients switched to a manic episode and around 6% switched to a hypomanic episode. Micro-longitudinal studies have also shown that sleep disturbance increases in the days or weeks leading up to the onset of a manic episode. More specifically, several studies have shown that shorter sleep duration, more so than the timing of sleep onset or offset, predicts greater severity of next-day manic symptoms.[49,50]

A limited number of longitudinal studies have been published to date that examined the association of disturbed sleep in healthy individuals drawn from a large community sample and subsequent onset of BD. In one study with a 10-year follow-up, controlling for age, sex, parental mood disorder, and lifetime cannabis or alcohol dependence, disturbed sleep at baseline was found to significantly increase the risk of BD (OR = 1.75;[11]). The median length of time between baseline assessment and conversion to BD was 1.9 years. In addition, in at least 2 studies of individuals at high familial risk of BD, sleep disturbances in early childhood emerged as a significant predictor of later onset of the disorder.[51,52]

Anxiety disorders

Anxiety is a response to a real or perceived threat, characterized by physiologic changes that increase alertness and arousal and, thus, prepares the body for action. This response interferes with sleep, which necessarily involves sufficient reduction of the arousal (cognitive, physical, and emotional) associated with normal waking activities, let alone the response to threat. Thus, one would expect that sleep disturbances are common in individuals with an anxiety disorder, and they are. Around 70% to 90% of individuals with an anxiety disorder report experiencing insomnia.[53–55] In turn there are higher rates of clinically significant anxiety[24] and presleep arousal[56] in individuals with sleep disturbances. Sleep disturbance occurs most commonly in GAD, which is characterized by excessive worry and hyperarousal, and is included in the diagnostic criteria for this disorder. For example, in a longitudinal study of 533 patients seen in primary care, those with a diagnosis of GAD at intake were 140% more likely than patients with another anxiety disorder diagnosis to report sleep disturbance.[57]

Based on objective measurement of sleep, those with GAD exhibit lower sleep duration and slow-wave sleep, and increased sleep onset latency and wakefulness after sleep onset, as compared with healthy controls.[8] At least one study has also shown increased REM latency.[58] Findings regarding the relationship between sleep disturbance and other anxiety disorders is more mixed. There is a clear indication that total sleep time is reduced in individuals with OCD and that this is related to symptom severity; however, evidence for disturbances in REM sleep are inconclusive.[8] Similarly, PD is associated with decreased total sleep time and sleep efficiency, as well as increased sleep onset latency, although evidence for alterations in sleep architecture is mixed.[59–61] No evidence has been found for objective sleep disturbance in those with SAD.

Both experimental and longitudinal studies suggest a causal relationship between sleep and anxiety. For example, Pires and colleagues[62] conducted a meta-analysis of the effects of sleep deprivation on state anxiety levels. They found that total experimental sleep deprivation, but not sleep restriction, significantly increased subsequent anxiety levels. Several studies have also examined the association between sleep disturbance or insomnia symptoms assessed at baseline and risk of developing clinically significant anxiety at a later time point. Both have been shown to increase the odds of developing anxiety up to 12 months later in most studies,[10,63,64] although there are exceptions (eg,[65]). A recent meta-analysis of 6 studies reported the odds ratio to be 2.92.[34] Sleep disturbance or insomnia has not, however, been shown to be associated with the persistence of anxiety over time.[10,57]

Posttraumatic stress disorder

PTSD is conceptualized as a disorder of nonrecovery following exposure to a traumatic event. The disorder is characterized by re-experiencing of the event, avoidance of reminders of the event, changes in mood and cognition, and heightened arousal and reactivity.[3] Individuals with PTSD exhibit 2 types of sleep disturbance: arousal-related insomnia-type symptoms, and intrusive nightmares that fragment and promote avoidance of sleep.[3] In one study of individuals in the general population, around 70% of those with PTSD reported sleep disturbance, including insomnia (40%) or nightmares (20%).[66] Across diverse samples, including veterans, sexual assault survivors, and mixed trauma, individuals with PTSD consistently report decreased sleep duration and greater sleep disruption than healthy controls or trauma-exposed individuals without PTSD (eg,[67,68]). There is some evidence to suggest that experiencing sexual assault, more severe trauma, and dissociative and hyperarousal symptoms following trauma are all more strongly associated with sleep disturbance.[69–72] Sleep disturbance, in turn, is associated with greater severity of PTSD symptoms.[13]

Polysomnographic studies generally show that individuals with PTSD have lower total sleep time, reduced slow-wave sleep, and more disrupted sleep as compared with healthy controls.[73] Reduced total sleep time and slow-wave sleep are also associated with PTSD severity.[73] REM sleep is of particular relevance to PTSD, given that it is the stage of sleep most associated with dreaming. One meta-analysis of 31 studies found no differences in REM sleep parameters, except in individuals younger than 30 who exhibited shorter duration of time spent in REM as compared with age-matched controls.[73] Several studies have compared objective sleep parameters between individuals with PTSD to trauma exposed individuals without PTSD, with mixed findings.[74–76] In addition, comparisons of individuals with PTSD and MDD have provided no conclusive evidence of objective differences in sleep continuity or sleep architecture.[72]

Previous night's sleep duration, quality, and difficulty falling and staying asleep have all been shown to predict next-day PTSD symptoms.[77,78] Longitudinal studies also demonstrate that sleep disturbances both before and following a trauma predict PTSD symptoms over time. For example, in a naturalistic, longitudinal study of 191 Hurricane Katrina survivors, general sleep disturbance 2 years later predicted PTSD symptom severity at 2.5 years, even after controlling for PTSD symptom severity at first assessment.[79] Similar findings were reported after the Wenchuan earthquake in Dujiangyan, China, whereby poor sleep quality 12 months after the disaster significantly increased the odds for PTSD at 24 months (OR = 1.80).[80] In that study, poor sleep quality also predicted persistence of PTSD over time. Moreover, among veterans, sleep disturbance before deployment has been shown to predict the onset of PTSD postdeployment.[81–83] Lastly, sleep disturbance after deployment significantly predicts PTSD symptoms up to 4 years later.[84–86]

Summary

Sleep disturbance across psychiatric disorders can present in several ways, including alterations in sleep architecture or deficient or fragmented sleep due to insomnia, nightmares, or other sleep disorders. The above-reviewed studies also provide evidence for a prospective association between sleep disturbance and the subsequent development of psychopathology, which implies shared causal and/or maintaining mechanisms. An explanation of these mechanisms is beyond the scope of the current paper; however, several comprehensive reviews are available that expand on this topic (eg,[87–90]). These reviews highlight several possible shared biological mechanisms, including common genetics, neuroinflammatory dysregulation, disturbances in circadian genes, and neurotransmitter dysfunction, among others.[87–89] Sleep disturbances might also contribute to the development of psychopathology through an increase in negative emotions, decrease in positive emotions, and greater difficulty with emotion regulation,[90–92] and/or through behavioral and cognitive mechanisms. Regarding the latter, daytime symptoms associated with sleep disturbance, such as fatigue and sleepiness, can contribute to reduced engagement in valued activities. Indeed, individuals with insomnia are more likely than good sleepers to call in sick to work or cancel appointments, meetings, and social activities when feeling fatigued or sleepy.[93,94] Unhelpful beliefs about sleep also directly contribute to arousal and can discourage engagement in behaviors that could help to manage emotional distress (eg, avoiding exercise or socializing to conserve energy;[93,94]), thereby increasing susceptibility to psychopathology. As our understanding of shared mechanisms and causal pathways increases, this will help to guide prevention and interventions initiatives.

Impact of Treatment for Psychopathology on Sleep

Unipolar depression

For patients with comorbid depression and sleep disturbance, treatment has historically focused on addressing depressive symptoms, while neglecting the treatment of disturbed sleep. Yet, several studies have now shown that targeting depression alone is insufficient, as insomnia is one of the most commonly reported residual symptoms following treatment (eg,[12,95–97]). For instance, a study by Carney and colleagues[12] found that in those whose depression successfully remitted following either cognitive behavioral therapy (CBT) or pharmacotherapy for depression, 22% reported residual sleep-onset insomnia, 26% reported sleep-maintenance insomnia, and 17% reported early morning awakenings; rates of residual insomnia symptoms did not differ significantly between the 2 treatment modalities. In a more recent study of 523 adults treated with cognitive therapy for depression, 64% of patients continued to report clinically significant sleep disturbance at posttreatment.[95]

In addition, sleep disturbance seems to moderate treatment response. For example, Thase and colleagues[98] showed that individuals with objectively determined abnormalities in sleep (ie, decreased REM latency, increased REM density, and reduced sleep efficiency) had poorer remission rates following the psychological treatment of depression than those without these abnormalities. More recently, prolonged sleep onset latency and shorter sleep duration (less than 6 hours) either alone or in combination with insomnia were shown to predict nonremission from depression after either pharmacotherapy or psychotherapy.[99]

Regarding the impact of sleep disturbance on the risk of relapse or recurrence to depression, findings are less clear. Several studies have documented a relationship between residual sleep disturbance and risk of relapse or recurrence (eg,[96,100–102]), whereas several studies have not (eg,[95,103]). Discrepant findings may be due to methodological differences, as well the time at which residual sleep disturbance is measured. For example, while most studies examine post-treatment sleep disturbance as a predictor of recurrence, Perlis and colleague[101] found that steadily worsening sleep disturbance occurred in the weeks before the recurrence of depression.

Bipolar disorder

Although limited evidence exists thus far to show sleep deficiency as a risk factor for the first onset of BD, a greater body of evidence demonstrates that residual sleep disturbance after the resolution of a (hypo)manic or depressive episode is associated with, and can even hasten, relapse to both. For example, in a sample of interepisode individuals, Gruber and colleagues[104] found that greater sleep variability (calculated as the maximum minus the minimum sleep hours) was associated with increased severity of both depression and mania across 12 months. In addition, Kaplan and colleagues[40] found that interepisode hypersomnia was associated with recurrence of depressive symptoms 6 months later in a sample of 56 individuals with BD. Finally, Cretu and colleagues[105] found that those with poor sleep quality during the interepisode period had earlier recurrence of any mood episode compared with those with good sleep quality, while Gershon and colleagues[106] found that abnormal sleep duration (total sleep time less than 6 hours or >9 hours) was associated with shorter time to recurrence of depression.

Evidence also exists suggesting a relationship between sleep disturbances and treatment outcomes in BD. One study found that, of patients admitted to the hospital with a BD diagnosis, those with a longer total sleep time at admission showed more improvement in symptoms and earlier discharge than those with a shorter total sleep time.[107] In addition, sleep disturbance might moderate response to treatment of BD, although findings in the few studies that have examined this have been mixed. For example, Sylvia and colleagues[108] showed that, when comparing quetiapine and lithium in the treatment of BD, individuals with sleep disturbance at baseline had a 45% lower probability of sustained response to treatment compared with individuals without sleep disturbance. In contrast, abnormal sleep duration was not found to moderate treatment response for individuals participating in the Systematic Treatment Enhancement Program for BD (STEP-BD) trial, a multi-site longitudinal study of CBT, interpersonal and social rhythms therapy, or family-focused therapy for BD.[109] As Kaplan[110] notes, this raises the possibility that there is a differential impact of sleep on treatment outcome for psychotherapy versus pharmacotherapy, or by different types of sleep disturbance.

Anxiety disorders

Like depression, psychological treatments for anxiety also result in improvements in sleep. For example, in 2010 Belleville and colleagues[111] published a meta-analysis of the effects of CBT for anxiety disorders on sleep outcomes. They found that the treatment of anxiety resulted in a moderate reduction in insomnia symptoms (hedge's $g = 0.527$). Furthermore, findings did not significantly differ depending on the type of sleep problem that was measured (eg, insomnia symptom severity, nightmares, etc.), or the anxiety disorder (GAD, PD, or PTSD;[111]).

However, numerous studies have shown sleep disturbance to be a common residual symptom after effective treatment of anxiety. For example, following 8 weeks of pharmacotherapy and psychotherapy for patients with PD, Cervena and colleagues[112] found that while anxiety significantly improved, there were no significant changes in multiple sleep parameters by either subjective or objective measurement. In a sample of 134 older adults with GAD who were randomized to either CBT or usual care, those who received CBT demonstrated greater improvement in a measure of sleep quality as compared with controls; however, scores remained in the clinically significant range.[113] Similar findings were reported by Ramsawh and colleagues[59] in a sample of 50 adults with either GAD or PD: sleep quality improved from pre to posttreatment, although remained clinically elevated. Furthermore, poorer sleep quality at baseline was significantly associated with worse treatment outcome.[59] This may be attributable, at least in part, to the fact that sleep seems to be necessary for fear extinction learning and memory consolidation.[114] In particular, insomnia symptoms and fragmentation of REM sleep can reduce the effectiveness of extinction learning and safety learning. Thus, sleep disturbance could interfere with exposure-based treatments.[115] To the best of this author's knowledge, the relationship between residual sleep disturbance and risk of relapse to anxiety disorders has not been examined.

Posttraumatic stress disorder

Psychological treatment of PTSD similarly results in clear improvements in sleep; yet, clinically significant insomnia symptoms remain for roughly half of the patients.[15,116–118] In a recent study, 108 active-duty US Army soldiers were randomized to complete 12 sessions of group cognitive processing therapy or an active control condition (group present-centered therapy) and were followed for 12 months posttreatment,[119] At pretreatment, almost the entire sample (92%) reported insomnia symptoms and over half (69%) reported nightmares. Both sleep complaints significantly improved following treatment, but overall remained elevated. At follow-up, 77% of the sample reported insomnia symptoms and 52% reported nightmares, regardless of treatment type. This was true even when the response to PTSD treatment was good, with 57% and 13% of patients no longer meeting criteria for PTSD at follow-up reporting continued insomnia symptoms or nightmares, respectively.[119] In a second study of adolescent rape survivors, nightmares and insomnia symptoms were reported by 72% and 86% of the sample, respectively.[120] Both sleep and PTSD symptom severity significantly improved following either prolonged exposure or client-centered therapy. Yet 55% of the sample continued to report clinically significant insomnia and 20% reported nightmares, and residual sleep disturbance predicted poorer functioning up to 12-months follow-up. As with anxiety disorders, whether or not residual sleep disturbance predicts relapse to PTSD is not yet clear.

Summary

There is a growing body of literature documenting the relationship between sleep deficiency and outcomes of treatment of various psychiatric disorders. While psychological treatments typically result in improvements in sleep, sleep disturbance often does not fully resolve. Furthermore, sleep disturbance before treatment is associated with poorer treatment response in some studies, and residual sleep disturbance can increase the risk of relapse to depression and (hypo)mania. Taken together, these findings corroborate the postulate that sleep is likely not a mere epiphenomenon of psychiatric disorders and that additional treatment is warranted to address comorbid sleep disturbance in patients with mental health disorders.

Impact of Sleep Treatment on Comorbid Psychopathology

Unipolar depression

Several meta-analyses have shown that cognitive behavioral therapy for insomnia (CBT-I) results in a decrease in the severity of depressive symptoms, with effect sizes in the small to medium range in comparison to control conditions.[18,121,122] When directly compared with depression-focused treatments, CBT-I has also been shown to result in comparable improvements in depressive symptoms (eg,[123,124]). Indeed, CBT-I seems to have a greater impact on insomnia symptoms and equal effect on depressive symptoms as CBT for depression; thus, CBT-I might be a more efficacious and cost-effective treatment option for those with comorbid diagnoses.

The above meta-analyses focused on the effects of CBT-I alone, rather than in combination with a depression-focused intervention. Two randomized controls trials to date have tested the efficacy of CBT-I (or a control condition) combined with pharmacotherapy for depression.[16,124] Neither study found an additive effect of CBT-I plus pharmacotherapy with respect to reducing depression symptom severity. However, Manber and colleagues[125] found that improvements in insomnia within the first half of treatment mediated remission from depression by the end of treatment in the CBT-I group only. Furthermore, those with the most rapid, early improvement in insomnia symptoms had the best response in terms of depression outcome.[126] A more recent study also found that improvement in depression severity after CBT-I occurred through a reduction in insomnia symptom severity.[127] Thus, improvement in depression seems to be dependent, at least in part, on a reduction in sleep disturbance, particularly early on in treatment. This holds important implications for real-time treatment planning for individuals with comorbid sleep disturbance and depression.

If sleep-focused treatment could help lower the risk of future development of depression, this could have a significant impact on individual distress and larger health care costs. In the only study conducted to date on this topic, Christensen and colleagues[128] tested whether an Internet CBT-I program delivered to individuals with insomnia and depressive symptomatology could reduce depressive symptoms up to 6 months posttreatment. Results showed that the CBT-I intervention was significantly more effective for reducing depressive symptoms at 6 months as compared with a control condition, even after accounting for differential dropout. Fewer participants developed a MDD in the CBT-I group (n = 9) than in the control (n = 13), although the difference was not statistically significant.[128] The lack of significant effect may have been attributable to the low total incidence of development of depression (4%) in the sample. Studies with longer follow-up periods are needed to clarify the effect of sleep-focused treatment on reducing the risk of developing subsequent depression.

Bipolar disorder

Only one clinical trial to date has tested the efficacy of a sleep-focused intervention in a sample of patients with BD. In this study, Harvey and colleagues[129] adapted CBT-I to include elements of evidence-based treatments for BD (CBTI-BP), such as interpersonal and social rhythms therapy. Although it was not a pure test of a sleep-focused intervention, it should be noted that interpersonal and social rhythms therapy seeks to regularize daytime and nighttime activity and, thus, likely helps to stabilize and strengthen the circadian rhythm. Interepisode patients with BD were randomized to either CBTI-BP or a psychoeducation control condition. Results showed that CBTI-BP significantly improved insomnia symptoms and resulted in a greater proportion of patients remitting from insomnia than the control condition. Moreover, the CBTI-BP group spent fewer days in any bipolar episode and exhibited lower (hypo) mania relapse rates at 6-month follow-up. There were no differences between groups with respect to relapse to depression, functional impairment, or quality of life.[129] Of note, sleep restriction and stimulus control, the two active components of CBT-I, were safe and did not increase the risk of (hypo)mania in the sample. This is important clinically, given the association between sleep deprivation and risk of onset or recurrence of (hypo) mania. Thus, findings show promise for the effect of successful sleep treatment on the prevention of future (hypo)manic episodes in patient with BD, although more studies are needed.

Anxiety disorders

A 2011 meta-analysis conducted by Belleville and colleagues[130] identified 50 controlled and uncontrolled studies of CBT-I that included anxiety as an outcome variable. Results showed a moderate effect of CBT-I on anxiety and anxiety-related constructs (eg, stress, worry; $g = 0.406$): the effect was small in comparison to controls. This is lower than typical effect sizes for CBT for anxiety, which tends to be in the large range.[131] Interestingly, studies that included treatment components specifically targeting anxiety did not increase the efficacy of CBT-I with respect to reducing anxiety. It is important to note, however, that only 4 studies included in the meta-analysis recruited individuals with an anxiety disorder diagnoses, as opposed to just anxiety symptoms.[130] A more recent meta-analysis of 8 controlled studies evaluated change in anxiety symptom severity following internet-based CBT-I.[132] The authors found a small effects size (SMD [standardized mean difference] = −0.35) for Internet CBT-I as compared with wait-list control. Similarly, in this meta-analysis, none of the included studies focused on patients with a comorbid anxiety disorder, highlighting the need for additional clinical trials including participants with a dual diagnosis of insomnia and an anxiety disorder.

Posttraumatic stress disorder

Several psychological interventions show promise for treating insomnia and PTSD-related nightmares, as well as non–sleep-related PTSD symptoms. In veterans, CBT-I with or without adjunctive nightmare-focused interventions improves sleep and PTSD symptoms more than a control condition.[133,134] A recent meta-analysis of 11 randomized controlled trials showed an overall moderate effect size for both self-reported and clinician-rated PTSD symptoms ($g = 0.6$).[19] This is comparable to effects sizes for PTSD treatments (eg, $d = 0.49$[135]; $d = 0.56$[136]), apart from prolonged exposure therapy, which has shown large effects ($g = 1.08$[137]). Thus, CBT-I seems to be similarly efficacious in the treatment of PTSD symptoms as most types of PTSD interventions. In addition, at least one study has shown that improvements in subjective sleep predict improvement in PTSD symptoms.[116]

With respect to nightmares, imagery rehearsal therapy (IRT) has been the most researched nonpharmacological intervention. IRT is an adapted CBT whereby a patient "rescripts" or rewrites a nightmare into a nondisturbing script and rehearses the new dream script during the day. When delivered alone, studies have shown that IRT results in significant improvements in subjective sleep quality and reduces nightmare frequency in individuals with PTSD (eg,[138–140]). Beyond sleep-related outcomes, meta-analyses have shown that IRT has a small ($g = 0.31$[140]) to moderate ($g = 0.58$[139]) effect on PTSD symptoms. Thus, extant clinical trials clearly show that improving sleep is one mechanism by which PTSD symptoms improve. It is still unclear, however, how best to incorporate sleep treatment into existing empirically supported PTSD therapies.[141]

Summary

The high co-occurrence of sleep deficiency and psychopathology, and the relationship between sleep deficiency and onset, course, and treatment of psychopathology, has important clinical implications. Recent evidence suggests that treating sleep disturbances can have a significant impact on symptoms of depression, BD, anxiety disorders, and PTSD. Furthermore, sleep-focused treatments seem to be at least as effective as treatments targeting comorbid depression and PTSD for reducing symptoms of these disorders. CBT-I has a moderate impact on comorbid anxiety, although does not seem to be as effective for reducing symptoms of anxiety disorders as anxiety-focused treatments are. Given that CBT for anxiety also has a moderate impact on comorbid sleep difficulties, clinicians can determine, based on patient preference and their own expertise, which should be targeted in treatment first. However, regardless of the treatment sequence, both problems should be given separate attention. The relative efficacy of sleep-focused treatment and treatments for BD is not yet established, although preliminary evidence suggests that sleep treatment may be promising for reducing the risk of relapse to mania.

CONCLUSION

Sleep deficiency is a common complaint of individuals with mental health disorders; often, sleep complaints are so common they are included in the diagnostic criteria for the disorder. Such complaints include too little (and occasionally too much) sleep, fragmented sleep, variability in sleep timing, and parasomnias. In addition to subjective complaints, sleep deficiency is apparent using objective measures of sleep. Accumulating evidence from longitudinal studies suggests that sleep deficiency, particularly when persistent, predicts the onset and maintenance of MDD, anxiety disorders, BD, and PTSD. There is also a relationship between the severity of sleep disturbance and comorbid psychopathology. These findings indicate a causal role of sleep deficiency in the development of psychopathology.

The fact that sleep problems persist after successful treatment of comorbid psychiatric disorders, and are associated with treatment outcomes, also contradicts the theory that sleep deficiency is an epiphenomenon. In addition, recent evidence indicates that sleep-focused treatment can effectively reduce symptoms of both sleep disturbance and comorbid psychopathology. Importantly, these findings suggest that addressing sleep deficiency may reduce the likelihood of developing mental health problems and/or buffer their severity. More research is needed to determine whether this is the case, as well as to establish how best to integrate sleep-focused interventions into existing evidence-based treatments for each psychiatric disorder.

From a clinical perspective, the extent literature on the psychiatric disorder-sleep relationship speaks to the need to not simply treat what is assumed to be an underlying psychiatric condition, but to concurrently address sleep disturbance. Therefore, it is recommended that sleep problems become part of the routine assessment for patients at initial presentation. When sleep problems are apparent, they should be appropriately treated with the recommended evidence-based treatments. Although additional research is needed to address gaps in the current body of literature, this work promises to improve our understanding of both sleep and psychiatric conditions and to provide better clinical care to patients with comorbid psychiatric and sleep disorders.

CLINICS CARE POINTS

- Individuals with a range of psychiatric disorders exhibit disturbances in sleep duration, continuity, and architecture as compared with healthy controls.
- Sleep deficiency has been shown to predict the onset of psychiatric disorders and is associated with severity and course of psychopathology.
- The assumption that the treatment of the psychiatric disorder will resolve sleep deficiency is unfounded, and there is increasing support for evidence-based treatments of sleep deficiency being integral to the successful management of psychopathology.
- Clinical practice should include the routine assessment of sleep disturbances and referral to appropriate treatment.

DISCLOSURE

The authors have nothing to disclose.

REFERENCES

1. National Institutes of Health. National institutes of health sleep disorders research plan. National Institutes of Health; 2011.
2. Chattu VK, Manzar MD, Kumary S, et al. The global problem of insufficient sleep and its serious public health implications. Healthcare (Basel) 2018;7(1):1.
3. American Psychiatric Association. Diagnostic and statistical manual of mental disorders. 5th edition. American Psychiatric Publishing; 2013.
4. Morin CM, Jarrin DC. Epidemiology of insomnia: prevalence, course, risk factors, and public health burden. Sleep *Med Clin* 2013;8(3):281–97.
5. Ohayon MM. Epidemiology of insomnia: what we know and what we still need to learn. Sleep Med Rev 2002;6(2):97–111.
6. Roth T. Insomnia: definition, prevalence, etiology, and consequences. J Clin Sleep Med 2007;3(5 Suppl):S7–10.
7. Iber C, Ancoli-Israel S, Chesson A, et al. The AASM manual for the scoring of sleep and associated events: rules, terminology, and technical specification. 1st edition. American Academy of Sleep Medicine; 2007.
8. Cox RC, Olatunji BO. A systematic review of sleep disturbance in anxiety and related disorders. J Anxiety Disord 2016;37:104–29.
9. Buysse DJ, Angst J, Gamma A, et al. Prevalence, course, and comorbidity of insomnia and depression in young adults. Sleep 2008;31(4):473–80.
10. Johansson M, Jansson-Fröjmark M, Norell-Clarke A, et al. Changes in insomnia as a risk factor for the incidence and persistence of anxiety and depression: a longitudinal community study. Sleep Sci Pract 2021;5(5).

11. Ritter PS, Hofler M, Wittchen H-U, et al. Disturbaned sleep as a risk factor for the subsequent onset of bipolar disorder: data from a 10-year prospective-longitudinal study among adolescents and young adults. J Psychiatr Res 2015;68:76–82.
12. Carney CE, Segal ZV, Edinger JD, et al. A comparison of rates of residual insomnia symptoms following pharmacotherapy or cognitive-behavioral therapy for major depressive disorder. J Clin Psychiatry 2007;68(2):254–60.
13. Belleville G, Guay S, Marchand A. Impact of sleep disturbances on PTSD symptoms and perceived health. J Nerv Ment Dis 2009;197(2):126–32.
14. Galovski TE, Monson C, Bruce SE, et al. Does cognitive– behavioral therapy for PTSD improve perceived health and sleep impairment? J Trauma Stress 2009;22(3):197–204.
15. Gutner CA, Casement MD, Gilbert KS, et al. Change in sleep symptoms across cognitive processing therapy and prolonged exposure: a longitudinal perspective. Behav Res Ther 2013;51(12): 817–22.
16. Carney CE, Edinger JD, Kuchibhatla M, et al. Cognitive behavioral insomnia therapy for those with insomnia and depression: a randomized controlled clinical trial. Sleep 2017;40(4):zsx019.
17. Espie CA, Emsley R, Kyle SD, et al. Effect of digital cognitive behavioral therapy for insomnia on health, psychological well-being, and sleep-related quality of life: a randomized clinical trial. JAMA Psychiatry. 2019;76(1):21–30.
18. Gee B, Orchard F, Clarke E, et al. The effect of non-pharmacological sleep interventions on depression symptoms: a meta-analysis of randomised controlled trials. Sleep Med Rev 2019;43:118–28.
19. Ho FY, Chan CS, Tang KN. Cognitive-behavioral therapy for sleep disturbances in treating posttraumatic stress disorder symptoms: a meta-analysis of randomized controlled trials. Clin Psychol Rev 2016;43:90–102.
20. Krystal AD. Psychiatric disorders and sleep. Neurol Clin 2012;30(4):1389–413.
21. Freeman D, Sheaves B, Waite F, et al. Sleep disturbance and psychiatric disorders. Lancet Psychiatry 2020;7(7):628–37.
22. Hasin DS, Sarvet AL, Meyers JL, et al. Epidemiology of adult *DSM-5* major depressive disorder and its specifiers in the United States. JAMA Psychiatry. 2018;75(4):336–46.
23. Geoffroy PA, Hoertel N, Etain B, et al. Insomnia and hypersomnia in major depressive episode: prevalence, sociodemographic characteristics and psychiatric comorbidity in a population-based study. J Affect Disord 2018;226:132–41.
24. Taylor DJ, Lichstein KL, Durrence HH, et al. Epidemiology of insomnia, depression, and anxiety. Sleep 2005;28:1457–64.
25. Murphy MJ, Peterson MJ. Sleep disturbances in depression. Sleep Med Clin 2015;10(1):17–23.
26. Nofzinger EA, Thase ME, Reynolds CF 3rd, et al. Hypersomnia in bipolar depression: a comparison with narcolepsy using the multiple sleep latency test. Am J Psychiatry 1991;148:1177–781.
27. Billiard M, Partinen M, Roth T, et al. Sleep and psychiatric disorders. J Psychosom Res 1994;38:1–2.
28. Plante DT, Finn LA, Hagen EW, et al. Subjective and objective measures of hypersomnolence demonstrate divergent associations with depression among participants in the Wisconsin sleep cohort study. J Clin Sleep Med 2016;12(4):571–8.
29. Dolenc L, Besset A, Billiard M. Hypersomnia in association with dysthymia in comparison with idiopathic hypersomnia and normal controls. Pflugers Arch 1996;431:R303–4.
30. Dauvilliers Y, Lopez R, Ohayon M, et al. Hypersomnia and depressive symptoms: methodological and clinical aspects. BMC Med 2013;11:78.
31. Baglioni C, Battagliese G, Feige B, et al. Insomnia as a predictor of depression: a meta-analytic evaluation of longitudinal epidemiological studies. J Affect Disord 2011;135(1–3):10–9.
32. Bao YP, Han Y, Ma J, et al. Cooccurrence and bidirectional prediction of sleep disturbances and depression in older adults: meta-analysis and systematic review. Neurosci Biobehav Rev 2017;75: 257–73.
33. Li L, Wu C, Gan Y, et al. Insomnia and the risk of depression: a meta-analysis of prospective cohort studies. BMC Psychiatry 2016;16(1):375.
34. Hertenstein E, Feige B, Gmeiner T, et al. Insomnia as a predictor of mental disorders: a systematic review and meta-analysis. Sleep Med Rev 2019;43: 96–105.
35. Harvey AG, Talbot LS, Gershon A. Sleep disturbance in bipolar disorder across the lifespan. Clin Psychol 2009;16(2):256–77 (New York).
36. Ng TH, Chung KF, Ho FY, et al. Sleep-wake disturbance in interepisode bipolar disorder and high-risk individuals: a systematic review and meta-analysis. Sleep Med Rev 2015;20:46–58.
37. Boland EM, Alloy LB. Sleep disturbance and cognitive deficits in bipolar disorder: toward an integrated examination of disorder maintenance and functional impairment. Clin Psychol Rev 2013; 33(1):33–44.
38. Eidelman P, Talbot LS, Gruber J, et al. Sleep, illness course, and concurrent symptoms in inter-episode bipolar disorder. J Behav Ther Exp Psychiatry 2010;41:145–9.
39. Harvey AG, Schmidt DA, Scarnà A, et al. Sleep-related functioning in euthymic patients with bipolar disorder, patients with insomnia, and subjects without sleep problems. Am J Psychiatry 2005; 162(1):50–7.

40. Kaplan KA, Gruber J, Eidelman P, et al. Hypersomnia in inter-episode bipolar disorder: does it have prognostic significance? J Affect Disord 2011; 132(3):438–44.
41. Huhne A, Welsh DK, Landgraf D. Prospects for circadian treatment of mood disorders. Ann Med 2018;50(8):637–54.
42. Takaesu Y, Inoue Y, Murakoshi A, et al. Prevalence of circadian rhythm sleep-wake disorders and associated factors in euthymic patients with bipolar disorder. PLoS One 2016;11(7):e0159578.
43. Levenson JC, Wallace ML, Anderson BP, et al. Social rhythm disrupting events increase the risk of recurrence among individuals with bipolar disorder. Bipolar Disord 2015;17(8):869–79.
44. Gold AK, Sylvia LG. The role of sleep in bipolar disorder. Nat Sci Sleep 2016;8:207–14.
45. Geoffroy PA, Scott J, Boudebesse C, et al. Sleep in patients with remitted bipolar disorders: a meta-analysis of actigraphy studies. Acta Psychiatr Scand 2015;131(2):89–99.
46. Jackson A, Cavanagh J, Scott J. A systematic review of manic and depressive prodromes. J Affect Disord 2003;74:209–17.
47. Wehr TA, Sack DA, Rosenthal NE. Sleep reduction as a final common pathway in the genesis of mania. Am J Psychiatry 1987;144:201–4.
48. Colombo C, Benedetti F, Barbini B, et al. Rate of switch from depression into mania after therapeutic sleep deprivation in bipolar depression. Psychiatry Res 1999;86:267–70.
49. Leibenluft E, Albert PS, Rosenthal NE, et al. Relationship between sleep and mood in patients with rapid-cycling bipolar disorder. Psychiatry Res 1996;63:161–8.
50. Barbini B, Bertelli S, Colombo C, et al. Sleep loss, a possible factor in augmenting manic episode. Psychiatry Res 1996;65:121–5.
51. Duffy A, Goodday S, Keown-Stoneman C, et al. The emergent course of bipolar disorder: observations over two decades from the Canadian high-risk offspring cohort. Am J Psychiatry 2019;176(9):720–9.
52. Levenson JC, Axelson DA, Merranko J, et al. Differences in sleep disturbances among offspring of parents with and without bipolar disorder: association with conversion to bipolar disorder. Bipolar Disord 2015;17(8):836–48.
53. Mellman TA. Sleep and anxiety disorders. Psychiatr Clin North Am 2006;29(4):1047–58.
54. Papadimitriou GN, Linkowski P. Sleep disturbance in anxiety disorders. Int Rev Psychiatry 2005; 17(4):229–36.
55. Uhde TW, Cortese BM, Vedeniapin A. Anxiety and sleep problems: emerging concepts and theoretical treatment implications. Curr Psychiatry Rep 2009;11(4):269–76.
56. Robertson JA, Broomfield NM, Espie CA. Prospective comparison of subjective arousal during the pre-sleep period in primary sleep-onset insomnia and normal sleepers. J Sleep Res 2007;16(2): 230–8.
57. Marcks BA, Weisberg RB, Edelen MO, et al. The relationship between sleep disturbance and the course of anxiety disorders in primary care patients. Psychiatry Res 2010;178:487–92.
58. Lund HG, Bech P, Eplov L, et al. An epidemiological study of REM latency and psychiatric disorders. J Affect Disord 1991;23(3):107–12.
59. Ramsawh HJ, Bomyea J, Stein MB, et al. Sleep quality improvement during cognitive behavioral therapy for anxiety disorders. Behav Sleep Med 2016;14(3):267–78.
60. Zalta AK, Dowd S, Rosenfield D, et al. Sleep quality predicts treatment outcome in CBT for social anxiety disorder. Depress Anxiety 2013;30(11): 1114–20.
61. Belleville G, Potočnik A. A meta-analysis of sleep disturbances in panic disorder., . Psychopathology: An international and interdisciplinary perspective. IntechOpen; 2019. https://doi.org/10.5772/intechopen.86306.
62. Pires GN, Bezerra AG, Tufik S, et al. Effects of acute sleep deprivation on state anxiety levels: a systematic review and meta-analysis. Sleep Med 2016;24:109–18.
63. Morphy H, Dunn KM, Lewis M, et al. Epidemiology of insomnia: a longitudinal study in a UK population. Sleep 2007;30(3):274–80.
64. Jansson-Fröjmark M, Lindblom K. A bidirectional relationship between anxiety and depression, and insomnia? A prospective study in the general population. J Psychosom Res 2008;64(4):443–9.
65. Johnson EO, Roth T, Breslau N. The association of insomnia with anxiety disorders and depression: exploration of the direction of risk. J Psychiatr Res 2006;40(8):700–8.
66. Ohayon MM, Shapiro CM. Sleep disturbances and psychiatric disorders associated with posttraumatic stress disorder in the general population. Compr Psychiatry 2000;41:469–78.
67. Straus LD, Drummond SPA, Nappi CM, et al. Sleep variability in military-related PTSD: a comparison to primary insomnia and healthy controls. J Trauma Stress 2015;28:8–16.
68. Wild J, Smith KV, Thompson E, et al. A prospective study of pre-trauma risk factors for post-traumatic stress disorder and depression. Psychol Med 2016;46:2571–82.
69. Armour C, Elklit A, Lauterbach D, et al. The DSM-5 dissociative-PTSD subtype: can levels of depression, anxiety, hostility, and sleeping difficulties differentiate between dissociative-PTSD and

PTSD in rape and sexual assault victims? J Anxiety Disord 2014;28:418–26.
70. Hall Brown TS, Akeeb A, Mellman TA. The role of trauma type in the risk for insomnia. J Clin Sleep Med 2015;11(7):735–9.
71. Graham J, Legarreta M, North L, et al. A preliminary study of DSM-5 PTSD symptom patterns in veterans by trauma type. Mil Psychol 2016; 28(2):115–22.
72. van Wyk M, Thomas KG, Solms M, et al. Prominence of hyperarousal symptoms explains variability of sleep disruption in posttraumatic stress disorder. Psychol Trauma 2016;8(6):688–96.
73. Zhang Y, Ren R, Sanford LD, et al. Sleep in posttraumatic stress disorder: a systematic review and meta-analysis of polysomnographic findings. Sleep Med Rev 2019;48:101210.
74. van Liempt S, Vermetten E, Lentjes E, et al. Decreased nocturnal growth hormone secretion and sleep fragmentation in combat-related posttraumatic stress disorder: potential predictors of impaired memory consolidation. Psychoneuroendocrinology 2011;36:1361–9.
75. van Liempt S, van Zuiden M, Westenberg H, et al. Impact of impaired sleep on the development of PTSD symptoms in combat veterans: a prospective longitudinal cohort study. Depress Anxiety 2013; 30:469–74.
76. Cohen DJ, Begley A, Alman JJ, et al. Quantitative electroencephalography during rapid eye movement (REM) and non-REM sleep in combat-exposed veterans with and without post-traumatic stress disorder. J Sleep Res 2013;22:76–82.
77. Dietch JR, Ruggero CJ, Schuler K, et al. Posttraumatic stress disorder symptoms and sleep in the daily lives of world trade center responders. J Occup Health Psychol 2019;24(6):689–702.
78. Biggs QM, Ursano RJ, Wang J, et al. Post traumatic stress symptom variation associated with sleep characteristics. BMC Psychiatry 2020;20:174.
79. Hall Brown T, Mellman TA, Alfano CA, et al. Sleep fears, sleep disturbance, and PTSD symptoms in minority youth exposed to Hurricane Katrina. J Trauma Stress 2011;24(5):575–80.
80. Fan F, Zhou Y, Liu X. Sleep disturbance predicts posttraumatic stress disorder and depressive symptoms: a cohort study of Chinese adolescents. J Clin Psychiatry 2017;78(7):882–8.
81. Acheson DT, Kwan B, Maihofer AX, et al. Sleep disturbance at pre-deployment is a significant predictor of post-deployment re-experiencing symptoms. Eur J Psychotraumatol 2019;10:1679964.
82. Koffel E, Polusny MA, Arbisi PA, et al. Pre-deployment daytime and nighttime sleep complaints as predictors of postdeployment PTSD and depression in National Guard troops. J Anxiety Disord 2013;27:512–9.
83. Gehrman P, Seelig AD, Jacobson, et al. Predeployment sleep duration and insomnia symptoms as risk factors for new-onset mental health disorders following military deployment. Sleep 2013;36(7): 1009–18.
84. Pigeon WR, Campbell CE, Possemato K, et al. Longitudinal relationships of insomnia, nightmares, and PTSD severity in recent combat veterans. J Psychosom Res 2013;75:546–50.
85. Wright KM, Britt TW, Bliese PD, et al. Insomnia as predictor versus outcome of PTSD and depression among Iraq combat veterans. J Clin Psychol 2011; 67:1240–58.
86. Rosen RC, Cikesh B, Fang S, et al. Posttraumatic stress disorder severity and insomnia-related sleep disturbance: longitudinal associations in a large, gender-based cohort of combat-exposed veterans. J Trauma Stress 2019;32(6):936–45.
87. Harvey AG, Murray G, Chandler RA, et al. Sleep disturbance as transdiagnostic: consideration of neurobiological mechanisms. Clin Psychol Rev 2011;31(2):225–35.
88. Pandi-Perumal SR, Monti JM, Burman D, et al. Clarifying the role of sleep in depression: a narrative review. Psychiatry Res 2020;291:113239.
89. Fang H, Tu S, Sheng J, et al. Depression in sleep disturbance: a review on a bidirectional relationship, mechanisms and treatment. J Cell Mol Med 2019;23(4):2324–32.
90. Richards A, Kanady JC, Neylan TC. Sleep disturbance in PTSD and other anxiety-related disorders: an updated review of clinical features, physiological characteristics, and psychological and neurobiological mechanisms. Neuropsychopharmacology 2020;45:55–73.
91. Palmer CA, Alfano CA. Sleep and emotion regulation: an organizing, integrative review. Sleep Med Rev 2017;31:6–16.
92. Gruber R, Cassoff J. The interplay between sleep and emotion regulation: conceptual framework empirical evidence and future directions. Curr Psychiatry Rep 2014;16(11):500.
93. Harvey AG. Identifying safety behaviors in insomnia. J Nerv Ment Dis 2002;190:16e21.
94. Hood HK, Carney CE, Harris AL. Rethinking safety behaviors in insomnia: examining the perceived utility of sleep-related safety behaviors. Behav Ther 2011;42(4):644–54.
95. Boland EM, Vittengl JR, Clark LA, et al. Is sleep disturbance linked to short- and long-term outcomes following treatments for recurrent depression? J Affect Disord 2020;262:323–32.
96. Taylor DJ, Walters HM, Vittengl JR, et al. Which depressive symptoms remain after response to cognitive therapy of depression and predict relapse and recurrence? J Affect Disord 2010; 123(1–3):181–7.

97. Schennach R, Feige B, Riemann D, et al. Pre- to post-inpatient treatment of subjective sleep quality in 5,481 patients with mental disorders: a longitudinal analysis. J Sleep Res 2019;28:e12842.
98. Thase ME, Fasiczka AL, Berman SR, et al. Electroencephalographic sleep profiles before and after cognitive behavior therapy of depression. Arch Gen Psychiatry 1998;55(2):138–44.
99. Troxel WM, Kupfer DJ, Reynolds CF 3rd, et al. Insomnia and objectively measured sleep disturbances predict treatment outcome in depressed patients treated with psychotherapy or psychotherapy-pharmacotherapy combinations. J Clin Psychiatry 2012;73(4):478–85.
100. Cho HJ, Lavretsky H, Olmstead R, et al. Sleep disturbance and depression recurrence in community-dwelling older adults: a prospective study. Am J Psychiatry 2008;165(12):1543–50.
101. Perlis ML, Giles DE, Buysee DJ, et al. Self-reported sleep disturbance as a prodormal symptom in recurrent depression. J Affect Disord 1997;42:209–12.
102. Inada K, Enomoto M, KYamato K, et al. Effect of residual insomnia and use of hypnotics on relapse of depression: a retrospective cohort study using a health insurance claims database. J Affect Disord 2021;281:539–46.
103. Nierenberg AA, Husain MM, Trivedi MH, et al. Residual symptoms after remission of major depressive disorder with citalopram and risk of relapse: a STAR*D report. Psychol Med 2010;40(1):41–50.
104. Gruber SA, Rogowska J, Yurgelun-Todd DA. Decreased activation of the anterior cingulate in bipolar patients: an fMRI study. J Affect Disord 2004;82:191–201.
105. Cretu JB, Culver JL, Goffin KC, et al. Sleep, residual mood symptoms, and time to relapse in recovered patients with bipolar disorder. J Affect Disord 2016;190:162–6.
106. Gershon A, Do D, Satyanarayana S, et al. Abnormal sleep duration associated with hastened depressive recurrence in bipolar disorder. J Affect Disord 2017;218:374–9.
107. Nowlin-Finch NL, Altshuler LL, Szuba MP, et al. Rapid resolution of first episodes of mania: sleep related? J Clin Psychiatry 1994;55:26–9.
108. Sylvia LG, Chang WC, Kamali M, et al. Sleep disturbance may impact treatment outcome in bipolar disorder: a preliminary investigation in the context of a large comparative effectiveness trial. J Affect Disord 2018;225:563–8.
109. Sylvia LG, Salcedo S, Peters AT, et al. Do sleep disturbances predict or moderate the response to psychotherapy in bipolar disorder? J Nerv Ment Dis 2017;205:196–202.
110. Kaplan KA. Sleep and sleep treatments in bipolar disorder. Curr Opin Psychol 2020;34:117–22.
111. Belleville G, Cousineau H, Levrier K, et al. The impact of cognitive-behavior therapy for anxiety disorders on concomitant sleep disturbances: a meta-analysis. J Anxiety Disord 2010;24(4):379–86.
112. Cervena K, Matousek M, Prasko J, et al. Sleep disturbances in patients treated for panic disorder. Sleep Med 2005;6(2):149–53.
113. Bush AL, Armento ME, Weiss BJ, et al. The pittsburgh sleep quality index in older primary care patients with generalized anxiety disorder: psychometrics and outcomes following cognitive behavioral therapy. Psychiatry Res 2012;199(1):24–30.
114. Pace-Schott EF, Germain A, Milad MR. Effects of sleep on memory for conditioned fear and fear extinction. Psychol Bull 2015;141(4):835–57.
115. Colvonen PJ, Straus LD, Acheson D, et al. A review of the relationship between emotional learning and memory, sleep, and PTSD. Curr Psychiatry Rep 2019;21(1):2.
116. Galovski TE, Harik JM, Blain LM, et al. Augmenting cognitive processing therapy to improve sleep impairment in PTSD: a randomized controlled trial. J Couns Psychol 2016;84(2):167–77.
117. Colvonen PJ, Straus LD, Stepnowsky C, et al. Recent advancements in treating sleep disorders in co-occurring PTSD. Curr Psychiatry Rep 2018;20(7):48.
118. Belleville G, Guay S, Marchand A. Persistence of sleep disturbances following cognitive-behavior therapy for posttraumatic stress disorder. J Psychosom Res 2011;7(4):318–27.
119. Pruiksma KE, Taylor DJ, Wachen JS, et al. Residual sleep disturbances following PTSD treatment in active duty military personnel. Psychol Trauma 2016;8(6):697–701.
120. Brownlow JA, McLean CP, Gehrman PR, et al. Influence of sleep disturbance on global functioning after posttraumatic stress disorder treatment. J Trauma Stress 2016;29(6):515–21.
121. Ballesio A, Aquino MRJV, Feige B, et al. The effectiveness of behavioural and cognitive behavioural therapies for insomnia on depressive and fatigue symptoms: a systematic review and network meta-analysis. Sleep Med Rev 2018;37:114–29.
122. Gebara MA, Siripong N, DiNapoli EA, et al. Effect of insomnia treatments on depression: a systematic review and meta-analysis. Depress Anxiety 2018;35(8):717–31.
123. Blom K, Jernelöv S, Kraepelien M, et al. Internet treatment addressing either insomnia or depression, for patients with both diagnoses: a randomized trial. Sleep 2015;38:267–77.
124. Manber R, Edinger JD, Gress JL, et al. Cognitive behavioral therapy for insomnia enhances depression outcome in patients with comorbid major

depressive disorder and insomnia. Sleep 2008; 31(4):489–95.

125. Manber R, Buysse DJ, Edinger J, et al. Efficacy of cognitive-behavioral therapy for insomnia combined with antidepressant pharmacotherapy in patients with comorbid depression and insomnia: a randomized controlled trial. J Clin Psychiatry 2016;77:e1316–23.

126. Bei B, Asarnow LD, Krystal A, et al. Treating insomnia in depression: insomnia related factors predict long-term depression trajectories. J Consult Clin Psychol 2018;86(3):282–93.

127. Norell-Clarke A, Tillfors M, Jansson-Fröjmark M, et al. Does mid-treatment insomnia severity mediate between cognitive behavioural therapy for insomnia and post-treatment depression? An investigation in a sample with comorbid insomnia and depressive symptomatology. Behav Cogn Psychother 2018;46(6):726–37.

128. Christensen H, Batterham PJ, Gosling JA, et al. Effectiveness of an online insomnia program (SHUTi) for prevention of depressive episodes (the GoodNight Study): a randomised controlled trial. Lancet Psychiatry 2016;3(4):333–41.

129. Harvey AG, Soehner AM, Kaplan KA, et al. Treating insomnia improves mood state, sleep, and functioning in bipolar disorder: a pilot randomized controlled trial. J Consult Clin Psychol 2015;83(3): 564–77.

130. Belleville G, Cousineau H, Levrier K, et al. Meta-analytic review of the impact of cognitive-behavior therapy for insomnia on concomitant anxiety. Clin Psychol Rev 2011;31(4):638–52.

131. Stewart RE, Chambless DL. Cognitive-behavioral therapy for adult anxiety disorders in clinical practice: a meta-analysis of effectiveness studies. J Consult Clin Psychol 2009;77(4):595–606.

132. Ye YY, Zhang YF, Chen J, et al. Internet-based cognitive behavioral therapy for insomnia (ICBT-i) improves comorbid anxiety and depression: a meta-analysis of randomized controlled trials. PLoS One 2015;10(11):e0142258.

133. Margolies SO, Rybarczyk B, Vrana SR, et al. Efficacy of a cognitive-behavioral treatment for insomnia and nightmares in Afghanistan and Iraq veterans with PTSD. J Clin Psychol 2013;69(10): 1026–42.

134. Talbot LS, Maguen S, Metzler TJ, et al. Cognitive behavioral therapy for insomnia in posttraumatic stress disorder: a randomized controlled trial. Sleep 2014;37(2):327–41.

135. Goodson J, Helstrom A, Halpern JM, et al. Treatment of posttraumatic stress disorder in US combat veterans: a meta-analytic review. Psychol Rep 2011;109:573–99.

136. Sloan DM, Feinstein BA, Gallagher MW, et al. Efficacy of group treatment for posttraumatic stress disorder symptoms: a meta-analysis. Psychol Trauma 2013;5:176–83.

137. Powers MB, Halpern JM, Ferenschak MP, et al. A meta-analytic review of prolonged exposure for posttraumatic stress disorder. Clin Psychol Rev 2010;30:635–41.

138. Casement MD, Swanson LM. A meta-analysis of imagery rehearsal for post-trauma nightmares: effects on nightmare frequency, sleep quality, and posttraumatic stress. Clin Psychol Rev 2012; 32(6):566–74.

139. Levrier K, Leathead C, Bourdon DE, et al. The impact of cognitive-behavioral therapies for nightmares and prazosin on the reduction of post-traumatic nightmares, sleep, and PTSD symptoms: a systematic review and meta-analysis of randomized and non-randomized studies. In: El-Baalbaki G, Fortin C, editors. A multidimensional approach to post-traumatic stress disorder – from theory to practice. In tech; 2016.

140. Yücel DE, van Emmerik AAP, Souama C, et al. Comparative efficacy of imagery rehearsal therapy and prazosin in the treatment of trauma-related nightmares in adults: a meta-analysis of randomized controlled trials. Sleep Med Rev 2020;50: 101248.

141. Colvonen PJ, Drummond SPA, Angkaw AC, et al. Piloting cognitive-behavioral therapy for insomnia integrated with prolonged exposure. Psychol Trauma 2019;11(1):107–13.

Sleep Deficiency and Cardiometabolic Disease

Roo Killick, MBBS, FRACP, PhD[a], Lachlan Stranks, MBBS[a,b], Camilla M. Hoyos, MPH, PhD[a,c,*]

KEYWORDS

• Sleep restriction • Sleep deprivation • Cardiovascular disease • Cardiometabolic outcomes • Metabolic health

KEY POINTS

- Short sleep duration has been associated with many negative cardiometabolic outcomes including mortality, coronary heart disease, and type 2 diabetes mellitus.
- Many underlying pathways have been proposed to link sleep deficiency and cardiometabolic dysfunction including oxidative stress, inflammation, endothelial dysfunction, and insulin resistance, which have been investigated in animal models and experimental human studies.
- Early evidence on whether sleep extension could reduce cardio-metabolic impacts of habitual sleep restriction is inconsistent and strategies on the implementation of such interventions still need to be developed.

INTRODUCTION

Sleep is a basic human need and lack of sleep disrupts many physiologic processes and health outcomes. Sleep loss has long been established to have widespread detrimental effects, with the earliest sleep deprivation experiments in rodents showing that the animals could not survive extreme durations of sleep deprivation, likely due to disturbances in cardiometabolic and immunologic control.[1] The National Sleep Foundation's most recent recommendations suggest that the ideal nightly duration of sleep for adults is between 7 and 9 h/night.[2] To date there have been numerous publications, suggesting that globally humans are sleeping less than previously, with a higher proportion of modern society curtailing their sleep due to various societal pressures.[3–5] Some have disputed this data due to discrepancies in how subjective sleep duration is assessed and the potential lack of correlation with objective sleep measurements.[6] Despite this, there is ample evidence, both experimental and at a population level, implicating sleep loss as a risk factor for negative cardiometabolic outcomes.[7,8] In this review we will summarize the main adverse cardiometabolic effects associated with sleep loss and discuss the mechanisms that are implicated within this relationship. For many of the outcomes, U-shaped relationships with sleep duration have been described; however, the associations with long sleep duration are outside the focus of this review. Furthermore, we will provide an overview of interventional studies examining the effect of short-term sleep extension on a variety of cardiometabolic outcomes.

CLINICAL OUTCOMES

Mortality, Cardiovascular Mortality, and Coronary Artery Disease

The association between sleep duration and overall mortality was first reported nearly 60 years ago[9] and has been confirmed in differing populations since that time, including various recent meta-analyses and systematic reviews of the ever-

[a] Centre for Sleep and Chronobiology, Woolcock Institute of Medical Research, University of Sydney, Sydney, Australia; [b] The University of Adelaide, Faculty of Health and Medical Sciences, Adelaide, Australia; [c] The University of Sydney, Faculty of Science, School of Psychology and Brain and Mind Centre, Sydney, Australia
* Corresponding author. Woolcock Institute of Medical Research, PO Box M77, Missenden Road, New South Wales 2050, Australia.
E-mail address: camilla.hoyos@sydney.edu.au

Clin Chest Med 43 (2022) 319–336
https://doi.org/10.1016/j.ccm.2022.02.011

growing literature in this area.[10–26] Many of these studies report a U-shaped relationship with sleep duration, and we will focus on the evidence that exists for short sleep duration for the purposes of this review. The associations with longer sleep duration could represent other pathophysiology, depending on the age and comorbidities of the population under investigation. Reports even suggest a gender difference in some of these relationships. Nonetheless most use 7 h/night as the reference point of so-called healthy sleep duration.

Coronary artery disease (CAD) is a significant cause of morbidity and mortality worldwide, and prevalence continues to rise.[27] Abnormal sleep duration has been identified as a risk factor for developing CAD in multiple epidemiologic studies,[28–30] and the U-shaped relationship once again is demonstrated in many, implicating both short and long sleep duration.[31–37] As an example of such data, a meta-analysis of 15 studies comprising 474,684 participants, demonstrated short sleep duration, defined as ≤5 to 6 h/night, was associated with an increased risk of developing or dying from CAD (relative risk (RR): 1.48, 95% confidence interval (CI): 1.22 to 1.80).[34] A prospective study of 60,586 Taiwanese adults similarly demonstrated that subjective sleep duration of less than 6 h/night significantly increased the risk of CAD in adults 40 years of age or older (hazards ratio (HR): 1.13, 95% CI: 1.04 to 1.23).[35] Interestingly, this study showed that individuals with subjective poor sleep quality were also at a higher risk of CAD compared with those who felt they had good quality sleep.[35] This finding is reflected in other work which demonstrated the risk of CAD was in fact highest in those with both short sleep duration and concurrent sleep disturbance (RR: 1.55, 95% CI: 1.33–1.81), with the risk being lower in people reporting only one of these anomalies.[36] It has been suggested that the higher incidence of type 2 diabetes mellitus found prospectively among short and long sleepers was one of, if not the primary, factor driving the paralleled increased risk of CAD in those with subjective short (<6 h/night) and long (>9 h/night) sleep duration in a cohort of 16,344 middle-aged men and women in the Malmö Diet Cancer Study followed for 14 to 16 years.[37] Diabetes is certainly an established risk factor for CAD; however, there are likely multiple pathophysiological mechanisms responsible for this positive association to which sleep restriction contributes. There is also an association between short sleep duration and risk of cardiac arrhythmias. In particular, the risk of atrial fibrillation has been shown to be higher in short sleepers in pooled observation studies.[38–41]

Hypertension

Sleep is associated with various physiologic alterations, including blood pressure control. Blood pressure is regulated through multiple mechanisms, including peripheral vascular resistance, cardiac contractility, and cardiac output. These mechanisms are largely regulated by the autonomic nervous system with 24h hemodynamic oscillations a result of fluctuating sympathetic and parasympathetic output.[42] During normal sleep, it is expected blood pressure will fall by at least 10% from daytime wake levels, a phenomenon referred to as the "nocturnal dip."[43,44] A pertinent finding in persistent short sleepers is the attenuation of this nocturnal blood pressure decline, and in turn increased daytime blood pressure.[43] As a result, there is increasing evidence, indicating that the blunting of the nocturnal blood pressure dip is associated with increased overall cardiovascular morbidity and mortality.[45] There are multiple physiologic processes likely responsible for this phenomenon, including increased sympathetic activity, increased catecholamine release,[46] an altered inflammatory response[44] and deranged circadian rhythm[47] which in turn could lead to increased daytime blood pressure.

Epidemiologic studies in well-established cohorts have demonstrated a relationship between short sleep duration and a higher prevalence of hypertension.[28,48–57] Some studies reported that the association between short sleep duration and hypertension was more pronounced in women and variable among different age groups. Results from the long-established, large Whitehall II cohort indicated only women were at higher risk of hypertension as a result of sleep deficiency, while no obvious pattern could be established in male subjects, when looking at cross-sectional analyses at the 12 to 14 year (phase 5) follow-up.[54] This finding was also reflected in a cohort of 3027 subjects in the Western New York Health Study showing women sleeping less than 6 h/night were at the highest risk of hypertension, with the effect being strongest in premenopausal women.[58] Interestingly, there may be a dose-dependent relationship between sleep duration and hypertension risk, with a shorter sleep duration more strongly associated with hypertension.[56] For instance, data from the Whitehall II study in their 5 year prospective analysis found those sleeping 6 h/night at 1.6 times (odds ratio (OR): 1.56 95% CI: 1.07–2.27), and those sleeping less than 5 h/night at nearly 2 times (OR: 1.94 95% CI: 1.08–3.50) greater risk of developing hypertension compared with those sleeping 7 h/night.[54]

A meta-analysis of 6 prospective and 17 cross-sectional studies confirmed the increased prevalence of hypertension (OR: 1.20, 95% CI: 1.09–1.32) with short sleep duration, especially in women and in subjects less than 65 years old.[52] As the collective data have grown in the past decade, further meta-analyses have been performed confirming that the relationship of short sleep duration holds with both prevalence and incidence of hypertension;[56,57,59] however, caution has been drawn to methodology when pooling results with regard to confounders and definitions of sleep duration cut-offs.[60]

Cerebrovascular Disease

Stroke is a significant cause of global morbidity and mortality. Numerous studies have investigated the relationship between short sleep duration and incidence of cerebrovascular disease.[28,61] For instance, results from a cohort of 266,848 Australian adults indicated a significantly increased risk of stroke in individuals sleeping less than 6 h/night (OR: 1.70, 95% CI: 1.50–1.92), compared with 7 h/night.[28] A recent meta-analysis of 20 studies assessing altered sleep duration and stroke risk demonstrated the lowest risk of stroke with a sleep duration of 6 to 7 h/night, and subsequent pooled relative risk of stroke of 1.05 (95% CI: 1.01–1.09) for every hour reduction of sleep beyond this.[62] This parallels a previous meta-analysis showing a J-shaped relationship between sleep duration and stroke or stroke mortality, with an increased relative risk of stroke events of 1.07 (95% CI: 1.02–1.12) for each hour reduction below 7 h/night. Interestingly, longer sleep duration was associated with a higher risk of stroke mortality, which may have different pathophysiologies in regard to those with significant illness and comorbidities.[63]

Obesity and Metabolic Syndrome

Sleep loss and its relationship with obesity have been long established, with ample epidemiologic data, suggesting that shorter sleepers have an increased risk of obesity across all age groups,[64–69] although there are likely differences between ethnicities.[70,71] A recent meta-analysis of prospective cohort studies found a reverse J-shape relationship with sleep duration; with a 9% increased risk of obesity seen for every hour reduction in sleep from 7 h/night.[72] Importantly with the growing obesity epidemic[73,74] and ever-increasing obesity rates,[75] there is particular interest in children and adolescences,[76,77] hoping that sleep could be a modifiable risk factor in the development of obesity. A systematic review and meta-analysis of prospective longitudinal data in children from infancy to adolescence found the association held firm across all age groups.[78] There was also an inverse relationship between sleep duration and change in BMI over time.[78] More specifically another meta-analysis examined this exclusively in preschool children and again found a robust relationship between short sleep and the risk of developing obesity (RR: 1.54; 95% CI: 1.33–1.77) in 42,878 children across 13 studies). Furthermore in 4 out of 5 intervention studies analyzed, improved outcomes were seen with sleep extension.[79]

When exploring the components that would lead to the development of an increased cardiovascular risk profile, aside from obesity alone, sound epidemiologic data of over 45 studies have shown a relationship between short sleep and the incidence of the metabolic syndrome, a collection of cardiometabolic markers including blood pressure, waist circumference, lipid and glucose parameters.[80,81] For instance the Quebec Family Study, a cross-sectional study of 810 adults, found short sleepers (<6 h/night) had an increased risk of metabolic syndrome (OR: 1.76, 95% CI: 1.08–2.84) compared with 7–8 h/night after adjustment for various confounders.[82] This relationship was also confirmed in the large NHANES surveys.[83] Other data have reiterated this finding that men seem to be at higher risk than women in some domains,[84] whereas some have only found this relationship in extreme short sleepers (<4 h/night).[85] A study examined children and adolescents with similar results,[86] and data looking across all ages have suggested heterogeneity across differing age groups.[87] Bringing these examples and the wealth of similar literature together, a recent meta-analysis of both 36 cross-sectional and 9 longitudinal studies (n = 164,799 subjects and 430,895 controls) confirmed the relationship, in both prevalence (OR: 1.11, 95% CI: 1.05–1.18) and incidence (RR: 1.16, 95% CI: 1.05–1.23) of metabolic syndrome.[88] This review followed many similar meta-analyses,[89–92] which reflects the scientific interest in this subject, reinforcing the significant risk of cardiometabolic disease and the global importance to find ways to reduce its mortality and morbidity.

Diabetes Mellitus and Insulin Resistance

Similar data exist when exploring the incidence of type 2 diabetes mellitus and short sleep duration. Once again, the field is abloom with meta-analyses in the past decade illustrating this relationship, examining cross-sectional and prospective datasets across multiple population groups,[93–97] and furthermore looking specifically at glycemic control.[98] Type 2 diabetes has had much of the attention, but there is also a relationship between short sleep duration and glycemic control in type 1 diabetes,[99,100] with a meta-analysis describing 22 studies showing that children with type 1 diabetes had subjective shorter sleep than controls without diabetes.[100] In adults, although subjective sleep duration was not different between subjects and controls, there was better glycemic control (as determined by lower HbA1C levels) in those who slept >6 h/night compared with <6 h/night. There was also a higher incidence of poor sleep quality reported in those with higher HbA1C levels and a higher incidence of OSA.[100] Furthermore, the relationship with sleep duration has also been demonstrated in meta-analyses looking at gestational diabetes.[101,102]

PATHWAYS AND EXPERIMENTAL DATA

In this section, some of the proposed mechanistic pathways that may contribute toward the associations between short sleep duration and poor cardiometabolic outcomes will be explored. These include endothelial dysfunction, oxidative stress, and inflammatory pathways. Much of this cellular evidence has been performed in animal models; however, experimental trials in humans under tightly controlled sleep conditions have provided specific associations between sleep and metabolic outcomes and these will also be reviewed.

Endothelial Dysfunction

There is increasing evidence linking sleep deprivation with endothelial dysfunction, a known risk factor for cardiovascular disease.[103] Impairment of endothelium-dependent vasodilation is the hallmark of endothelial dysfunction, and while its pathogenesis in sleep restriction is likely multifactorial, sympathetic activation and reduced bioavailability of nitric oxide are likely critical. Animal studies have demonstrated that persistent sleep fragmentation in mice results in endothelial dysfunction and structural vascular change.[104] Doppler flow through the dorsal tail vein of mice was observed to alter after 8 to 9 weeks of persistent sleep disturbance, with reduction in peak blood flow from baseline, and increased duration of postocclusive hyperemic changes. Histologically, significant aortic structural changes were also found with elastic fiber disruption and disorganization, and immune cell infiltration, without significant change in wall thickness.[104] Experimental studies of sleep restriction in humans have also demonstrated impairment in markers of endothelial function mostly measured by flow-mediated brachial artery vasodilation (FMD).[105–107]

Oxidative Stress

Oxidative stress occurs when pro-oxidative pathways saturate antioxidant systems, resulting in an increased production of damaging reactive oxygen species (ROS). When this imbalance between these 2 systems generates an excess of these free radicals, a cascade of pro-inflammatory pathways can be initiated, leading to cellular damage and, over time, inflammation and subsequently, disease states can ensue. One proposed function of sleep is to remove ROS from the brain and other organs, and thus protect against oxidative injury.[108] Hence, sleep restriction may allow the accumulation of ROS and predispose to cellular injury.[109]

Experimental studies in this area are mostly described in animal models, as they are difficult to perform in humans. A meta-analysis of 44 animal studies supports that experimental sleep restriction in rodents promotes oxidative stress.[110] Furthermore, data demonstrate that sleep deprivation results in intestinal ROS accumulation in both flies and mice and may result in early mortality. It was suggested that this could be a consequence of alterations in the gut microbiota and modulation of gut immunity, disorders of which are also becoming increasingly implicated in human disease states.[111]

Studies in humans have similarly explored whether sleep deprivation contributes to the production of markers of oxidative stress, with some of the literature in this area performed in the context of intense physical activity. A study of 23 male students showed that after 36h of survival training, levels of lipid hydroperoxides and creatine kinase were elevated, but subsequently recovered after a single 12h period (only incorporating 7.5 h available sleep time).[112] In contrast, in a subsequent study of 15 soldiers who completed 48h of military survival training incorporating sleep deprivation (total sleep deprivation within first 24h and 3h sleep maximum in second 24h) showed reduced levels of glutathione peroxidase activity (that is reduced antioxidant activity), but no changes in the activity of other biochemical markers of oxidative stress, including lipid hydroperoxides, creatine kinase, and superoxide dismutase.[113]

Arrhythmogenicity

Experimental studies have also attempted to investigate the relationship between sleep duration, cardiac function, and arrhythmias. In a study of 27 healthy young adults subjected to acute sleep deprivation, echocardiographic assessment demonstrated reduced left atrial early diastolic strain rate,[114] suggesting that chronic sleep deprivation may produce more permanent alterations in the left atrium, and so predispose to atrial fibrillation and other atrial tachyarrhythmias.[114] Similarly, one night of sleep deprivation in healthy young individuals was associated with the prolongation of the QT interval, a phenomenon associated with higher risk of sudden cardiac death and ventricular tachyarrhythmias.[115] Intervention studies in humans have looked at cardiac autonomic changes with sleep deprivation. Sixty subjects had continuous ambulatory electrocardiogram monitoring and underwent 24h total sleep deprivation.[116] Significantly lower vagal activity and elevated sympathetic activity were found using heart rate variability, which improved after treatment with metoprolol. Furthermore, a randomized, placebo-controlled study of 72 healthy, young participants examined the effect of a statin on heart rate variability (as a marker of cardiac autonomic control) using a well-controlled in-laboratory study of 48h of total sleep deprivation. The addition of a statin led to a significant decrease in premature atrial and ventricular complexes, hence the authors promoted the concept of possible preventative cardiovascular treatment of those individuals at risk of sleep deprivation.[117]

Metabolomics and Transcriptomics

At a molecular level, there is much interest in the interaction between oxidative stress, metabolic markers, clock genes, and subsequent dysregulation by sleep loss. To attempt to understand the molecular mechanisms between sleep loss and metabolic dysregulation, studies have conducted metabolite profiling in the context of sleep loss to elucidate any markers of interest. In the first study which examined 12 healthy young male subjects undergoing 24h of total sleep deprivation, 27 out of a total of 171 metabolites had increased levels in the context of sleep loss, with 78 (out of 109) showing decreased amplitude in their circadian rhythmicity.[118] In a study investigating sleep restriction as opposed to total sleep deprivation, 2 metabolites (oxalic acid and diacylglycerol 36:3) were reduced following sleep restriction and restored following recovery in both rats and humans, suggesting a potential use as biomarkers of oxidative stress during sleep loss. Furthermore, higher levels of phospholipids were seen in both rodents and humans in this study, providing evidence of an oxidative environment.[119]

A landmark paper provided a comprehensive analysis of the effect of sleep loss on the human transcriptome.[120] Blood RNA samples were examined from 26 participants before and after a week of partial sleep deprivation (5.7 h/night (experimental arm) v 8.5 h/night (control arm)). This showed that an impressive 711 genes were up- or down-regulated by sleep loss, and these genes were associated with circadian rhythm, sleep homeostasis, metabolism, and oxidative stress, providing evidence that there are close relationships between all these circadian and physiologic processes.[120]

Inflammatory pathways

Various inflammatory pathways are upregulated in response to sleep deprivation, with effects on proinflammatory gene expression and increased levels of circulating inflammatory mediators.[121] Atherosclerosis is acknowledged as an inflammatory condition driven by circulating lipids and leukocytes and is a critical pathologic mechanism behind myocardial infarction and cerebrovascular disease through the formation of unstable arterial plaques.[122] Leukocytosis is a recognized predictor of cardiovascular events through white blood cells' role in the formation of these arterial lesions.[123]

A study demonstrated the relationship between sleep restriction and accelerated atherosclerosis in a population of mice predisposed to atherosclerotic disease. Compared with control mice, sleep-deprived mice were found to have more severe and extensive atherosclerotic disease despite no differences in body weight, glucose tolerance, or plasma cholesterol, but with higher levels of circulating leukocytes, particularly atherosclerosis-forming monocytes. Interestingly, reduced levels of hypocretin, the wakefulness-promoting protein, were found. This neuropeptide normally inhibits and regulates the release of colony-stimulating factor-1 (CSF-1) from neutrophil precursors, thus its deficiency results in increased production of CSF-1, and subsequently leukocytosis from the bone marrow.[124] Genetically altered mice who were unable to produce hypocretin similarly demonstrated more severe atherosclerosis, with reversal of this phenomenon following hypocretin administration, thus it was postulated sleep restriction results in signaling to the bone marrow to increase white blood cell production, ultimately damaging blood vessels.[124]

Increasing carotid intima-media thickness (CIMT) is a marker for subclinical coronary atherosclerosis and predictor of cardiac and cerebrovascular events in humans, given it reflects arterial inflammation.[125] In an observational cohort of

617 middle-aged adults, shorter sleep duration, measured objectively by actigraphy, was associated with increased CIMT in men but not women.[125] A subsequent systematic review explored the association between subjectively and objectively measured sleep duration and subclinical measures of cardiovascular disease including coronary artery calcium, carotid intima-media thickness, arterial stiffness, and endothelial dysfunction.[126] The association between short sleep duration (both subjective and objective) with CIMT had been consistently reported; however, the association with other surrogate markers was variable. The authors concluded, however, that despite the mixed results between the surrogate markers, there is a relationship between sleep duration at both extremes and subclinical cardiovascular burden.[126]

Small experimental human studies have investigated the relationship between partial sleep deprivation and circulating markers of inflammation and have demonstrated increased upstream proinflammatory activity and signaling in sleep restriction.[121,127] Conversely, a recent meta-analysis did not demonstrate an association between short sleep duration (<7 h/night) and elevated downstream systemic inflammatory markers, including C-reactive protein (CRP) and interleukin-6 (IL-6), suggesting that other mechanisms may also be contributing, or longer-term sleep restriction is required to demonstrate an elevation in measurable levels of proinflammatory markers.[128]

Insulin resistance, energy expenditure, weight gain

Several mechanisms to explain the relationship between short sleep duration, obesity and diabetes have been proposed, including higher calorific intake due to increased time awake, differences in energy expenditure, differences in eating behaviors, or changes in metabolic markers leading to cardiometabolic derangement. To investigate these mechanisms individually requires experimental studies with a high level of control of confounders. This ultimately translates to small, expensive to run, mainly in-laboratory studies, with strict sleep and environmental conditions.

A landmark paper was the first to establish that experimental sleep restriction led to reduced glucose tolerance in 11 healthy men sleep restricted to 4 h/night over 6 nights compared with post 6 nights of recovery sleep of 12 h/night.[129] As then many have replicated these findings, using different protocols and durations of sleep restriction,[130–137] which we and others have previously reviewed.[66,138,139] Data from our group explored whether this effect was also seen in those individuals who catch-up on sleep at weekends and self-restrict during the working week, which is a prevalent sleep pattern in modern society.[140] Indeed, a similar reduction in insulin sensitivity was seen after extended partial sleep restriction compared with a weekend of sleep extension.[140]

Energy expenditure has also been examined under certain conditions to see whether that would explain the association of short sleep with weight gain. One such study under strict conditions in 16 individuals showed that after 5 days of sleep restriction, although energy expenditure increased by 5%, energy intake increased in excess of this leading to a positive energy balance and weight gain, particularly in women.[141] A study which measured energy expenditure by whole room calorimetry concurred with these findings.[142] Other data found similar changes in energy intake, but no change in energy expenditure.[143] A larger study also showed that food intake increased and weight was gained after 5 nights of sleep restriction, with higher intake of fat during the extra night time hours awake.[144] As those data were published, more studies followed, providing data for 2 meta-analyses of up to 18 studies.[145,146] One of these reports confirmed that increased energy intake occurs following sleep restriction without finding a change in energy expenditure, leading to an overall positive energy balance,[146] whereas the other meta-analysis showed that both energy expenditure and energy intake increased and the net result was less clear.[145] This ambiguity is not altogether surprising, as there are various ways to measure many of the variables in these experiments, alongside the small numbers of participants in the studies, encompassing both genders which may also cause differences in appetite regulation.[147] Indeed, there are also likely individual differences in energy metabolism.[148] However, taken overall these findings may postulate that there are likely both physiologic and behavioral components which lead to the increased food intake under conditions of sleep restriction,[149,150] and mechanistically these will lead to weight gain over time.

SLEEP EXTENSION STUDIES

With the mounting evidence of the association between short sleep duration and an increased risk of cardiometabolic health outcomes, interventions to reverse these complications need to be developed. Studies have investigated the effect of sleep extension; however, to date these have been of small sample size, with varying study designs and outcomes **Table 1**..[151–155]

Table 1
Sleep extension studies

	N; Age; Description	Design	Intervention	Outcomes	Findings (Reporting TST and Cardiometabolic Outcomes Only)
Al Khatib, 2018[1]	42; 18–64y; short sleep duration (5 to <7h-actigraphy)	RCT parallel, free-living	Sleep extension: 4 wk, behavioral consultation session on sleep hygiene Control: 4 wk, maintained habitual short sleep	Primary: feasibility and sugar intake Secondary: energy expenditure (RMR), body composition (bioelectric impedance), physical activity, anthropometry, lipids, appetite hormones, and HRV	Sleep extension ↑ TST by 21 mins (mean of 7 nights actigraphy). Sleep extension reduced intake of free sugars compared with control (Cohen's d = 0.79). No significant differences between groups in any secondary outcomes.
Baron, 2019[2]	16; 30–65y; pre/stage 1 hypertension (blood pressure ≥ 120–159/80–99 mm Hg on 24h ABPM) and < 7h sleep duration (actigraphy)	RCT parallel (2:1 ratio), free-living	Sleep extension (n = 11): 6 wk, technology-assisted intervention Control (n = 5): 6 wk, self-management	Feasibility, 24h blood pressure	90% completion rate of coaching sessions, with enjoyment rated as 4 or 5/5. Sleep extension ↑ TST by 0.57 h and control ↑ by 0.08 h (actigraphy). Overall 24h SBP and DBP had greater reductions with sleep extension compared with the control. No other differences in other ABPM outcomes. No changes in BMI or office blood pressure measures.

(*continued on next page*)

Table 1
(continued)

	N; Age; Description	Design	Intervention	Outcomes	Findings (Reporting TST and Cardiometabolic Outcomes Only)
Haack, 2013[3]	22; 25–65y; h pre/stage 1 hypertension (120–159/ 80–99 mm Hg) and sleep duration <7h or sleep duration >1h shorter than self-estimated sleep need (sleep diaries and actigraphy)	RCT parallel, free-living	Sleep extension: 6 wk, bedtimes 30 min earlier and 30 min later than usual lights out/lights on times Control: 6 wk, continue habitual bedtimes	Primary: Beat to beat BP over 24h (digital photoplethysmography) Secondary: Nutrient intake (food records), weight, body fat (bioelectric impedance)[1], BMI, IL-6, hs-CRP, urinary creatinine, and norepinephrine	Sleep extension ↑ TST by 31 mins cf to control (actigraphy), SBP/DBP reduction of 14/8 mm Hg. No change in BMI, body fat, calorific intake, WBC, IL-6, CRP, norepinephrine.
Hartescu, 2021[4]	18; 25–55y; BMI >25 kg/m^2, sleep duration ≤6.5 h(actigraphy)	RCT parallel, free-living	Sleep extension: 6 wk, n = 10, program based on cognitive-behavioral principles Control: 6 wk, n = 8	Primary: TST (actigraphy) Secondary: Fasting plasma insulin, insulin resistance (HOMA-IR), blood pressure, appetite-related hormones from a mixed-meal tolerance test, continuous glucose levels.	Sleep extension ↑ TST by 72 min cf to controls (actigraphy). Sleep extension improved SBP, DBP, fasting insulin, HOMA-IR. No changes seen in weight, mean continuous glucose levels, fasting glucose, glucose AUC, fasting ghrelin, ghrelin AUC, fasting leptin levels.

Leproult, 2015[5]	16; 20–50y; BMI <30 kg/m^2, sleep duration <7h weekdays (sleep diaries and actigraphy)	Within-participant (before and after intervention), free-living	2 wk of habitual TIB, then 6 wk sleep extension (increasing TIB by 1 h/night with sleep hygiene information and individual schedules)	TST (PSG, actigraphy), weight, fasting glucose, fasting insulin, insulin resistance (insulin-to-glucose ratio and HOMA), insulin sensitivity (QUICKI).	Sleep extension ↑ TST by 49 min (PSG, actigraphy). No changes in weight, glucose, or insulin levels. Correlations (n = 15) found associations between change in sleep time (actigraphy) and fasting glucose (r = +0.65, *P* = .017) insulin (r = −0.57, *P* = .053), insulin-to-glucose ratio (r = −0.66, *P* = .019) and QUICKI (r = 0.57, *P* = .053).
Moreno-Frais, 2020[6]	52; 14–18y; BMI <30 kg/m^2	RCT Parallel, free-living	All calorie restricted by 500 cal/d. Sleep extension: 4 wk, (n = 25), personalised sleep plan to increase TST by 1h. Control: 4 wk (n = 27)	TST (sleep diaries), weight, glucose, insulin, insulin resistance (HOMA), lipid profile, leptin.	Weight decreased in both groups with diet. Sleep extension: ↑TST by 66 min (+36 min cf to controls), ↓weight, ↓waist circumference, ↓insulin, ↓IL6 cf to controls. No change in leptin, HOMA-IR.
Reutrakal, 2020[7] (sub-analysis of Son-ngern)	See later in discussion	See later in discussion	See later in discussion	Gut microbiota	No changes associated with sleep extension.

(*continued on next page*)

Table 1
(continued)

	N; Age; Description	Design	Intervention	Outcomes	Findings (Reporting TST and Cardiometabolic Outcomes Only)
Reynold, 2014[8]	14; 18–55y, sleep duration 6–9h (self-report)	RCT, parallel, free-living	Sleep extension: 1 wk, n = 8, fixed sleep schedule whereby TIB was 3 h/night longer than the median baseline TIB (actigraphy) Control: 1 wk, n = 6	Physical activity (pedometer), blood pressure, heart rate, IL-6, TNF-α, CRP, and adiponectin	Sleep extension ↑TIB 127 min, TST 120 min Controls ↓TIB 27 min, TST 16 min (actigraphy). No changes between groups in blood pressure, heart rate, blood, except IL-6 which increased with extension but not control. Physical activity increased in both groups.
So-ngern, 2019[9]	21; 20–55y, self-reported ≤6h weekdays; nondiabetic (screening OGTT)	Cross-over (alternate order), free-living	Sleep extension: 2 wk, modifying bedtime earlier with individualized information. Control: 2 wk	Primary: OGTT -glucose metabolism (FBG, AUC glucose, insulin resistance [HOMA-IR], early insulin secretion [insulinogenic index], insulin sensitivity [Matsuda index], β-cell function [disposition index]) Secondary outcomes: self-reported sleep assessment (ESS, PSQI), dietary intake, weight.	Sleep extension ↑TST 36 mins (actigraphy). No changes in any outcomes with sleep extension cf to control. No order effect seen for glucose outcomes or the change in sleep duration itself. In those who slept >6h (n = 8) significant improvements seen in insulin resistance, early insulin secretion, and β-cell function.

Stock, 2020[10]	53; 18–23y, undergraduate students; sleep duration 6–8h (actigraphy)	Within-participant (before and after intervention), free-living	Sleep extension: 1 wk, ↑TIB by 1h Control: 1 wk	Blood pressure, heart rate.	Sleep extension ↑TST 43 mins (actigraphy). Systolic BP ↓ sitting (−7.0 mm Hg ± 3.0, $P < .5$) and standing (−8.8 ± 2.7, $P < .1$). No changes in diastolic BP or heart rate.
Tasali, 2014[11]	10; 21–40y, BMI 25-<30 kg/m^2, sleep duration <6.5 h (self-report)	Within-participant (before and after intervention), free-living	Baseline: 1 wk, habitual TIB, followed by Sleep extension: 2 wk, ↑ TIB to 8.5 h, individualized behavioral counseling on sleep hygiene, with individual recommendations.	Appetite (visual analog scale), food desire (self-reported scales for different food items). Sleepiness (ESS),	Sleep extension ↑ TST 1.6 h (actigraphy). Sleep extension ↓overall appetite by 14% and desire for sweet/salty foods by 62%. Desire for fruit, vegetables, and protein-rich nutrients were not changed. Sleep extension ↓sleepiness, ↑vigor ratings.

[1] ABPM: ambulatory blood pressure monitoring; AUC: area under the curve; BMI: body mass index; CRP: C-reactive protein; DBP: diastolic blood pressure; ESS: Epworth sleep scale; FBG: fasting blood glucose; h: hours; HOMA-IR: HOMA-IR (Homeostatic Model Assessment for Insulin Resistance); HRV: heart rate variability; IL-6: Interleukin 6; min: minute; mmHg: millimetre of mercury; OGTT: oral glucose tolerance test; PSG: polysomnography; PSQI: Pittsburgh sleep quality index; QUICKI: quantitative insulin sensitivity check index; RCT: randomised controlled trial; RMR: resting metabolic rate; SBP: systolic blood pressure; TIB: time in bed; TNF: tumour necrosis factor; TST: total sleep time; WBC: white blood cells; wk: week; y: years.

Depending on the methodology chosen, some earlier experimental studies could be considered sleep extension studies relative to prior sleep deprivation; however, in general in many of those studies the individuals were often recruited as "normal" sleepers. This provides useful information with regards to putative target outcomes but may not physiologically be the same as trying to extend the sleep in habitual short sleepers, a population whom, as we have discussed in this review, are already at higher risk of cardiometabolic comorbidities.

Therefore, more recent studies (see **Table 1**) have specifically recruited the target population of habitual short sleepers and examined the feasibility of promoting and achieving longer sleep times. These have included advising earlier bedtimes or later wake-up times, sleep hygiene education, individualized sleep schedules, or even CBT techniques.[156–166] Many of the studies are still small in numbers and to our knowledge, there have not yet been large scale field studies to determine whether sleep extension interventions are practical and achievable at a population level. Using everyday technology such as activity monitors, and other wearables, now so widely available at relatively low cost, may be a way to provide this on a broader platform and in home environments.[164] While the results of these trials demonstrate variable and at times conflicting results, the intervention period in most of these studies has tended to be of relatively short duration (days to weeks). It is encouraging that all have used objective sleep measurements to document the increase in sleep duration, rather than self-report. Furthermore, these studies have all been in free-living conditions, not in sleep laboratories. Despite this meaning some confounders will be less controlled for, these studies are now very valuable to see if meaningful outcomes can be achieved in real-life settings. Thus, it remains to be seen whether longer-term sleep extension in larger sample sizes can reverse the negative effects of sleep restriction and improve cardiometabolic health outcomes.

SUMMARY

The cardiometabolic effects of short sleep duration are widely acknowledged and have been thoroughly examined in the literature over the past decade with ample meta-analyses of the available data encompassing many fields. The next step is how to broaden sleep extension studies to larger sample sizes so that any consistent benefits derived from lengthening sleep can help deliver sleep health recommendations at a population level.

CLINICS CARE POINTS

Sleep deprivation is associated with negative cardiometabolic outcomes.

- Asking about sleep duration should be incorporated into clinical discussions by health professions with individuals.
- Educating individuals about the importance of sleep as an overall general health measure is a clinical priority.

DISCLOSURES

The authors have no disclosure to declare.

FUNDING

Dr C. Hoyos is supported by a National Heart Foundation Future Leader Fellowship.

REFERENCES

1. Everson CA, Bergmann BM, Rechtschaffen A. Sleep deprivation in the rat: III. Total sleep deprivation. Sleep 1989;12(1):13–21.
2. Hirshkowitz M, Whiton K, Albert SM, et al. National Sleep Foundation's sleep time duration recommendations: methodology and results summary. Sleep Health 2015;1(1):40–3.
3. Jean-Louis G, Williams NJ, Sarpong D, et al. Associations between inadequate sleep and obesity in the US adult population: analysis of the national health interview survey (1977-2009). BMC Public Health 2014;14:290.
4. Basner M, Fomberstein KM, Razavi FM, et al. American time use survey: sleep time and its relationship to waking activities. Sleep 2007;30(9): 1085–95.
5. Statistics NCfH. Quick-Stats: percentage of adults who reported an average of <6 hrs sleep per 24-hr period, by sex and age group- United States, 1985 and 2004. MMWR Morb Mort Wkly Rep 2005;54:933.
6. Bin YS, Marshall NS, Glozier N. Sleeping at the limits: the changing prevalence of short and long sleep durations in 10 countries. Am J Epidemiol 2013;177(8):826–33.
7. Cappuccio FP, Miller MA. Sleep and cardiometabolic disease. Curr Cardiol Rep 2017;19(11): 110.

8. St-Onge MP, Grandner MA, Brown D, et al. Sleep duration and quality: impact on lifestyle behaviors and cardiometabolic health: a scientific statement from the american heart association. Circulation 2016;134(18):e367–86.
9. Hammond EC. Some preliminary findings on physical complaints from a prospective study of 1,064,004 men and women. Am J Public Health Nations Health 1964;54:11–23.
10. Gangwisch JE, Heymsfield SB, Boden-Albala B, et al. Sleep duration associated with mortality in elderly, but not middle-aged, adults in a large US sample. Sleep 2008;31(8):1087–96.
11. Patel SR, Ayas NT, Malhotra MR, et al. A prospective study of sleep duration and mortality risk in women. Sleep 2004;27(3):440–4.
12. Grandner MA, Hale L, Moore M, et al. Mortality associated with short sleep duration: the evidence, the possible mechanisms, and the future. Sleep Med Rev 2010;14(3):191–203.
13. Wingard DL, Berkman LF. Mortality risk associated with sleeping patterns among adults. Sleep 1983; 6(2):102–7.
14. Tamakoshi A, Ohno Y. Self-reported sleep duration as a predictor of all-cause mortality: results from the JACC study, Japan. Sleep 2004;27(1):51–4.
15. Shankar A, Koh WP, Yuan JM, et al. Sleep duration and coronary heart disease mortality among Chinese adults in Singapore: a population-based cohort study. Am J Epidemiol 2008;168(12): 1367–73.
16. Kripke DF, Garfinkel L, Wingard DL, et al. Mortality associated with sleep duration and insomnia. Arch Gen Psychiatry 2002;59(2):131–6.
17. Kaplan GA, Seeman TE, Cohen RD, et al. Mortality among the elderly in the Alameda county study: behavioral and demographic risk factors. Am J Public Health 1987;77(3):307–12.
18. Ferrie JE, Shipley MJ, Cappuccio FP, et al. A prospective study of change in sleep duration: associations with mortality in the Whitehall II cohort. Sleep 2007;30(12):1659–66.
19. Hublin C, Partinen M, Koskenvuo M, et al. Sleep and mortality: a population-based 22-year follow-up study. Sleep 2007;30(10):1245–53.
20. Lan TY, Lan TH, Wen CP, et al. Nighttime sleep, Chinese afternoon nap, and mortality in the elderly. Sleep 2007;30(9):1105–10.
21. Gallicchio L, Kalesan B. Sleep duration and mortality: a systematic review and meta-analysis. J Sleep Res 2009;18(2):148–58.
22. Cappuccio FP, D'Elia L, Strazzullo P, et al. Sleep duration and all-cause mortality: a systematic review and meta-analysis of prospective studies. Sleep 2010;33(5):585–92.
23. Pienaar PR, Kolbe-Alexander TL, van Mechelen W, et al. Associations between self-reported sleep duration and mortality in employed individuals: systematic review and meta-analysis. Am J Health Promot 2021;35(6):853–65.
24. da Silva AA, de Mello RG, Schaan CW, et al. Sleep duration and mortality in the elderly: a systematic review with meta-analysis. BMJ Open 2016;6(2): e008119.
25. He M, Deng X, Zhu Y, et al. The relationship between sleep duration and all-cause mortality in the older people: an updated and dose-response meta-analysis. BMC Public Health 2020;20(1): 1179.
26. Liu TZ, Xu C, Rota M, et al. Sleep duration and risk of all-cause mortality: a flexible, non-linear, meta-regression of 40 prospective cohort studies. Sleep Med Rev 2017;32:28–36.
27. Khan MA, Hashim MJ, Mustafa H, et al. Global epidemiology of ischemic heart disease: results from the global burden of disease study. Cureus 2020;12(7):e9349.
28. Magee CA, Kritharides L, Attia J, et al. Short and long sleep duration are associated with prevalent cardiovascular disease in Australian adults. J Sleep Res 2012;21(4):441–7.
29. Ayas NT, White DP, Manson JE, et al. A prospective study of sleep duration and coronary heart disease in women. Arch Intern Med 2003;163(2):205–9.
30. Hoevenaar-Blom MP, Spijkerman AM, Kromhout D, et al. Sleep duration and sleep quality in relation to 12-year cardiovascular disease incidence: the MORGEN study. Sleep 2011;34(11):1487–92.
31. Aggarwal S, Loomba RS, Arora RR, et al. Associations between sleep duration and prevalence of cardiovascular events. Clin Cardiol 2013;36(11): 671–6.
32. Kwok CS, Kontopantelis E, Kuligowski G, et al. Self-reported sleep duration and quality and cardiovascular disease and mortality: a dose-response meta-analysis. J Am Heart Assoc 2018;7(15): e008552.
33. Krittanawong C, Tunhasiriwet A, Wang Z, et al. Association between short and long sleep durations and cardiovascular outcomes: a systematic review and meta-analysis. Eur Heart J Acute Cardiovasc Care 2019;8(8):762–70.
34. Cappuccio FP, Cooper D, D'Elia L, et al. Sleep duration predicts cardiovascular outcomes: a systematic review and meta-analysis of prospective studies. Eur Heart J 2011;32(12):1484–92.
35. Lao XQ, Liu X, Deng HB, et al. Sleep quality, sleep duration, and the risk of coronary heart disease: a prospective cohort study with 60,586 adults. J Clin Sleep Med 2018;14(1):109–17.
36. Chandola T, Ferrie JE, Perski A, et al. The effect of short sleep duration on coronary heart disease risk is greatest among those with sleep disturbance: a

prospective study from the Whitehall II cohort. Sleep 2010;33(6):739–44.
37. Svensson AK, Svensson T, Kitlinski M, et al. Incident diabetes mellitus may explain the association between sleep duration and incident coronary heart disease. Diabetologia 2018;61(2): 331–41.
38. Chokesuwattanaskul R, Thongprayoon C, Sharma K, et al. Associations of sleep quality with incident atrial fibrillation: a meta-analysis. Intern Med J 2018;48(8):964–72.
39. Khawaja O, Sarwar A, Albert CM, et al. Sleep duration and risk of atrial fibrillation (from the Physicians' Health Study). Am J Cardiol 2013;111(4): 547–51.
40. Zhao J, Yang F, Zhuo C, et al. Association of sleep duration with atrial fibrillation and heart failure: a mendelian randomization analysis. Front Genet 2021;12:583658.
41. Morovatdar N, Ebrahimi N, Rezaee R, et al. Sleep duration and risk of atrial fibrillation: a systematic review. J Atr Fibrillation 2019;11(6):2132.
42. Mancia G, Grassi G. The autonomic nervous system and hypertension. Circ Res 2014;114(11): 1804–14.
43. Thomas SJ, Calhoun D. Sleep, insomnia, and hypertension: current findings and future directions. J Am Soc Hypertens 2017;11(2):122–9.
44. Tobaldini E, Costantino G, Solbiati M, et al. Sleep, sleep deprivation, autonomic nervous system and cardiovascular diseases. Neurosci Biobehav Rev 2017;74(Pt B):321–9.
45. Yano Y, Kario K. Nocturnal blood pressure and cardiovascular disease: a review of recent advances. Hypertens Res 2012;35(7):695–701.
46. Tochikubo O, Ikeda A, Miyajima E, et al. Effects of insufficient sleep on blood pressure monitored by a new multibiomedical recorder. Hypertension 1996; 27(6):1318–24.
47. Goncharuk VD, van Heerikhuize J, Dai JP, et al. Neuropeptide changes in the suprachiasmatic nucleus in primary hypertension indicate functional impairment of the biological clock. J Comp Neurol 2001;431(3):320–30.
48. Fang J, Wheaton AG, Keenan NL, et al. Association of sleep duration and hypertension among US adults varies by age and sex. Am J Hypertens 2012;25(3):335–41.
49. Knutson KL, Van Cauter E, Rathouz PJ, et al. Association between sleep and blood pressure in midlife: the CARDIA sleep study. Arch Intern Med 2009;169(11):1055–61.
50. Gangwisch JE, Heymsfield SB, Boden-Albala B, et al. Short sleep duration as a risk factor for hypertension: analyses of the first National Health and Nutrition Examination Survey. Hypertension 2006; 47(5):833–9.
51. Gottlieb DJ, Redline S, Nieto FJ, et al. Association of usual sleep duration with hypertension: the sleep heart health study. Sleep 2006;29(8):1009–14.
52. Wang Q, Xi B, Liu M, et al. Short sleep duration is associated with hypertension risk among adults: a systematic review and meta-analysis. Hypertens Res 2012;35(10):1012–8.
53. Shulman R, Cohen DL, Grandner MA, et al. Sleep duration and 24-hour ambulatory blood pressure in adults not on antihypertensive medications. J Clin Hypertens (Greenwich) 2018;20(12):1712–20.
54. Cappuccio FP, Stranges S, Kandala NB, et al. Gender-specific associations of short sleep duration with prevalent and incident hypertension: the Whitehall II Study. Hypertension 2007;50(4): 693–700.
55. Li C, Shang S. Relationship between sleep and hypertension: findings from the NHANES (2007-2014). Int J Environ Res Public Health 2021;18(15).
56. Li H, Ren Y, Wu Y, et al. Correlation between sleep duration and hypertension: a dose-response meta-analysis. J Hum Hypertens 2019;33(3):218–28.
57. Wang L, Hu Y, Wang X, et al. The association between sleep duration and hypertension: a meta and study sequential analysis. J Hum Hypertens 2021;35(7):621–6.
58. Stranges S, Dorn JM, Cappuccio FP, et al. A population-based study of reduced sleep duration and hypertension: the strongest association may be in premenopausal women. J Hypertens 2010;28(5):896–902.
59. Guo X, Zheng L, Wang J, et al. Epidemiological evidence for the link between sleep duration and high blood pressure: a systematic review and meta-analysis. Sleep Med 2013;14(4):324–32.
60. Kawada T. The definition of sleep duration and the risk for hypertension: caution for meta-analysis. Sleep Med 2013;14(12):1431.
61. McDermott M, Brown DL, Chervin RD. Sleep disorders and the risk of stroke. Expert Rev Neurother 2018;18(7):523–31.
62. Yin J, Jin X, Shan Z, et al. Relationship of sleep duration with all-cause mortality and cardiovascular events: a systematic review and dose-response meta-analysis of prospective cohort studies. J Am Heart Assoc 2017;6(9):e005947.
63. Li W, Wang D, Cao S, et al. Sleep duration and risk of stroke events and stroke mortality: a systematic review and meta-analysis of prospective cohort studies. Int J Cardiol 2016;223:870–6.
64. Cappuccio FP, Taggart FM, Kandala NB, et al. Meta-analysis of short sleep duration and obesity in children and adults. Sleep 2008;31(5):619–26.
65. Marshall NS, Glozier N, Grunstein RR. Is sleep duration related to obesity? A critical review of the epidemiological evidence. Sleep Med Rev 2008;12(4):289–98.

66. Killick R, Banks S, Liu PY. Implications of sleep restriction and recovery on metabolic outcomes. J Clin Endocrinol Metab 2012;97(11):3876–90.
67. Wu Y, Zhai L, Zhang D. Sleep duration and obesity among adults: a meta-analysis of prospective studies. Sleep Med 2014;15(12):1456–62.
68. Patel SR, Hu FB. Short sleep duration and weight gain: a systematic review. Obesity (Silver Spring) 2008;16(3):643–53.
69. Patel SR, Blackwell T, Redline S, et al. The association between sleep duration and obesity in older adults. Int J Obes (Lond) 2008;21:21.
70. Stamatakis KA, Kaplan GA, Roberts RE. Short sleep duration across income, education, and race/ethnic groups: population prevalence and growing disparities during 34 years of follow-up. Ann Epidemiol 2007;17(12):948–55.
71. Jean-Louis G, Youngstedt S, Grandner M, et al. Unequal burden of sleep-related obesity among black and white Americans. Sleep Health 2015;1(3):169–76.
72. Zhou Q, Zhang M, Hu D. Dose-response association between sleep duration and obesity risk: a systematic review and meta-analysis of prospective cohort studies. Sleep Breath 2019;23(4):1035–45.
73. Kelly T, Yang W, Chen CS, et al. Global burden of obesity in 2005 and projections to 2030. Int J Obes (Lond) 2008;32(9):1431–7.
74. Wang Y, Beydoun MA, Liang L, et al. Will all Americans become overweight or obese? estimating the progression and cost of the US obesity epidemic. Obesity (Silver Spring) 2008;16(10):2323–30.
75. Liu B, Du Y, Wu Y, et al. Trends in obesity and adiposity measures by race or ethnicity among adults in the United States 2011-18: population based study. BMJ 2021;372:n365.
76. Simon SL, Higgins J, Melanson E, et al. A model of adolescent sleep health and risk for type 2 diabetes. Curr Diab Rep 2021;21(2):4.
77. Guo Y, Miller MA, Cappuccio FP. Short duration of sleep and incidence of overweight or obesity in Chinese children and adolescents: a systematic review and meta-analysis of prospective studies. Nutr Metab Cardiovasc Dis 2021;31(2):363–71.
78. Miller MA, Kruisbrink M, Wallace J, et al. Sleep duration and incidence of obesity in infants, children, and adolescents: a systematic review and meta-analysis of prospective studies. Sleep 2018;41(4):zsy018.
79. Miller MA, Bates S, Ji C, et al. Systematic review and meta-analyses of the relationship between short sleep and incidence of obesity and effectiveness of sleep interventions on weight gain in preschool children. Obes Rev 2021;22(2):e13113.
80. Chaput JP, McNeil J, Despres JP, et al. Short sleep duration as a risk factor for the development of the metabolic syndrome in adults. Prev Med 2013;57(6):872–7.
81. Hall MH, Muldoon MF, Jennings JR, et al. Self-reported sleep duration is associated with the metabolic syndrome in midlife adults. Sleep 2008;31(5):635–43.
82. Chaput JP, McNeil J, Despres JP, et al. Seven to eight hours of sleep a night is associated with a lower prevalence of the metabolic syndrome and reduced overall cardiometabolic risk in adults. PLoS One 2013;8(9):e72832.
83. Smiley A, King D, Bidulescu A. The association between sleep duration and metabolic syndrome: the NHANES 2013/2014. Nutrients 2019;11(11):2582.
84. Kim CE, Shin S, Lee HW, et al. Association between sleep duration and metabolic syndrome: a cross-sectional study. BMC Public Health 2018;18(1):720.
85. Stefani KM, Kim HC, Kim J, et al. The influence of sex and age on the relationship between sleep duration and metabolic syndrome in Korean adults. Diabetes Res Clin Pract 2013;102(3):250–9.
86. Duan Y, Sun J, Wang M, et al. Association between short sleep duration and metabolic syndrome in Chinese children and adolescents. Sleep Med 2020;74:343–8.
87. Arora A, Pell D, van Sluijs EMF, et al. How do associations between sleep duration and metabolic health differ with age in the UK general population? PLoS One 2020;15(11):e0242852.
88. Xie J, Li Y, Zhang Y, et al. Sleep duration and metabolic syndrome: an updated systematic review and meta-analysis. Sleep Med Rev 2021;59:101451.
89. Hua J, Jiang H, Wang H, et al. Sleep duration and the risk of metabolic syndrome in adults: a systematic review and meta-analysis. Front Neurol 2021;12:635564.
90. Iftikhar IH, Donley MA, Mindel J, et al. Sleep duration and metabolic syndrome. an updated dose-risk metaanalysis. Ann Am Thorac Soc 2015;12(9):1364–72.
91. Zhao JJ, Zhang TT, Liu XH, et al. [A Meta-analysis on the association between sleep duration and metabolic syndrome in adults]. Zhonghua Liu Xing Bing Xue Za Zhi 2020;41(8):1272–9.
92. Xi B, He D, Zhang M, et al. Short sleep duration predicts risk of metabolic syndrome: a systematic review and meta-analysis. Sleep Med Rev 2014;18(4):293–7.
93. Cappuccio FP, D'Elia L, Strazzullo P, et al. Quantity and quality of sleep and incidence of type 2 diabetes: a systematic review and meta-analysis. Diabetes Care 2010;33(2):414–20.
94. Itani O, Jike M, Watanabe N, et al. Short sleep duration and health outcomes: a systematic review, meta-analysis, and meta-regression. Sleep Med 2017;32:246–56.

95. Anothaisintawee T, Reutrakul S, Van Cauter E, et al. Sleep disturbances compared to traditional risk factors for diabetes development: systematic review and meta-analysis. Sleep Med Rev 2016;30:11–24.
96. Shan Z, Ma H, Xie M, et al. Sleep duration and risk of type 2 diabetes: a meta-analysis of prospective studies. Diabetes Care 2015;38(3):529–37.
97. Holliday EG, Magee CA, Kritharides L, et al. Short sleep duration is associated with risk of future diabetes but not cardiovascular disease: a prospective study and meta-analysis. PLoS One 2013;8(11):e82305.
98. Lee SWH, Ng KY, Chin WK. The impact of sleep amount and sleep quality on glycemic control in type 2 diabetes: a systematic review and meta-analysis. Sleep Med Rev 2017;31:91–101.
99. Ji X, Wang Y, Saylor J. Sleep and type 1 diabetes mellitus management among children, adolescents, and emerging young adults: a systematic review. J Pediatr Nurs 2021;61:245–53.
100. Reutrakul S, Thakkinstian A, Anothaisintawee T, et al. Sleep characteristics in type 1 diabetes and associations with glycemic control: systematic review and meta-analysis. Sleep Med 2016;23:26–45.
101. Zhang X, Zhang R, Cheng L, et al. The effect of sleep impairment on gestational diabetes mellitus: a systematic review and meta-analysis of cohort studies. Sleep Med 2020;74:267–77.
102. Reutrakul S, Anothaisintawee T, Herring SJ, et al. Short sleep duration and hyperglycemia in pregnancy: aggregate and individual patient data meta-analysis. Sleep Med Rev 2018;40:31–42.
103. Kohansieh M, Makaryus AN. Sleep deficiency and deprivation leading to cardiovascular disease. Int J Hypertens 2015;2015:615681.
104. Carreras A, Zhang SX, Peris E, et al. Chronic Sleep fragmentation induces endothelial dysfunction and structural vascular changes in mice. Sleep 2014;37(11):1817–24.
105. Sauvet F, Drogou C, Bougard C, et al. Vascular response to 1 week of sleep restriction in healthy subjects. A metabolic response? Int J Cardiol 2015;190:246–55.
106. Calvin AD, Covassin N, Kremers WK, et al. Experimental sleep restriction causes endothelial dysfunction in healthy humans. J Am Heart Assoc 2014;3(6):e001143.
107. Hall MH, Mulukutla S, Kline CE, et al. Objective sleep duration is prospectively associated with endothelial health. Sleep 2017;40(1):zsw003.
108. Reimund E. The free radical flux theory of sleep. Med Hypotheses 1994;43(4):231–3.
109. Atrooz F, Salim S. Sleep deprivation, oxidative stress and inflammation. Adv Protein Chem Struct Biol 2020;119:309–36.
110. Villafuerte G, Miguel-Puga A, Rodríguez EM, et al. Sleep deprivation and oxidative stress in animal models: a systematic review. Oxid Med Cell Longev 2015;2015:234952.
111. Vaccaro A, Kaplan Dor Y, Nambara K, et al. Sleep Loss can cause death through accumulation of reactive oxygen species in the gut. Cell 2020;181(6):1307–28.e1315.
112. Jowko E, Rozanski P, Tomczak A. Effects of a 36-h survival training with sleep deprivation on oxidative stress and muscle damage biomarkers in young healthy men. Int J Environ Res Public Health 2018;15(10):2066.
113. Rozanski P, Jowko E, Tomczak A. Assessment of the levels of oxidative stress, muscle damage, and psychomotor abilities of special force soldiers during military survival training. Int J Environ Res Public Health 2020;17(13):4886.
114. Açar G, Akçakoyun M, Sari I, et al. Acute sleep deprivation in healthy adults is associated with a reduction in left atrial early diastolic strain rate. Sleep Breath 2013;17(3):975–83.
115. Cakici M, Dogan A, Cetin M, et al. Negative effects of acute sleep deprivation on left ventricular functions and cardiac repolarization in healthy young adults. Pacing Clin Electrophysiol 2015;38(6):713–22.
116. Chen WR, Shi XM, Yang TS, et al. Protective effect of metoprolol on arrhythmia and heart rate variability in healthy people with 24 hours of sleep deprivation. J Interv Card Electrophysiol 2013;36(3):267–72 [discussion: 272].
117. Chen WR, Liu HB, Sha Y, et al. Effects of statin on arrhythmia and heart rate variability in healthy persons with 48-hour sleep deprivation. J Am Heart Assoc 2016;5(11):e003833.
118. Davies SK, Ang JE, Revell VL, et al. Effect of sleep deprivation on the human metabolome. Proc Natl Acad Sci U S A 2014;111(29):10761–6.
119. Weljie AM, Meerlo P, Goel N, et al. Oxalic acid and diacylglycerol 36:3 are cross-species markers of sleep debt. Proc Natl Acad Sci U S A 2015;112(8):2569–74.
120. Moller-Levet CS, Archer SN, Bucca G, et al. Effects of insufficient sleep on circadian rhythmicity and expression amplitude of the human blood transcriptome. Proc Natl Acad Sci U S A 2013;110(12):E1132–41.
121. Irwin MR, Wang M, Ribeiro D, et al. Sleep loss activates cellular inflammatory signaling. Biol Psychiatry 2008;64(6):538–40.
122. Geovanini GR, Libby P. Atherosclerosis and inflammation: overview and updates. Clin Sci (Lond) 2018;132(12):1243–52.
123. Swirski FK, Nahrendorf M. Leukocyte behavior in atherosclerosis, myocardial infarction, and heart failure. Science 2013;339(6116):161–6.

124. McAlpine CS, Kiss MG, Rattik S, et al. Sleep modulates haematopoiesis and protects against atherosclerosis. Nature 2019;566(7744):383–7.
125. Sands MR, Lauderdale DS, Liu K, et al. Short sleep duration is associated with carotid intima-media thickness among men in the Coronary Artery Risk Development in Young Adults (CARDIA) Study. Stroke 2012;43(11):2858–64.
126. Aziz M, Ali SS, Das S, et al. Association of subjective and objective sleep duration as well as sleep quality with non-invasive markers of subclinical cardiovascular disease (CVD): a systematic review. J Atheroscler Thromb 2017;24(3):208–26.
127. Irwin MR, Wang M, Campomayor CO, et al. Sleep deprivation and activation of morning levels of cellular and genomic markers of inflammation. Arch Intern Med 2006;166(16):1756–62.
128. Irwin MR, Olmstead R, Carroll JE. Sleep disturbance, sleep duration, and inflammation: a systematic review and meta-analysis of cohort studies and experimental sleep deprivation. Biol Psychiatry 2016;80(1):40–52.
129. Spiegel K, Leproult R, Van Cauter E. Impact of sleep debt on metabolic and endocrine function. Lancet 1999;354(9188):1435–9.
130. Nedeltcheva AV, Kessler L, Imperial J, et al. Exposure to recurrent sleep restriction in the setting of high caloric intake and physical inactivity results in increased insulin resistance and reduced glucose tolerance. J Clin Endocrinol Metab 2009;94(9):3242–50.
131. Donga E, van Dijk M, van Dijk JG, et al. A single night of partial sleep deprivation induces insulin resistance in multiple metabolic pathways in healthy subjects. J Clin Endocrinol Metab 2010;95(6):2963–8.
132. Zielinski MR, Kline CE, Kripke DF, et al. No effect of 8-week time in bed restriction on glucose tolerance in older long sleepers. J Sleep Res 2008;5:5.
133. van Leeuwen WM, Hublin C, Sallinen M, et al. Prolonged sleep restriction affects glucose metabolism in healthy young men. Int J Endocrinol 2010;2010:108641.
134. Bosy-Westphal A, Hinrichs S, Jauch-Chara K, et al. Influence of partial sleep deprivation on energy balance and insulin sensitivity in healthy women. Obes Facts 2008;1(5):266–73.
135. Schmid SM, Jauch-Chara K, Hallschmid M, et al. Mild sleep restriction acutely reduces plasma glucagon levels in healthy men. J Clin Endocrinol Metab 2009;94(12):5169–73.
136. Buxton OM, Pavlova M, Reid EW, et al. Sleep restriction for 1 week reduces insulin sensitivity in healthy men. Diabetes 2010;59(9):2126–33.
137. St-Onge MP, O'Keeffe M, Roberts AL, et al. Short sleep duration, glucose dysregulation and hormonal regulation of appetite in men and women. Sleep 2012;35(11):1503–10.
138. Morselli LL, Guyon A, Spiegel K. Sleep and metabolic function. Pflugers Archiv 2012;463(1):139–60.
139. Morselli L, Leproult R, Balbo M, et al. Role of sleep duration in the regulation of glucose metabolism and appetite. Best Pract Res Clin Endocrinol Metab 2010;24(5):687–702.
140. Killick R, Hoyos CM, Melehan K, et al. Metabolic and hormonal effects of 'catch-up' sleep in men with chronic, repetitive, lifestyle-driven sleep restriction. Clin Endocrinol (Oxf) 2015;83(4):498–507.
141. Markwald RR, Melanson EL, Smith MR, et al. Impact of insufficient sleep on total daily energy expenditure, food intake, and weight gain. Proc Natl Acad Sci U S A 2013;110(14):5695–700.
142. Shechter A, Rising R, Albu JB, et al. Experimental sleep curtailment causes wake-dependent increases in 24-h energy expenditure as measured by whole-room indirect calorimetry. Am J Clin Nutr 2013;98(6):1433–9.
143. St-Onge MP, Roberts AL, Chen J, et al. Short sleep duration increases energy intakes but does not change energy expenditure in normal-weight individuals. Am J Clin Nutr 2011;94(2):410–6.
144. Spaeth AM, Dinges DF, Goel N. Effects of experimental sleep restriction on weight gain, caloric intake, and meal timing in healthy adults. Sleep 2013;36(7):981–90.
145. Capers PL, Fobian AD, Kaiser KA, et al. A systematic review and meta-analysis of randomized controlled trials of the impact of sleep duration on adiposity and components of energy balance. Obes Rev 2015;16(9):771–82.
146. Al Khatib HK, Harding SV, Darzi J, et al. The effects of partial sleep deprivation on energy balance: a systematic review and meta-analysis. Eur J Clin Nutr 2017;71(5):614–24.
147. Gallegos JV, Boege HL, Zuraikat FM, et al. Does sex influence the effects of experimental sleep curtailment and circadian misalignment on regulation of appetite? Curr Opin Endocr Metab Res 2021;17:20–5.
148. McNeil J, St-Onge MP. Increased energy intake following sleep restriction in men and women: a one-size-fits-all conclusion? Obesity (Silver Spring) 2017;25(6):989–92.
149. St-Onge MP, McReynolds A, Trivedi ZB, et al. Sleep restriction leads to increased activation of brain regions sensitive to food stimuli. Am J Clin Nutr 2012;95(4):818–24.
150. St-Onge MP, Wolfe S, Sy M, et al. Sleep restriction increases the neuronal response to unhealthy food in normal-weight individuals. Int J Obes (Lond) 2014;38(3):411–6.

151. Hoddy KK, Potts KS, Bazzano LA, et al. Sleep extension: a potential target for obesity treatment. Curr Diab Rep 2020;20(12):81.
152. Zhu B, Yin Y, Shi C, et al. Feasibility of sleep extension and its effect on cardiometabolic parameters in free-living settings: a systematic review and meta-analysis of experimental studies. Eur J Cardiovasc Nurs 2022;21(1):9–25.
153. Pizinger TM, Aggarwal B, St-Onge MP. Sleep extension in short sleepers: an evaluation of feasibility and effectiveness for weight management and cardiometabolic disease prevention. Front Endocrinol (Lausanne) 2018;9:392.
154. Kothari V, Cardona Z, Chirakalwasan N, et al. Sleep interventions and glucose metabolism: systematic review and meta-analysis. Sleep Med 2021;78: 24–35.
155. Henst RHP, Pienaar PR, Roden LC, et al. The effects of sleep extension on cardiometabolic risk factors: a systematic review. J Sleep Res 2019; 28(6):e12865.
156. Al Khatib HK, Hall WL, Creedon A, et al. Sleep extension is a feasible lifestyle intervention in free-living adults who are habitually short sleepers: a potential strategy for decreasing intake of free sugars? A randomized controlled pilot study. Am J Clin Nutr 2018;107(1):43–53.
157. So-Ngern A, Chirakalwasan N, Saetung S, et al. Effects of two-week sleep extension on glucose metabolism in chronically sleep-deprived individuals. J Clin Sleep Med 2019;15(5):711–8.
158. Reutrakul S, So-Ngern A, Chirakalwasan N, et al. No changes in gut microbiota after two-week sleep extension in chronically sleep-deprived individuals. Sleep Med 2020;68:27–30.
159. Stock AA, Lee S, Nahmod NG, et al. Effects of sleep extension on sleep duration, sleepiness, and blood pressure in college students. Sleep Health 2020;6(1):32–9.
160. Tasali E, Chapotot F, Wroblewski K, et al. The effects of extended bedtimes on sleep duration and food desire in overweight young adults: a home-based intervention. Appetite 2014;80:220–4.
161. Leproult R, Deliens G, Gilson M, et al. Beneficial impact of sleep extension on fasting insulin sensitivity in adults with habitual sleep restriction. Sleep 2015;38(5):707–15.
162. Haack M, Serrador J, Cohen D, et al. Increasing sleep duration to lower beat-to-beat blood pressure: a pilot study. J Sleep Res 2013;22(3): 295–304.
163. Reynold AM, Bowles ER, Saxena A, et al. Negative effects of time in bed extension: a pilot study. J Sleep Med Disord 2014;1(1):1002.
164. Baron KG, Duffecy J, Richardson D, et al. Technology assisted behavior intervention to extend sleep among adults with short sleep duration and prehypertension/stage 1 hypertension: a randomized pilot feasibility study. J Clin Sleep Med 2019;15(11): 1587–97.
165. Moreno-Frias C, Figueroa-Vega N, Malacara JM. Sleep extension increases the effect of caloric restriction over body weight and improves the chronic low-grade inflammation in adolescents with obesity. J Adolesc Health 2020;66(5):575–81.
166. Hartescu I, Stensel DJ, Thackray AE, et al. Sleep extension and metabolic health in male overweight/obese short sleepers: a randomised controlled trial. J Sleep Res 2022;31(2):e13469.

Sleep Deficiency, Sleep Apnea, and Chronic Lung Disease

Bernie Y. Sunwoo, MBBS[a], Robert L. Owens, MD[a,*]

KEYWORDS

• Chronic lung disease • Sleep deficiency • Obstructive sleep apnea • Overlap syndrome • Chronic obstructive pulmonary disease • Sleep • Breathing

KEY POINTS

- Poor sleep is a common complaint among those with chronic lung disease.
- Multiple factors contribute to sleep deficiency in chronic lung disease.
- In patients with chronic lung disease, primary sleep disorders such as obstructive sleep apnea (OSA) and restless leg syndrome can co-exist and need specific treatment.
- Treatment of OSA in those with chronic lung disease is associated with improved morbidity and mortality.

INTRODUCTION

Chronic lung diseases are diseases of the airways and other structures of the lung, and are leading causes of morbidity and mortality worldwide.[1] In 2017, 545 million people worldwide had a chronic lung disease, representing an increase of 40% compared with 1990.[2] Sleep disturbances leading to sleep deficiency are common in chronic lung disease and associated with adverse outcomes including reduced quality of life. Yet little attention is often given to the sleep period in chronic lung disease.

Multiple factors contribute to sleep deficiency in chronic lung disease (**Fig. 1**). Disease-specific symptoms can disrupt sleep. Lung function displays circadian variation and normal physiologic changes in respiration during sleep can result in more profound hypoxemia and hypercapnia in patients with chronic lung disease. Coexisting sleep disorders, especially obstructive sleep apnea (OSA), and medical comorbidities associated with poor sleep themselves, like depression and anxiety, are common in chronic lung disease adding to sleep deficiency. Additionally, various pharmacologic therapeutics used to treat chronic lung disease may interrupt sleep.

The acute and chronic effects of sleep deficiency are not unique to patients with chronic lung disease but a complex and likely bidirectional relationship exists between sleep deficiency and chronic lung disease. As the prevalence of chronic lung diseases increases and in light of the known negative health consequences of poor sleep, it is essential to address sleep in patients with chronic lung disease. We focus on sleep deficiency in the more common chronic lung diseases including chronic obstructive pulmonary disease (COPD) and asthma, but many of the principles likely hold true for other chronic lung diseases such as cystic fibrosis (CF) and interstitial lung diseases (ILD). Additional research is needed to better understand the determinants of sleep deficiency in chronic lung diseases, thereby providing targets for optimizing sleep and overall health in this patient population.

[a] Division of Pulmonary, Critical Care and Sleep Medicine, University of California San Diego, 9300 Campus Point Drive, La Jolla, CA 92037, USA
* Corresponding author.
E-mail address: rowens@health.ucsd.edu

Clin Chest Med 43 (2022) 337–352
https://doi.org/10.1016/j.ccm.2022.02.012

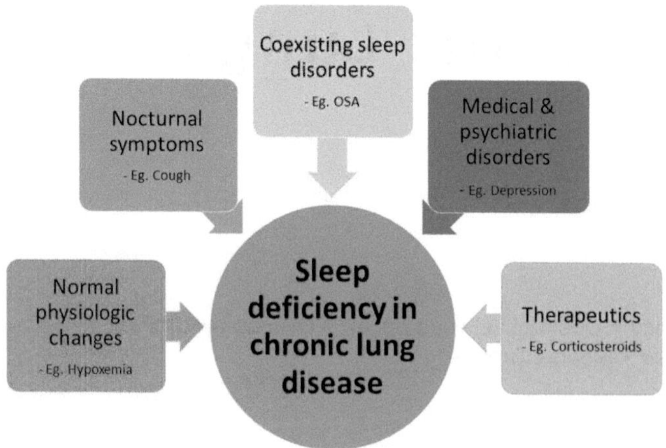

Fig. 1. Multiple factors contribute to sleep deficiency seen in chronic lung disease.

SLEEP AND BREATHING

Normal human sleep is associated with stage-specific changes in ventilatory control. There is a decrease in minute ventilation largely driven by a reduction in the tidal volume, reduced respiratory muscle contractility, increased upper airway resistance, and blunted hypoxic and hypercapnic ventilatory responses during sleep.[3,4] These physiologic changes result in hypoventilation and make sleep a potentially vulnerable period for patients with chronic lung disease.

Furthermore, pulmonary function displays endogenous circadian variability. Spengler and colleagues examined pulmonary function in 10 healthy adults for more than 41 hours in a state of relaxed wakefulness. A diurnal rhythm in lung function with significant circadian variations in forced expiratory volume in 1 second (FEV_1), ratio of FEV_1 to forced vital capacity (FVC), cortisol and core body temperature was observed (**Fig. 2**).[5] The peak to trough of mean circadian changes in spirometric variables was 2% to 3.2% of the mesor. The same group also documented circadian variation in respiratory control, drawing attention to the potential relevance of the phase of the circadian cycle when scheduling medications for patients with chronic lung disease.[6]

Chronic Obstructive Pulmonary Disease

COPD is a preventable and treatable disease characterized by persistent respiratory symptoms and airflow obstruction. It is usually caused by major exposure to noxious particles or gases (eg, cigarette smoking or burning of biofuels) and influenced by host factors including abnormal lung development.[7] Diagnosis requires demonstration of persistent airflow obstruction by the presence of a postbronchodilator FEV_1/FVC less than 0.70 on spirometry. This chronic airflow limitation is caused by a mixture of small airways disease and parenchymal destruction or emphysema, the relative contributions of which vary from person to person.

Prevalence data vary widely depending on analytical approaches used but COPD is estimated to affect 10% of adults.[7–10] COPD is a leading cause of morbidity and currently the fourth leading cause of death among adults in the world.[7] The prevalence and burden of COPD is only expected to increase with an aging population and worsening exposure to COPD risk factors including air pollution. By 2060 there may be more than 5.4 million deaths annually from COPD and related conditions.[7]

Sleep in Chronic Obstructive Pulmonary Disease

Sleep-related complaints are common in COPD.[11–20] In 2011, an expert panel found a prevalence of nocturnal symptoms and symptomatic sleep disturbance in excess of 75% in patients.[11] However, lack of a universally agreed definition of night-time symptoms in chronic lung disease was identified as a major limitation to research in this area. This limitation remains today, and studies have used variable measures to assess sleep deficiency in COPD. Nonetheless, subjective complaints of difficulties falling and staying asleep are common. In 146 patients with COPD asked to rate the frequency of 89 symptoms and experiences, sleep difficulties ranked third, after dyspnea and fatigue, which might itself relate to poor or insufficient sleep.[21] Patients with COPD clearly struggle with sleep, and have reported two times more regular hypnotic use for insomnia at 28% compared with 10% of patients without COPD.[15]

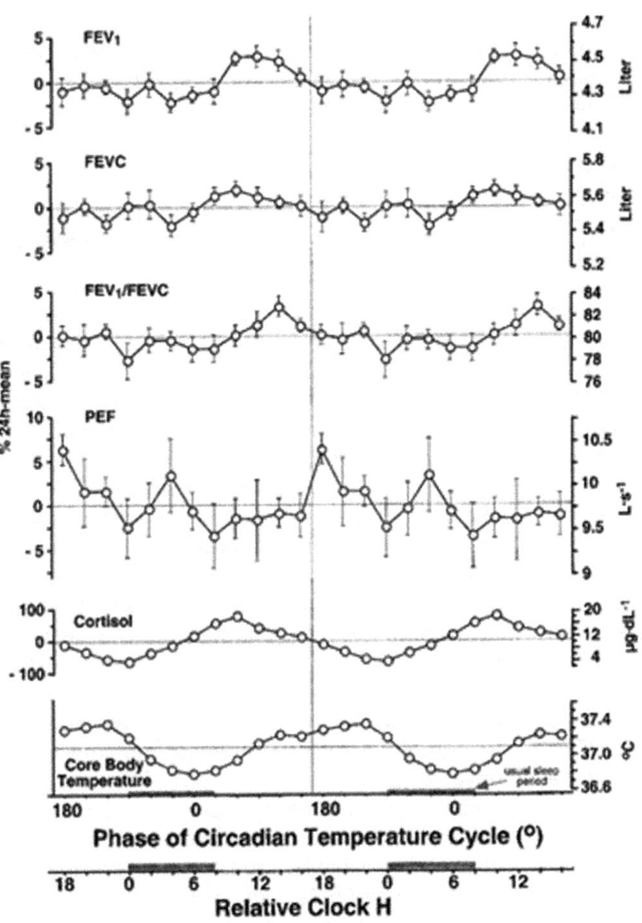

Fig. 2. Circadian rhythms of pulmonary function. Shown are the group mean levels of FEV_1, forced expiratory vital capacity (FEVC), FEV_1/FEVC, peak expiratory flow (PEF), plasma cortisol concentration, and core body temperature, aligned with respect to the reference circadian rhythm. The ordinate is expressed as deviation from the 24-h mean (left) and absolute units (right). The abscissa is expressed in degrees (with CBT_{min} assigned a phase of zero degrees) and in relative clock hour. The gray bars on the abscissa represent the time of the subjects' usual sleep episode (although sleep did not occur during this constant routine). (*From* Spengler CM, Shea SA. Endogenous circadian rhythm of pulmonary function in healthy humans. *Am J Respir Crit Care Med*. Sep 2000;162(3 Pt 1):1038-46.)

Overnight polysomnography in patients with COPD corroborates subjective complaints of disturbed sleep and sleep deficiency. Patients with COPD have reduced sleep efficiency with delayed sleep onset, reduced total sleep time, a lower arousal threshold, increased periods of wakefulness, and changes in sleep architecture with increased N1 and decreased rapid eye movement (REM) sleep compared with those without COPD.[15,17,18,22,23]

Sleep deficiency resulting from sleep disturbance in COPD is likely multifactorial in etiology, including disease-specific symptoms, comorbid sleep disorders and medical conditions, and pharmacotherapy (see **Fig. 1**). Dyspnea, cough, and wheeze are the most common symptoms of COPD. Like lung function, diurnal variation of symptoms has been described in COPD with worse symptoms in the early morning, but in patients with severe COPD, the night period was reported as the next worst time of day for experiencing symptoms.[24,25] The Tucson Epidemiologic Study of Chronic Lung Disease showed a significant relationship between respiratory symptoms including cough and/or wheeze and sleep complaints.[26] With one symptom, 29.1% reported insomnia whereas with both symptoms, 52.8% reported insomnia. Difficulty initiating or maintaining sleep was more strongly associated with the presence of respiratory symptoms than with either specific diagnoses of lung disease or pulmonary function. Similarly, in a cross-sectional European survey investigating the prevalence of night-time symptoms in COPD, 78% of 2807 patients with COPD reported night-time symptoms.[27] The presence of nocturnal symptoms was associated with sleep disturbance and poorer quality of life.

Night-time symptoms may indicate uncontrolled disease but studies to date have not consistently shown a clear association between sleep disturbance and COPD severity.[16,17,26–32] Hynninen and colleagues examined the association of symptoms of insomnia and objectively measured sleep parameters using polysomnography to the BODE index, a multidimensional index of COPD severity incorporating *b*ody mass index, airflow *o*bstructive, *d*yspnea and *e*xercise capacity, in 73 patients with COPD.[16] COPD severity, as measured using the BODE index was not associated with objectively measured sleep variables including total sleep time and, in multivariate analysis, insomnia symptoms were not independently associated with BODE scores. In contrast, in a study of 25 patients with severe emphysema undergoing evaluation for lung volume reduction surgery who completed in-laboratory polysomnography, sleep efficiency and total sleep time were decreased and total sleep time correlated with FEV_1% predicted (r = 0.5, P = .02) and FVC% predicted (r = 0.4, 0 = 0.03).[29] There was no correlation between total sleep time and measures of nocturnal oxygenation.

Nocturnal Oxygen Desaturation

The normal physiologic changes in sleep as discussed typically result in a small decrease in the partial pressure of oxygen (Pa_{O_2}) compared with the waking state. While usually not of clinical significance in normal healthy individuals, in patients with COPD, nocturnal oxygen desaturation (NOD) is common and has been associated with worse outcomes among patients with COPD.[33–35] Depending on where the patient lies on the oxyhemoglobin dissociation curve, the degree of NOD can be pronounced.[15,36,37] NOD is particularly evident during REM sleep for several reasons. First, the hypercapnic ventilatory response is further attenuated during REM compared with NREM sleep, leading to a further reduction in ventilation. Second, in COPD, there is often hyperinflation, flattening of the diaphragm, and reliance on accessory muscles of respiration to maintain ventilation. This contribution from the accessory muscles is lost during the skeletal muscle hypotonia that occurs during REM sleep. Ventilation-perfusion mismatch and a reduced functional residual capacity, exaggerated in the supine position, further contribute to NOD. Mulloy and colleagues compared ventilation and gas exchange in 19 patients with severe stable COPD during sleep and incremental treadmill exercise and SaO_2 fell twice as much during sleep as during maximum exercise, 13 versus 6% (P < .01).[38] Oxygen desaturation during sleep in COPD is primarily determined by the daytime SpO_2.[15,39–41] Hypoxemia has been implicated as one mechanism for sleep disruption in COPD, but like other measures of COPD severity, studies have not shown a consistent association between sleep efficiency and hypoxemia.[15,17,29,41] Hypoxia is a poor arousal stimulus in humans, both in nonrapid eye movements (NREM) and REM sleep.[42] In a study measuring arousal responses to progressive eucapnic hypoxia during wakefulness, NREM and REM sleep in 9 healthy adults, half failed to awaken to a SaO_2 of 70% in either NREM or REM sleep.[42]

Obstructive Sleep Apnea and Chronic Obstructive Pulmonary Disease: The Overlap Syndrome

Nocturnal hypoxemia is not unique to COPD and may signal an alternative or secondary sleep disorder, especially OSA that may be causing sleep deficiency. Like COPD, OSA is common, and is estimated to affect one billion adults globally.[43] Readers are directed to the article on sleep deficiency in OSA for a comprehensive review. In 1985, David Flenley described a unique pattern of sleep hypoxemia in patients with concomitant OSA and COPD, characterized by more profound hypoxemia, particularly during REM sleep, and a distinctive swinging pattern of nocturnal desaturation even outside REM sleep.[44] He coined the term "overlap syndrome" for the co-existence of OSA and COPD, but in his cardinal 1985 paper, he recognized this unique pattern of nocturnal hypoxemia was likely to occur with OSA and other chronic lung diseases including CF.

Prevalence data on the overlap syndrome are also widely variable, ranging from less than 1% to as high as 65%, depending on the population studied and the differing definitions used to diagnose both OSA and COPD.[45–51] Nonetheless, both OSA and COPD are common and even by chance alone the overlap syndrome is bound to occur. In his original description of the overlap syndrome, Flenley recognized that the blue bloater phenotype was particularly prone to hypoxemia when compared with the pink puffer phenotype and recently researchers have revisited the question of whether COPD phenotype matters. For example, Krachman and colleagues investigated lung inflation using spirometry and volumetric chest computed tomography (CT) in 51 smokers in the Genetic Epidemiology of COPD project who underwent full-night polysomnography for suspected OSA.[52] 57% had OSA and there was an inverse correlation between the apnea–hypopnea index (AHI) and CT-derived measures of emphysema and air trapping. The emphysema phenotype with air trapping and hyperinflation was proposed as potentially exerting tracheal traction to stiffen and stabilize the upper airway, thereby providing a possible protective mechanism for OSA in patients with more advanced COPD. But, note again the very high prevalence of OSA in this study.

One significant challenge to OSA research in chronic lung disease is uncertainty regarding the optimal diagnostic criteria for OSA in chronic lung disease. Currently, diagnosis of OSA relies on the calculation of the average number of apneas or hypopneas per hour of sleep or monitoring time. The scoring of hypopneas is dependent on oxyhemoglobin desaturation but there has been an ongoing debate regarding the degree of desaturation required. This issue is of particular relevance in patients with chronic lung disease who sit on the steep portion of the oxyhemoglobin dissociation curve whereby even a small drop in arterial oxygen tension can result in a major difference in SaO_2. Consequently, hypopneas may be scored more readily in patients with chronic lung disease for the same degree of upper airway collapse. In contrast, the use of supplemental oxygen eliminates one of the main criteria for scoring hypopneas and the AHI may be under-estimated in patients on supplemental oxygen. Regardless, caution must be exercised attributing NOD to COPD alone and a sleep study for the evaluation of OSA should be considered when NOD is seen in COPD.[53–55] (**Fig. 3**).

Timely and accurate diagnosis of OSA in chronic lung disease is essential as the overlap syndrome has been associated with worse outcomes when compared with OSA or COPD alone.[56–62] The overlap syndrome is associated with greater sleep-related hypoxemia and hypercapnia than OSA alone or patients with COPD with the same degree of airflow obstruction. Pulmonary hypertension is more common and more severe and quality of life is worse. Marin and colleagues compared 213 patients with the overlap syndrome to 210 patients with COPD without OSA for a median follow-up of 9.4 years and found higher mortality (relative risk 1.79, 95% confidence interval 1.21–2.38) and likelihood of COPD exacerbation leading to hospitalization (relative risk 1.70, 95% confidence interval 1.21–2.38) in patients with the overlap syndrome compared with patients with COPD without OSA.[58] Despite these adverse outcomes, little data exist specifically studying sleep duration and quality in the overlap syndrome. Fortunately, effective therapies for the overlap syndrome exist and in the same study by Marin and colleagues showing worse outcomes in patients with the overlap syndrome, CPAP treatment was associated with improved survival and decreased hospitalizations in these patients. Konikkara and colleagues screened for OSA in all patients hospitalized and consulted for a COPD exacerbation who had a BMI greater than 30 kg/m^2 and showed reduced readmissions with early recognition and treatment of OSA.[63]

Other Sleep Disorders in Chronic Obstructive Pulmonary Disease

There are few studies exploring the contribution of other sleep disorders to sleep deficiency in COPD. Some evidence exists for restless leg syndrome (RLS) or Willis–Ekbom disease (WED). WED is characterized by an unpleasant need or urge to move the legs at night time that can interfere with sleep thereby causing sleep deficiency. A higher prevalence of WED has been reported in COPD than in the general population, ranging between 26% and 37%.[64–67] During COPD exacerbations, the prevalence is even higher at 54%.[68] WED is thought to be caused by complex genetic and environmental interactions, but the reason for the increased frequency of WED in COPD is unknown with no consistent association shown between WED and lung function severity.[69] WED can be disabling and is associated with poor sleep quality. All patients with COPD should be specifically asked about symptoms of WED, especially given the availability of effective therapeutics.

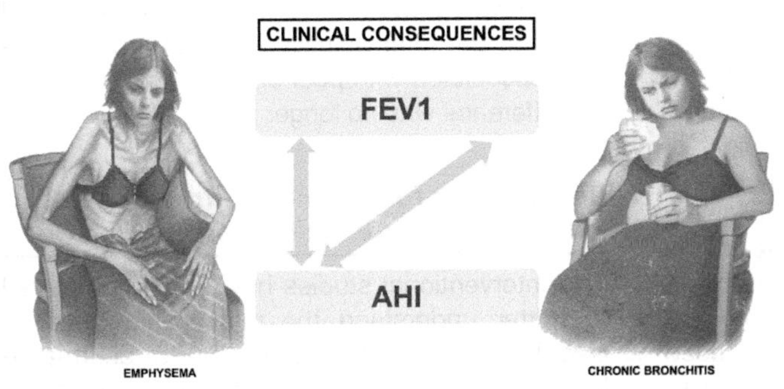

Fig. 3. The co-existence of OSA (elevated AHI) and COPD (reduced FEV1) has been associated with worse clinical outcomes, but it remains unknown which combination of OSA and COPD is associated with which clinical outcomes. Both disorders have varying phenotypes and a wide range of severity, For example, both a patient with severe emphysema (eg FEV_1 30% predicted) and mild OSA (eg AHI 7 events per hour) and a patient with mild chronic bronchitis (eg FEV_1 72% predicted) and severe OSA (eg AHI 60 events per hour) meet diagnostic criteria for the overlap syndrome, but the clinical presentation and outcomes of these 2 patients are likely to be very different.

Patients should also be asked about chronic medical and psychiatric comorbidities commonly seen in COPD that are also associated with poor sleep, in particular pain, depression, and anxiety[7,70–73] Depression and anxiety are more prevalent in COPD than the general population, with prevalence estimates ranging between 10% to 42% and 10% to 19% respectively.[71] In a recent systematic review, patients with COPD were 1.9 times more likely to commit suicide than patients without COPD.[74] Yet, the nature of the relationship between COPD, depression/anxiety, and sleep is complicated with overlap between symptoms. In fact, sleep complaints form part of the diagnostic and statistical manual (DSM) criteria for depression and anxiety. A meta-analysis of 34 prospective cohort studies showed that insomnia more than doubled risk of depression.[75] Consequently, comorbid depression and anxiety can add to sleep deficiency in COPD and have a major impact on health outcomes.[7,70–72,76] The combination of mental disorders with insomnia symptoms increased by five times the likelihood of hospitalization in COPD.[76] Yet, less than one-third of patients with COPD with comorbid depression or anxiety symptoms are receiving appropriate treatment.[72] Given the bidirectional relationship between sleep and depression, addressing depression and anxiety are essential in improving sleep in COPD.

Sleep deficiency is known to have a negative impact on a range of clinical outcomes and this holds true for COPD. Poor sleep quality in COPD has been associated with worse quality of life. In the SPIROMICS study evaluating the impact of patient-reported sleep quality and sleep apnea risk on disease-specific and overall quality of life in patients with COPD, poor sleep quality per se accounted for 9% to 14% of the variance in quality of life measures.[11,14,77–79]

Sleep Deficiency and Impact on Chronic Obstructive Pulmonary Disease

Once again, a bidirectional relationship between sleep disturbance and COPD likely exists. In 1987 Phillips et al studied 15 adults with stable COPD following a night of sleep or one night of sleep deprivation.[80] Small but statistically significant falls in FEV_1 and FVC were seen following sleep deprivation. There was no change in the FEV_1/FVC or ventilatory responsiveness to inhaled CO_2 but an accompanying fall in the maximal inspiratory pressure that was felt to reflect reduced muscular performance, either from actual weakness or a reduction in voluntary effort. In a study measuring respiratory muscle and pulmonary function in 30 normal males following 30 hours of sleep deprivation, significant decrements in inspiratory muscle endurance and maximal voluntary ventilation were seen after sleep loss.[81] In a separate study assessing the effect of sleep deprivation on respiratory motor output in 20 healthy subjects, one night of sleep deprivation was also associated with decreased cortical respiratory motor output and consequent inspiratory endurance decrement.[82] Interestingly, the sleep deprivation group more commonly used descriptors of breathlessness in relation to air hunger compared with controls, suggesting that sleep deprivation may influence the sensory perception of dyspnea itself.[83] The effects of sleep deprivation on ventilatory responses to hypercapnia and hypoxia in normal subjects have been more mixed with some concerns that initial studies suggesting reduced ventilatory responses to hypercapnia and hypoxia may have been affected by uncontrolled activities or environmental influences during sleep deprivation.[81,84–86]

Even less data on sleep deficiency and ventilatory control exist in COPD. COPD exacerbations negatively impact health status, rates of hospitalization, and disease progression. Poor baseline sleep quality assessed using the PSQI was associated with increased risk of COPD exacerbations in 480 adults with COPD followed more than 18 months.[87] Similarly, Omachi et al showed sleep disturbance longitudinally predicted both incident COPD exacerbations (odds ratio (OR) = 4.7, P = .018) and respiratory-related emergency utilization (OR = 11.5, P = .0004) in 98 adults with COPD followed for a median 2.4 years.[30] Sleep disturbance was also associated with poorer survival, even after controlling for baseline FEV_1. Poor sleep quality has been shown to be an independent predictor of functional exercise capacity in COPD.[88] However, again the relationship between sleep and COPD outcomes is complex. This was highlighted by Geiger-Brown et al who also demonstrated greater exacerbation rates in poor sleepers with COPD compared with good sleepers, but after adjusting for comorbid conditions associated with poor sleep and medications, the difference was no longer significant.[89]

Do Therapies for Chronic Obstructive Pulmonary Disease Improve Sleep?

Few interventional studies have been completed to better understand the relationship between sleep deficiency and COPD. COPD pharmacologic treatment is centered around bronchodilators and anti-inflammatory drugs. They have been shown to reduce symptoms, reduce the frequency and severity of exacerbations and improve health status and exercise tolerance. Given the relationship between respiratory symptoms and sleep-related complaints, it would naturally seem that reducing the severity of respiratory symptoms will improve sleep. Yet, studies to date have not confirmed this. Long-acting bronchodilators have been shown to improve FEV_1 and hypoxemia during sleep in COPD but a consistent improvement in sleep quality has not been shown.[90–94]

Similarly, studies administering supplemental oxygen in COPD have shown mixed results in sleep quality despite improvements in oxygenation, further highlighting the inconsistent association between hypoxemia and sleep.[95–98] Long-term administration of oxygen greater than 15 h/d improves survival in patients with COPD and severe daytime resting hypoxemia.[99,100] However, randomized controlled trials have failed to demonstrate clinically significant benefits in patients with less severe hypoxemia.[101] The International Nocturnal Oxygen (INOX) study was a multicenter randomized placebo-controlled trial designed to assess the efficacy of oxygen therapy in patients with COPD with isolated nocturnal arterial oxygen saturation, defined as an SO2 less than 90% for at least 30% of recording time on nocturnal oximetry.[102] However, recruitment was stopped prematurely limiting interpretation, and the evidence to date does not support the routine use of nocturnal oxygen for isolated sleep hypoxemia. Similarly, supplemental oxygen alone is not recommended as primary treatment of OSA or the overlap syndrome. Alford and colleagues studied 20 men with the overlap syndrome with polysomnography on 2 separate nights, with and without nocturnal supplemental oxygen at 4 L/min.[103] Supplemental oxygen administration again improved oxygenation but it also increased the mean duration of obstructive events by 5.7 seconds and increased end-apneic partial pressure of carbon dioxide by 9.5 mm Hg.

Pulmonary rehabilitation has many benefits in COPD, improving symptoms, exercise tolerance, and quality of life. The impact of pulmonary rehabilitation on sleep quality has again been mixed with very little data on objective sleep duration.[104–106] However, pulmonary rehabilitation has been shown to effectively reduce symptoms of anxiety and depression, and given the other clearly demonstrated benefits of pulmonary rehabilitation it should be integrated routinely into the management of COPD.[70,107]

Does Treatment of Sleep Problems Improve Chronic Obstructive Pulmonary Disease?

For those patients with the overlap syndrome, CPAP has been shown to be very effective in the treatment of OSA and overlap syndrome.[58,63,108] When comparing patients with the overlap syndrome adherent to CPAP treatment to those nonadherent, CPAP treatment has been associated with improved survival and decreased hospitalizations.[58,63] Screening for and treatment of OSA in patients admitted with a COPD exacerbation has also been associated with reduced 6-month hospital readmission rates and emergency room visits.[63] The survival benefit of CPAP in the overlap syndrome may be particularly true for hypercapnic patients.[109]

Increasing evidence supports the benefits of nocturnal noninvasive ventilation (NIV) in stable patients with COPD with persistent hypercapnia.[110–113] There are currently no studies on NIV in the overlap syndrome and it remains unknown whether NIV offers additional benefits over CPAP in the management of the overlap syndrome, especially in the subset of patients who are hypercapnic. Likely more important than the mode of positive airway pressure is adherence. Stanchina and colleagues showed a clear association between CPAP usage and mortality in patients with the overlap syndrome.[114]

Multicomponent cognitive behavioral therapy for insomnia (CBT-I) has been shown to improve sleep latency and wake after sleep onset and is recommended by the American Academy of Sleep Medicine as first-line treatment of chronic insomnia in adults.[115] Studies suggest CBT-I is also feasible in COPD with comparable favorable outcomes, and CBT-I should be discussed with every COPD patient reporting insomnia.[115–117] This is particularly true as hypnotic medications like benzodiazepines have the potential for respiratory depression, which is clearly of concern in patients with chronic lung disease and limited pulmonary reserve. Benzodiazepines have been associated with increased risk of exacerbations, respiratory failure, risk of suicide, and mortality with short term use in COPD, and should generally be avoided, especially among older patients.[20,118,119] While few studies have suggested a better safety profile with nonbenzodiazepine hypnotics like the nonbenzodiazepine benzodiazepine receptor agonists in COPD, there are limited data on the efficacy and safety of long-term hypnotic use in this group and CBT-I remains the preferred treatment of insomnia.[120]

In summary, sleep symptoms are common in COPD for many reasons. Treatments for COPD may not directly improve sleep symptoms. However, sleep-specific therapies like CBT-I for insomnia and PAP therapy for OSA are useful and can improve quality of life. PAP therapy for OSA might also reduce COPD exacerbations.

Finally, NIV should be considered for those with stable chronic hypercapnic COPD.

ASTHMA

Asthma is now recognized to be a heterogeneous disease caused by complex gene-environment interactions and is usually characterized by airway inflammation.[121,122] It is one of the most common chronic, noncommunicable diseases affecting all age groups. Prevalence varies between countries and is highest in developed countries, but in the United States, according to the 2018 Center for Disease Control (CDC) data, asthma is estimated to occur in approximately 7.7% of adults. Asthma is defined by a history of respiratory symptoms such as wheeze, shortness of breath, chest tightness, and cough that vary over time and in intensity, together with variable expiratory flow limitation.

Sleep in Asthma

Like COPD, complaints of difficulties falling and staying asleep are common in asthma and have been associated with worse quality of life.[123–126] Lal and colleagues used the National Health and Nutritional Examination Survey (NHANES) to examine the association between self-reported sleep problems among 3204 adults with obstructive lung diseases, 5.2% with asthma alone.[126] All obstructive lung diseases were associated with a higher prevalence of sleep problems, defined as any complaints which affect or involve sleep, but there was a stronger association between asthma and sleep problems as compared with COPD and asthma–COPD overlap. The authors speculated that the nocturnal burden of asthma contributes to sleep problems. As many as 74% of asthmatics are awakened by asthma symptoms at least once per week.[127]

Normal diurnal variations in lung function have been recognized for centuries and can lead to worsening symptoms at night or in the early morning.[128] In a study of 20 adults with stable asthma, there was a good correlation between nocturnal or awakening symptoms and the overnight fall in peak expiratory flow rate (PEFR).[129] The overnight decrement in lung function was related to daytime severity of asthma as determined by daytime measures of airflow limitation and bronchial responsiveness as well as the circadian variation in bronchial responsivity.[129] Very few studies have looked at the effects of sleep duration on this endogenous circadian variation, but no clear association between sleep deprivation or sleep efficiency and circadian variation has been shown.[5,129]

Nocturnal Asthma

Nocturnal asthma is defined by a greater than 15% reduction in the morning FEV_1 when compared with the evening FEV_1.[130–132] It is associated with increased morbidity and impaired quality of life, and treatment of nocturnal airway obstruction has been shown to improve daytime cognitive performance, a finding of particular importance in children with asthma.[133,134] Regrettably, few providers ask about nighttime symptoms.[135] Circadian variations in airway inflammation and physiologic variables including airflow limitation and airways hyperresponsiveness are accompanied by alterations in β_2-adrenergic and glucocorticoid receptors.[130,131] The number and physiologic function of β_2-adrenergic receptors is decreased between 4:00 PM and 4:00 AM leading to a reduced response to bronchodilators, while the binding affinity of glucocorticoid receptors is reduced at 4:00 AM versus 4:00 PM, contributing to airway inflammation. For example, Kraft M et al. performed bronchoscopic biopsies in asthmatic subjects and showed an increase in eosinophils in transbronchial specimens from nocturnal asthmatics, and a subsequent study showed a greater proportion of CD4+ cells in alveolar samples in nocturnal asthmatics.[136] Studies have also suggested altered hypothalamic–pituitary–adrenal interactions in nocturnal asthma. Reduced serum cortisol has been reported in nighttime sampling in asthmatic children, and another study reported increased corticotropin levels in nocturnal asthma, but without a commensurate increase in serum cortisol levels, suggesting that adrenal responsiveness to corticotropin may be blunted in nocturnal asthma. Sutherland ER has also investigated the possible role of melatonin as a proinflammatory mediator and demonstrated higher levels of melatonin, a hormone produced by the pineal gland in the dark cycle, in patients with nocturnal asthma compared to both non-nocturnal asthmatic and healthy controls. Both small airway and alveolar tissue inflammation are seen in nocturnal asthma.[137,138] Finally, gastroesophageal reflux disease (GERD) can be an important comorbidity that can worsen asthma in general and nocturnal asthma in particular. GERD is common among patients with asthma and can exacerbate airflow limitation although the exact mechanism remains unclear. These investigations highlight the range of potential mechanisms that can contribute to sleep-related symptoms in asthmatics.

Does the Timing of Asthma Treatment Matter? – The Concept of Chronotherapy

Consequently, the timing of therapeutics in asthma may influence clinical response. Chronooptimized therapy aims to synchronize medication levels in time with reference to need. Studies comparing dosing strategies have suggested greater improvement in nocturnal symptoms using dosing strategies aimed to optimize therapeutic drug levels during periods of nocturnal worsening.[139–143] Early evening administration of inhaled corticosteroids was shown to be preferable to morning dosing with regard to morning or evening peak flow.[141] In a double-blind, placebo-controlled, crossover trial, Beam WR et al compared spirometry, blood eosinophilic counts and bronchoalveolar lavage (BAL) cytology in 7 asthmatics administered a single 50 mg oral dose of prednisone variably at 8:00 AM, 3:00 PM or 8:00 PM Administration of prednisone at 3:00 PM resulted in a decrease in the overnight percentage fall in FEV_1, improvement in the 4:00 AM FEV_1, reduction in blood eosinophil counts, and pancellular reduction in BAL cytology, while the 8:00 AM and 8:00 PM dosing schedule did not.[139]

Obstructive Sleep Apnea and Asthma: Another Overlap

It is important to recognize that all that wheezes are not asthma and nocturnal symptoms perceived as asthma may be due to OSA.[144,145] With asthma and OSA both being among the most common chronic respiratory disorders, the co-existence of both is not surprising. Most epidemiologic studies support a higher prevalence of OSA in patients with asthma, and a meta-analysis of 26 studies estimated the prevalence of OSA in adults with asthma at 50%.[126,146–155] An even higher prevalence has been reported in patients with severe asthma and in a study of 22 adults with severe, poorly controlled asthma requiring oral corticosteroids, all but one had OSA diagnosed by polysomnography.[156,157] A sleep study should be considered in any patient with asthma describing poorly controlled symptoms.

Asthma has been also associated with an increased risk of new-onset OSA and it remains unclear whether the association between asthma and OSA represents correlation (ie, shared risk factors including obesity, rhinitis and gastroesophageal reflux), chance, or causation.[153,155] Confounders, like obesity, make it difficult to ascertain the relationship between asthma and OSA and likely a bidirectional relationship exists. Regardless, the co-existence of asthma and OSA has been associated with worse clinical outcomes including asthma control and exacerbations, greater FEV_1 decline, worse quality of life, and increased health resource utilization, highlighting the importance of diagnosing OSA in patients with asthma.[154,158–161]

This is especially true as very effective therapies for OSA are available. While randomized controlled studies are needed to better understand the impact of CPAP on asthmatics with OSA, observational studies have shown improved asthma symptom control and quality of life with CPAP in patients with asthma and OSA overlap.[125,157,162–166] Studies on lung function with CPAP use in asthmatics with OSA have been more mixed.[160,166] In a study of 77 adults with asthma and varying severities of OSA, FEV_1 decline was greatest among asthmatics with severe OSA as compared with those with mild to moderate OSA, and decline of FEV_1 significantly decreased after CPAP treatment.[160] Yet, other studies have failed to demonstrate FEV_1 improvement with CPAP use and CPAP has not been shown to improve objective measures of bronchial responsiveness, such as the provocative concentration causing a 20% fall in FEV_1 (PC_{20})[162,164,165]. Interestingly, some research looking at the effects of CPAP in asthmatics without coexisting OSA exists. By increasing stretch of the airway during sleep, CPAP has been proposed to suppress airway smooth muscle contractility.[167–170] Small animal and human studies have suggested improvement in bronchial hyperreactivity in asthmatics without OSA with CPAP use but these results have not been reproduced in a larger clinical study[125,167,168,171–174]

In summary, asthma may worsen at night and suggests overall poor asthma control. These nighttime symptoms also have daytime consequences. Like COPD, not all that wheezes at night is asthma and comorbid sleep disorders such as OSA should be considered. Like the COPD–OSA overlap syndrome, treatment of moderate to severe OSA with PAP therapy can improve quality of life. Finally, more work needs to be conducted to understand the impact of the timing of therapy to improve effectiveness and potentially reduce side effects.

SUMMARY

With sleep occupying up to one-third of every adult's life, addressing sleep is essential to overall health. Sleep disturbance and deficiency are common in patients with chronic lung diseases and associated with worse clinical outcomes and poor quality of life. A detailed history incorporating nocturnal respiratory symptoms, symptoms of OSA and restless legs syndrome, symptoms of anxiety and depression, and medications is the first step in identifying and addressing the multiple factors often contributing to sleep deficiency in chronic lung disease. Additional research is needed to better understand the relationship between sleep deficiency and the spectrum of chronic lung diseases.

CLINICS CARE POINTS

- In patients with chronic lung disease, ask about nocturnal symptoms as they are associated with sleep disturbance and worse quality of life.
- Obtain a comprehensive sleep history in all patients with chronic lung disease to identify potential co-existing sleep disorders including insomnia, sleep disordered breathing and RLS, that could be therapeutic targets.
- Recognize that normal circadian variability in pulmonary function and sleep-stage specific ventilatory changes during sleep, make sleep a potentially vulnerable period for worsening hypoxemia and hypercapnia in patients with chronic lung disease.
- Caution must be exercised attributing nocturnal respiratory symptoms and oxygen desaturation to chronic lung disease alone, and testing for obstructive sleep apnea should be considered.
- A bidirectional relationship likely exists between sleep deficiency and chronic lung disease and optimal management should address both sides.

DISCLOSURE

The authors have nothing to disclose.

REFERENCES

1. Bousquet J, Kaltaev N. Global surveillance, prevention and control of chronic respiratory diseases : a comprehensive approach / edited by Jean Bousquet and Nikolai Khaltaev. World Health Organization. 2007. Available at: https://apps.who.int/iris/handle/10665/43776ISBN9789241563468.
2. Collaborators GBDCRD. Prevalence and attributable health burden of chronic respiratory diseases, 1990-2017: a systematic analysis for the Global Burden of Disease Study 2017. Lancet Respir Med 2020;8(6):585–96.
3. Douglas NJ, White DP, Pickett CK, et al. Respiration during sleep in normal man. Thorax 1982; 37(11):840–4.
4. Douglas NJ, White DP, Weil JV, et al. Hypoxic ventilatory response decreases during sleep in normal men. Am Rev Respir Dis 1982;125(3):286–9.
5. Spengler CM, Shea SA. Endogenous circadian rhythm of pulmonary function in healthy humans. Am J Respir Crit Care Med 2000;162(3 Pt 1):1038–46.
6. Spengler CM, Czeisler CA, Shea SA. An endogenous circadian rhythm of respiratory control in humans. J Physiol 2000;526(Pt 3):683–94.
7. Disease GIfCOL. Globla strategy for the diagnosis, management, and prevention of chronic obstructive pulmonary disease. 2020 Report. 2020:1-141.
8. Adeloye D, Chua S, Lee C, et al. Global and regional estimates of COPD prevalence: systematic review and meta-analysis. J Glob Health 2015;5(2):020415.
9. Collaborators GBDCRD. Global, regional, and national deaths, prevalence, disability-adjusted life years, and years lived with disability for chronic obstructive pulmonary disease and asthma, 1990-2015: a systematic analysis for the Global Burden of Disease Study 2015. Lancet Respir Med 2017; 5(9):691–706.
10. Halbert RJ, Natoli JL, Gano A, et al. Global burden of COPD: systematic review and meta-analysis. Eur Respir J 2006;28(3):523–32.
11. Agusti A, Hedner J, Marin JM, et al. Night-time symptoms: a forgotten dimension of COPD. Eur Respir Rev 2011;20(121):183–94.
12. Budhiraja R, Roth T, Hudgel DW, et al. Prevalence and polysomnographic correlates of insomnia comorbid with medical disorders. Sleep 2011;34(7): 859–67.
13. Chang CH, Chuang LP, Lin SW, et al. Factors responsible for poor sleep quality in patients with chronic obstructive pulmonary disease. BMC Pulm Med 2016;16(1):118.
14. Zeidler MR, Martin JL, Kleerup EC, et al. Sleep disruption as a predictor of quality of life among patients in the subpopulations and intermediate outcome measures in COPD study (SPIROMICS). Sleep 2018; 41(5). https://doi.org/10.1093/sleep/zsy044.
15. Cormick W, Olson LG, Hensley MJ, et al. Nocturnal hypoxaemia and quality of sleep in patients with chronic obstructive lung disease. Thorax 1986; 41(11):846–54.
16. Hynninen MJ, Pallesen S, Hardie J, et al. Insomnia symptoms, objectively measured sleep, and disease severity in chronic obstructive pulmonary disease outpatients. Sleep Med 2013;14(12):1328–33.
17. McSharry DG, Ryan S, Calverley P, et al. Sleep quality in chronic obstructive pulmonary disease. Respirology 2012;17(7):1119–24.
18. Valipour A, Lavie P, Lothaller H, et al. Sleep profile and symptoms of sleep disorders in patients with stable mild to moderate chronic obstructive pulmonary disease. Sleep Med 2011;12(4):367–72.

19. Klink M, Quan SF. Prevalence of reported sleep disturbances in a general adult population and their relationship to obstructive airways diseases. Chest 1987;91(4):540–6.
20. Bellia V, Catalano F, Scichilone N, et al. Sleep disorders in the elderly with and without chronic airflow obstruction: the SARA study. Sleep 2003; 26(3):318–23.
21. Kinsman RA, Yaroush RA, Fernandez E, et al. Symptoms and experiences in chronic bronchitis and emphysema. Chest 1983;83(5):755–61.
22. Yamaguchi Y, Shiota S, Kusunoki Y, et al. Polysomnographic features of low arousal threshold in overlap syndrome involving obstructive sleep apnea and chronic obstructive pulmonary disease. Sleep Breath 2019;23(4):1095–100.
23. Parish JM. Sleep-related problems in common medical conditions. Chest 2009;135(2):563–72.
24. Kessler R, Partridge MR, Miravitlles M, et al. Symptom variability in patients with severe COPD: a pan-European cross-sectional study. Eur Respir J 2011; 37(2):264–72.
25. Partridge MR, Karlsson N, Small IR. Patient insight into the impact of chronic obstructive pulmonary disease in the morning: an internet survey. Curr Med Res Opin 2009;25(8):2043–8.
26. Klink ME, Dodge R, Quan SF. The relation of sleep complaints to respiratory symptoms in a general population. Chest 1994;105(1):151–4.
27. Price D, Small M, Milligan G, et al. Impact of night-time symptoms in COPD: a real-world study in five European countries. Int J Chron Obstruct Pulmon Dis 2013;8:595–603.
28. Donovan LM, Rise PJ, Carson SS, et al. Sleep disturbance in smokers with preserved pulmonary function and with chronic obstructive pulmonary disease. Ann Am Thorac Soc 2017;14(12): 1836–43.
29. Krachman SL, Chatila W, Martin UJ, et al. Physiologic correlates of sleep quality in severe emphysema. COPD 2011;8(3):182–8.
30. Omachi TA, Blanc PD, Claman DM, et al. Disturbed sleep among COPD patients is longitudinally associated with mortality and adverse COPD outcomes. Sleep Med 2012;13(5):476–83.
31. Sanders MH, Newman AB, Haggerty CL, et al. Sleep and sleep-disordered breathing in adults with predominantly mild obstructive airway disease. Am J Respir Crit Care Med 2003;167(1):7–14.
32. Antonelli-Incalzi R, Imperiale C, Bellia V, et al. Do GOLD stages of COPD severity really correspond to differences in health status? Eur Respir J 2003; 22(3):444–9.
33. Fletcher EC, Donner CF, Midgren B, et al. Survival in COPD patients with a daytime PaO2 greater than 60 mm Hg with and without nocturnal oxyhemoglobin desaturation. Chest 1992;101(3):649–55.
34. Macrea MM, Owens RL, Martin T, et al. The effect of isolated nocturnal oxygen desaturations on serum hs-CRP and IL-6 in patients with chronic obstructive pulmonary disease. Clin Respir J 2019;13(2): 120–4.
35. Sergi M, Rizzi M, Andreoli A, et al. Are COPD patients with nocturnal REM sleep-related desaturations more prone to developing chronic respiratory failure requiring long-term oxygen therapy? Respiration 2002;69(2):117–22.
36. Koo KW, Sax DS, Snider GL. Arterial blood gases and pH during sleep in chronic obstructive pulmonary disease. Am J Med 1975;58(5):663–70.
37. Trask CH, Cree EM. Oximeter studies on patients with chronic obstructive emphysema, awake and during sleep. N Engl J Med 1962;266:639–42.
38. Mulloy E, McNicholas WT. Ventilation and gas exchange during sleep and exercise in severe COPD. Chest 1996;109(2):387–94.
39. Chaouat A, Weitzenblum E, Kessler R, et al. Sleep-related O2 desaturation and daytime pulmonary haemodynamics in COPD patients with mild hypoxaemia. Eur Respir J 1997;10(8):1730–5.
40. Connaughton JJ, Catterall JR, Elton RA, et al. Do sleep studies contribute to the management of patients with severe chronic obstructive pulmonary disease? Am Rev Respir Dis 1988;138(2):341–4.
41. Lewis CA, Fergusson W, Eaton T, et al. Isolated nocturnal desaturation in COPD: prevalence and impact on quality of life and sleep. Thorax 2009; 64(2):133–8.
42. Berthon-Jones M, Sullivan CE. Ventilatory and arousal responses to hypoxia in sleeping humans. Am Rev Respir Dis 1982;125(6):632–9.
43. Benjafield AV, Ayas NT, Eastwood PR, et al. Estimation of the global prevalence and burden of obstructive sleep apnoea: a literature-based analysis. Lancet Respir Med 2019;7(8):687–98.
44. Flenley DC. Sleep in chronic obstructive lung disease. Clin Chest Med 1985;6(4):651–61.
45. Bednarek M, Maciejewski J, Wozniak M, et al. Prevalence, severity and underdiagnosis of COPD in the primary care setting. Thorax 2008;63(5):402–7.
46. Greenberg-Dotan S, Reuveni H, Tal A, et al. Increased prevalence of obstructive lung disease in patients with obstructive sleep apnea. Sleep Breath 2014;18(1):69–75.
47. Lopez-Acevedo MN, Torres-Palacios A, Elena Ocasio-Tascon M, et al. Overlap syndrome: an indication for sleep studies?: a pilot study. Sleep Breath 2009;13(4):409–13.
48. Owens RL, Macrea MM, Teodorescu M. The overlaps of asthma or COPD with OSA: a focused review. Respirology 2017;22(6):1073–83.
49. Schreiber A, Cemmi F, Ambrosino N, et al. Prevalence and Predictors of obstructive sleep apnea in patients with chronic obstructive pulmonary

disease undergoing inpatient pulmonary rehabilitation. COPD 2018;15(3):265–70.
50. Shawon MS, Perret JL, Senaratna CV, et al. Current evidence on prevalence and clinical outcomes of co-morbid obstructive sleep apnea and chronic obstructive pulmonary disease: a systematic review. Sleep Med Rev 2017;32:58–68.
51. Soler X, Gaio E, Powell FL, et al. High prevalence of obstructive sleep apnea in patients with moderate to severe chronic obstructive pulmonary disease. Ann Am Thorac Soc 2015;12(8):1219–25.
52. Krachman SL, Tiwari R, Vega ME, et al. Effect of emphysema severity on the apnea-hypopnea index in smokers with obstructive sleep apnea. Ann Am Thorac Soc 2016;13(7):1129–35.
53. Chang Y, Xu L, Han F, et al. Validation of the Nox-T3 portable monitor for diagnosis of obstructive sleep apnea in patients with chronic obstructive pulmonary disease. J Clin Sleep Med 2019; 15(4):587–96.
54. Jen R, Orr JE, Li Y, et al. Accuracy of WatchPAT for the diagnosis of obstructive sleep apnea in patients with chronic obstructive pulmonary disease. COPD 2020;17(1):34–9.
55. Oliveira MG, Nery LE, Santos-Silva R, et al. Is portable monitoring accurate in the diagnosis of obstructive sleep apnea syndrome in chronic pulmonary obstructive disease? Sleep Med 2012; 13(8):1033–8.
56. Chaouat A, Weitzenblum E, Krieger J, et al. Association of chronic obstructive pulmonary disease and sleep apnea syndrome. Am J Respir Crit Care Med 1995;151(1):82–6.
57. Kessler R, Chaouat A, Schinkewitch P, et al. The obesity-hypoventilation syndrome revisited: a prospective study of 34 consecutive cases. Chest 2001;120(2):369–76.
58. Marin JM, Soriano JB, Carrizo SJ, et al. Outcomes in patients with chronic obstructive pulmonary disease and obstructive sleep apnea: the overlap syndrome. Am J Respir Crit Care Med 2010;182(3):325–31.
59. Mermigkis C, Kopanakis A, Foldvary-Schaefer N, et al. Health-related quality of life in patients with obstructive sleep apnoea and chronic obstructive pulmonary disease (overlap syndrome). Int J Clin Pract 2007;61(2):207–11.
60. Weitzenblum E, Chaouat A, Kessler R, et al. Overlap syndrome: obstructive sleep apnea in patients with chronic obstructive pulmonary disease. Proc Am Thorac Soc 2008;5(2):237–41.
61. Zohal MA, Yazdi Z, Kazemifar AM, et al. Sleep quality and quality of life in COPD patients with and without suspected obstructive sleep apnea. Sleep Disord 2014;2014:508372.
62. Donovan LM, Feemster LC, Udris EM, et al. Poor outcomes among patients with chronic obstructive pulmonary disease with higher risk for undiagnosed obstructive sleep apnea in the LOTT cohort. J Clin Sleep Med 2019;15(1):71–7.
63. Konikkara J, Tavella R, Willes L, et al. Early recognition of obstructive sleep apnea in patients hospitalized with COPD exacerbation is associated with reduced readmission. Hosp Pract (1995) 2016; 44(1):41–7.
64. Cavalcante AG, de Bruin PF, de Bruin VM, et al. Restless legs syndrome, sleep impairment, and fatigue in chronic obstructive pulmonary disease. Sleep Med 2012;13(7):842–7.
65. Ding Z, Stehlik R, Hedner J, et al. Chronic pulmonary disease is associated with pain spreading and restless legs syndrome in middle-aged women-a population-based study. Sleep Breath 2019;23(1):135–42.
66. Kaplan Y, Inonu H, Yilmaz A, et al. Restless legs syndrome in patients with chronic obstructive pulmonary disease. Can J Neurol Sci 2008;35(3): 352–7.
67. Lo Coco D, Mattaliano A, Lo Coco A, et al. Increased frequency of restless legs syndrome in chronic obstructive pulmonary disease patients. Sleep Med 2009;10(5):572–6.
68. Aras G, Kadakal F, Purisa S, et al. Are we aware of restless legs syndrome in COPD patients who are in an exacerbation period? Frequency and probable factors related to underlying mechanism. COPD 2011;8(6):437–43.
69. Mandal T, Aydin S, Kanmaz D, et al. To what extent and why are COPD and Willis-Ekbom disease associated? Sleep Breath 2016;20(3):1021–7.
70. Coventry PA, Bower P, Keyworth C, et al. The effect of complex interventions on depression and anxiety in chronic obstructive pulmonary disease: systematic review and meta-analysis. PLoS One 2013; 8(4):e60532.
71. Maurer J, Rebbapragada V, Borson S, et al. Anxiety and depression in COPD: current understanding, unanswered questions, and research needs. Chest 2008;134(4 Suppl):43S–56S.
72. Yohannes AM, Lavoie KL. Overseeing anxiety and depression in patients with physical illness. Chest 2013;144(3):726–8.
73. Hanania NA, Mullerova H, Locantore NW, et al. Determinants of depression in the ECLIPSE chronic obstructive pulmonary disease cohort. Am J Respir Crit Care Med 2011;183(5):604–11.
74. Sampaio MS, Vieira WA, Bernardino IM, et al. Chronic obstructive pulmonary disease as a risk factor for suicide: a systematic review and meta-analysis. Respir Med 2019;151:11–8.
75. Li L, Wu C, Gan Y, et al. Insomnia and the risk of depression: a meta-analysis of prospective cohort studies. BMC Psychiatry 2016;16(1):375.
76. Ohayon MM. Chronic Obstructive Pulmonary Disease and its association with sleep and mental

disorders in the general population. J Psychiatr Res 2014;54:79–84.

77. Akinci B, Aslan GK, Kiyan E. Sleep quality and quality of life in patients with moderate to very severe chronic obstructive pulmonary disease. Clin Respir J 2018;12(4):1739–46.
78. Nunes DM, Mota RM, de Pontes Neto OL, et al. Impaired sleep reduces quality of life in chronic obstructive pulmonary disease. Lung 2009; 187(3):159–63.
79. Scharf SM, Maimon N, Simon-Tuval T, et al. Sleep quality predicts quality of life in chronic obstructive pulmonary disease. Int J Chron Obstruct Pulmon Dis 2010;6:1–12.
80. Phillips BA, Cooper KR, Burke TV. The effect of sleep loss on breathing in chronic obstructive pulmonary disease. Chest 1987;91(1):29–32.
81. Chen HI, Tang YR. Sleep loss impairs inspiratory muscle endurance. Am Rev Respir Dis 1989; 140(4):907–9.
82. Rault C, Sangare A, Diaz V, et al. Impact of sleep deprivation on respiratory motor output and endurance. A Physiological Study. Am J Respir Crit Care Med 2020;201(8):976–83.
83. Rault C, Heraud Q, Ragot S, et al. Sleep deprivation increases air hunger rather than breathing effort. Am J Respir Crit Care Med 2021;203(5):642–5.
84. Schiffman PL, Trontell MC, Mazar MF, et al. Sleep deprivation decreases ventilatory response to CO2 but not load compensation. Chest 1983; 84(6):695–8.
85. Spengler CM, Shea SA. Sleep deprivation per se does not decrease the hypercapnic ventilatory response in humans. Am J Respir Crit Care Med 2000;161(4 Pt 1):1124–8.
86. White DP, Douglas NJ, Pickett CK, et al. Sleep deprivation and the control of ventilation. Am Rev Respir Dis 1983;128(6):984–6.
87. Shorofsky M, Bourbeau J, Kimoff J, et al. Impaired sleep quality in COPD is associated with exacerbations: the CanCOLD cohort study. Chest 2019; 156(5):852–63.
88. Chen R, Tian JW, Zhou LQ, et al. The relationship between sleep quality and functional exercise capacity in COPD. Clin Respir J 2016;10(4):477–85.
89. Geiger-Brown J, Lindberg S, Krachman S, et al. Self-reported sleep quality and acute exacerbations of chronic obstructive pulmonary disease. Int J Chron Obstruct Pulmon Dis 2015;10:389–97.
90. Martin RJ, Bartelson BL, Smith P, et al. Effect of ipratropium bromide treatment on oxygen saturation and sleep quality in COPD. Chest 1999; 115(5):1338–45.
91. McNicholas WT, Calverley PM, Lee A, et al. Long-acting inhaled anticholinergic therapy improves sleeping oxygen saturation in COPD. Eur Respir J 2004;23(6):825–31.
92. Ryan S, Doherty LS, Rock C, et al. Effects of salmeterol on sleeping oxygen saturation in chronic obstructive pulmonary disease. Respiration 2010; 79(6):475–81.
93. Calverley PM, Lee A, Towse L, et al. Effect of tiotropium bromide on circadian variation in airflow limitation in chronic obstructive pulmonary disease. Thorax 2003;58(10):855–60.
94. Doherty DE, Tashkin DP, Kerwin E, et al. Effects of mometasone furoate/formoterol fumarate fixed-dose combination formulation on chronic obstructive pulmonary disease (COPD): results from a 52-week Phase III trial in subjects with moderate-to-very severe COPD. Int J Chron Obstruct Pulmon Dis 2012;7:57–71.
95. Calverley PM, Brezinova V, Douglas NJ, et al. The effect of oxygenation on sleep quality in chronic bronchitis and emphysema. Am Rev Respir Dis 1982;126(2):206–10.
96. Fleetham J, West P, Mezon B, et al. Sleep, arousals, and oxygen desaturation in chronic obstructive pulmonary disease. The effect of oxygen therapy. Am Rev Respir Dis 1982;126(3):429–33.
97. McKeon JL, Murree-Allen K, Saunders NA. Supplemental oxygen and quality of sleep in patients with chronic obstructive lung disease. Thorax 1989; 44(3):184–8.
98. Goldstein RS, Ramcharan V, Bowes G, et al. Effect of supplemental nocturnal oxygen on gas exchange in patients with severe obstructive lung disease. N Engl J Med 1984;310(7):425–9.
99. Continuous or nocturnal oxygen therapy in hypoxemic chronic obstructive lung disease: a clinical trial. Nocturnal Oxygen Therapy Trial Group. Ann Intern Med 1980;93(3):391–8.
100. Long term domiciliary oxygen therapy in chronic hypoxic cor pulmonale complicating chronic bronchitis and emphysema. Report of the Medical Research Council Working Party. Lancet 1981; 1(8222):681–6.
101. Long-Term Oxygen Treatment Trial Research G, Albert RK, Au DH, et al. A randomized trial of long-term oxygen for COPD with moderate desaturation. N Engl J Med 2016;375(17):1617–27.
102. Lacasse Y, Series F, Corbeil F, et al. Randomized trial of nocturnal oxygen in chronic obstructive pulmonary disease. N Engl J Med 2020;383(12):1129–38.
103. Alford NJ, Fletcher EC, Nickeson D. Acute oxygen in patients with sleep apnea and COPD. Chest 1986;89(1):30–8.
104. Cox NS, Pepin V, Burge AT, et al. Pulmonary rehabilitation does not improve objective measures of sleep quality in people with chronic obstructive pulmonary disease. COPD 2019;16(1):25–9.
105. Soler X, Diaz-Piedra C, Ries AL. Pulmonary rehabilitation improves sleep quality in chronic lung disease. COPD 2013;10(2):156–63.

106. Lan CC, Huang HC, Yang MC, et al. Pulmonary rehabilitation improves subjective sleep quality in COPD. Respir Care 2014;59(10):1569–76.
107. Harrison SL, Greening NJ, Williams JE, et al. Have we underestimated the efficacy of pulmonary rehabilitation in improving mood? Respir Med 2012; 106(6):838–44.
108. Machado MC, Vollmer WM, Togeiro SM, et al. CPAP and survival in moderate-to-severe obstructive sleep apnoea syndrome and hypoxaemic COPD. Eur Respir J 2010;35(1):132–7.
109. Jaoude P, Kufel T, El-Solh AA. Survival benefit of CPAP favors hypercapnic patients with the overlap syndrome. Lung 2014;192(2):251–8.
110. Duiverman ML. Noninvasive ventilation in stable hypercapnic COPD: what is the evidence? ERJ Open Res 2018;4(2). https://doi.org/10.1183/23120541.00012-2018.
111. Murphy PB, Rehal S, Arbane G, et al. Effect of home noninvasive ventilation with oxygen therapy vs oxygen therapy alone on hospital readmission or death after an acute COPD exacerbation: a randomized clinical trial. JAMA 2017;317(21):2177–86.
112. Struik FM, Lacasse Y, Goldstein RS, et al. Nocturnal noninvasive positive pressure ventilation in stable COPD: a systematic review and individual patient data meta-analysis. Respir Med 2014;108(2): 329–37.
113. Macrea M, Oczkowski S, Rochwerg B, et al. Long-term noninvasive ventilation in chronic stable hypercapnic chronic obstructive pulmonary disease. An Official American Thoracic Society Clinical Practice Guideline. Am J Respir Crit Care Med 2020;202(4):e74–87.
114. Stanchina ML, Welicky LM, Donat W, et al. Impact of CPAP use and age on mortality in patients with combined COPD and obstructive sleep apnea: the overlap syndrome. J Clin Sleep Med 2013; 9(8):767–72.
115. Edinger JD, Arnedt JT, Bertisch SM, et al. Behavioral and psychological treatments for chronic insomnia disorder in adults: an American Academy of Sleep Medicine clinical practice guideline. J Clin Sleep Med 2021;17(2):255–62.
116. Kapella MC, Herdegen JJ, Perlis ML, et al. Cognitive behavioral therapy for insomnia comorbid with COPD is feasible with preliminary evidence of positive sleep and fatigue effects. Int J Chron Obstruct Pulmon Dis 2011;6:625–35.
117. Wu JQ, Appleman ER, Salazar RD, et al. Cognitive behavioral therapy for insomnia comorbid with psychiatric and medical conditions: a meta-analysis. JAMA Intern Med 2015;175(9):1461–72.
118. Donovan LM, Malte CA, Spece LJ, et al. Risks of benzodiazepines in chronic obstructive pulmonary disease with comorbid posttraumatic stress disorder. Ann Am Thorac Soc 2019;16(1):82–90.
119. Vozoris NT, Fischer HD, Wang X, et al. Benzodiazepine drug use and adverse respiratory outcomes among older adults with COPD. Eur Respir J 2014; 44(2):332–40.
120. Girault C, Muir JF, Mihaltan F, et al. Effects of repeated administration of zolpidem on sleep, diurnal and nocturnal respiratory function, vigilance, and physical performance in patients with COPD. Chest 1996;110(5):1203–11.
121. GINA) GIfA. Global Strategy for Asthma Management and Prevention. 2020. Available at: https://ginasthma.org/gina-reports/.
122. Papi A, Brightling C, Pedersen SE, et al. Asthma. Lancet 2018;391(10122):783–800.
123. Auckley D, Moallem M, Shaman Z, et al. Findings of a Berlin Questionnaire survey: comparison between patients seen in an asthma clinic versus internal medicine clinic. Sleep Med 2008;9(5):494–9.
124. Janson C, De Backer W, Gislason T, et al. Increased prevalence of sleep disturbances and daytime sleepiness in subjects with bronchial asthma: a population study of young adults in three European countries. Eur Respir J 1996;9(10): 2132–8.
125. Kavanagh J, Jackson DJ, Kent BD. Sleep and asthma. Curr Opin Pulm Med 2018;24(6):569–73.
126. Lal C, Kumbhare S, Strange C. Prevalence of self-reported sleep problems amongst adults with obstructive airway disease in the NHANES cohort in the United States. Sleep Breath 2019. https://doi.org/10.1007/s11325-019-01941-0.
127. Turner-Warwick M. Epidemiology of nocturnal asthma. Am J Med 1988;85(1B):6–8.
128. Hetzel MR, Clark TJ. Comparison of normal and asthmatic circadian rhythms in peak expiratory flow rate. Thorax 1980;35(10):732–8.
129. Martin RJ, Cicutto LC, Ballard RD. Factors related to the nocturnal worsening of asthma. Am Rev Respir Dis 1990;141(1):33–8.
130. Sutherland ER. Nocturnal asthma. J Allergy Clin Immunol 2005;116(6):1179–86 [quiz: 1187].
131. Sutherland ER. Nocturnal asthma: underlying mechanisms and treatment. Curr Allergy Asthma Rep 2005;5(2):161–7.
132. Shigemitsu H, Afshar K. Nocturnal asthma. Curr Opin Pulm Med 2007;13(1):49–55.
133. Calhoun WJ. Nocturnal asthma. Chest 2003;123(3 Suppl):399S–405S.
134. Weersink EJ, van Zomeren EH, Koeter GH, et al. Treatment of nocturnal airway obstruction improves daytime cognitive performance in asthmatics. Am J Respir Crit Care Med 1997;156(4 Pt 1):1144–50.
135. Raherison C, Abouelfath A, Le Gros V, et al. Underdiagnosis of nocturnal symptoms in asthma in general practice. J Asthma 2006;43(3): 199–202.

136. Kraft M, Martin RJ, Wilson S, et al. Lymphocyte and eosinophil influx into alveolar tissue in nocturnal asthma. Am J Respir Crit Care Med 1999;159(1): 228–34.
137. Kraft M, Djukanovic R, Wilson S, et al. Alveolar tissue inflammation in asthma. Am J Respir Crit Care Med 1996;154(5):1505–10.
138. Martin RJ. Small airway and alveolar tissue changes in nocturnal asthma. Am J Respir Crit Care Med 1998;157(5 Pt 2):S188–90.
139. Beam WR, Weiner DE, Martin RJ. Timing of prednisone and alterations of airways inflammation in nocturnal asthma. Am Rev Respir Dis 1992; 146(6):1524–30.
140. D'Alonzo GE, Smolensky MH, Feldman S, et al. Twenty-four hour lung function in adult patients with asthma. Chronoptimized theophylline therapy once-daily dosing in the evening versus conventional twice-daily dosing. Am Rev Respir Dis 1990;142(1):84–90.
141. Pincus DJ, Humeston TR, Martin RJ. Further studies on the chronotherapy of asthma with inhaled steroids: the effect of dosage timing on drug efficacy. J Allergy Clin Immunol 1997;100(6 Pt 1):771–4.
142. Reinberg A, Gervais P, Chaussade M, et al. Circadian changes in effectiveness of corticosteroids in eight patients with allergic asthma. J Allergy Clin Immunol 1983;71(4):425–33.
143. Reinberg A, Halberg F, Falliers CJ. Circadian timing of methylprednisolone effects in asthmatic boys. Chronobiologia 1974;1(4):333–47.
144. Senaratna CV, Walters EH, Hamilton G, et al. Nocturnal symptoms perceived as asthma are associated with obstructive sleep apnoea risk, but not bronchial hyper-reactivity. Respirology 2019;24(12):1176–82.
145. BY Sunwoo, Owens RL. All that wheezes at night is not asthma. Respirology 2019;24(12):1127–8.
146. Ioachimescu OC, Janocko NJ, Ciavatta MM, et al. Obstructive lung disease and obstructive sleep apnea (OLDOSA) cohort study: 10-year assessment. J Clin Sleep Med 2020;16(2):267–77.
147. Damianaki A, Vagiakis E, Sigala I, et al. Tauhe coexistence of obstructive sleep apnea and bronchial asthma: revelation of a new asthma phenotype? J Clin Med 2019;8(9). https://doi.org/10.3390/jcm8091476.
148. Davies SE, Bishopp A, Wharton S, et al. The association between asthma and obstructive sleep apnea (OSA): a systematic review. J Asthma 2019; 56(2):118–29.
149. Kong DL, Qin Z, Shen H, et al. Association of obstructive sleep apnea with asthma: a meta-analysis. Sci Rep 2017;7(1):4088.
150. Larsson LG, Lindberg A, Franklin KA, et al. Symptoms related to obstructive sleep apnoea are common in subjects with asthma, chronic bronchitis and rhinitis in a general population. Respir Med 2001;95(5):423–9.
151. Shen TC, Lin CL, Wei CC, et al. Risk of obstructive sleep apnea in adult patients with asthma: a population-based cohort study in Taiwan. PLoS One 2015;10(6):e0128461.
152. Sweeney J, Patterson CC, Menzies-Gow A, et al. Comorbidity in severe asthma requiring systemic corticosteroid therapy: cross-sectional data from the optimum patient care research database and the british thoracic difficult asthma registry. Thorax 2016;71(4):339–46.
153. Teodorescu M, Barnet JH, Hagen EW, et al. Association between asthma and risk of developing obstructive sleep apnea. JAMA 2015;313(2): 156–64.
154. Teodorescu M, Broytman O, Curran-Everett D, et al. Obstructive sleep apnea risk, asthma burden, and lower airway inflammation in adults in the Severe Asthma Research Program (SARP) II. J Allergy Clin Immunol Pract 2015;3(4): 566–75.e1.
155. Prasad B, Nyenhuis SM, Imayama I, et al. Asthma and obstructive sleep apnea overlap: what has the evidence taught us? Am J Respir Crit Care Med 2019. https://doi.org/10.1164/rccm.201810-1838TR.
156. Julien JY, Martin JG, Ernst P, et al. Prevalence of obstructive sleep apnea-hypopnea in severe versus moderate asthma. J Allergy Clin Immunol 2009;124(2):371–6.
157. Yigla M, Tov N, Solomonov A, et al. Difficult-to-control asthma and obstructive sleep apnea. J Asthma 2003;40(8):865–71.
158. Becerra MB, Becerra BJ, Teodorescu M. Healthcare burden of obstructive sleep apnea and obesity among asthma hospitalizations: results from the U.S.-based Nationwide Inpatient Sample. Respir Med 2016;117:230–6.
159. Kim MY, Jo EJ, Kang SY, et al. Obstructive sleep apnea is associated with reduced quality of life in adult patients with asthma. Ann Allergy Asthma Immunol 2013;110(4):253–7, 257.e1.
160. Wang TY, Lo YL, Lin SM, et al. Obstructive sleep apnoea accelerates FEV1 decline in asthmatic patients. BMC Pulm Med 2017;17(1):55.
161. Wang Y, Liu K, Hu K, et al. Impact of obstructive sleep apnea on severe asthma exacerbations. Sleep Med 2016;26:1–5.
162. Ciftci TU, Ciftci B, Guven SF, et al. Effect of nasal continuous positive airway pressure in uncontrolled nocturnal asthmatic patients with obstructive sleep apnea syndrome. Respir Med 2005;99(5):529–34.
163. Kauppi P, Bachour P, Maasilta P, et al. Long-term CPAP treatment improves asthma control in patients with asthma and obstructive sleep apnoea. Sleep Breath 2016;20(4):1217–24.

164. Lafond C, Series F, Lemiere C. Impact of CPAP on asthmatic patients with obstructive sleep apnoea. Eur Respir J 2007;29(2):307–11.
165. Ng SSS, Chan TO, To KW, et al. Continuous positive airway pressure for obstructive sleep apnoea does not improve asthma control. Respirology 2018;23(11):1055–62.
166. Serrano-Pariente J, Plaza V, Soriano JB, et al. Asthma outcomes improve with continuous positive airway pressure for obstructive sleep apnea. Allergy 2017;72(5):802–12.
167. Busk M, Busk N, Puntenney P, et al. Use of continuous positive airway pressure reduces airway reactivity in adults with asthma. Eur Respir J 2013; 41(2):317–22.
168. Holbrook JT, Sugar EA, Brown RH, et al. Effect of continuous positive airway pressure on airway reactivity in asthma. A randomized, sham-controlled clinical trial. Ann Am Thorac Soc 2016; 13(11):1940–50.
169. Irvin CG, Pak J, Martin RJ. Airway-parenchyma uncoupling in nocturnal asthma. Am J Respir Crit Care Med 2000;161(1):50–6.
170. Skloot G, Permutt S, Togias A. Airway hyperresponsiveness in asthma: a problem of limited smooth muscle relaxation with inspiration. J Clin Invest 1995;96(5):2393–403.
171. Xue Z, Yu Y, Gao H, et al. Chronic continuous positive airway pressure (CPAP) reduces airway reactivity in vivo in an allergen-induced rabbit model of asthma. J Appl Physiol (1985) 2011;111(2): 353–7.
172. Xue Z, Zhang L, Liu Y, et al. Chronic inflation of ferret lungs with CPAP reduces airway smooth muscle contractility in vivo and in vitro. J Appl Physiol (1985) 2008;104(3):610–5.
173. Xue Z, Zhang L, Ramchandani R, et al. Respiratory system responsiveness in rabbits in vivo is reduced by prolonged continuous positive airway pressure. J Appl Physiol (1985) 2005;99(2): 677–82.
174. Owens RL, Campana LM, Foster AM, et al. Nocturnal bilevel positive airway pressure for the treatment of asthma. Respir Physiolo Neurobiol 2020;274:103355.

Sleep Deficiency in Obstructive Sleep Apnea

Olurotimi Adekolu, MD[a], Andrey Zinchuk, MD, MHS[b,*]

KEYWORDS

• Sleep deficiency • Obstructive sleep apnea (OSA) • Insomnia • COMISA • Circadian misalignment • Periodic limb movements of sleep (PLMS) • Cognitive behavioral therapy for insomnia (CBT-I)

KEY POINTS

- Sleep deficiency in patients with obstructive sleep apnea includes abnormal quality, timing, and duration of sleep, and the presence of other sleep disorders.
- Obstructive sleep apnea occurring alongside insomnia is termed comorbid insomnia and obstructive sleep apnea and affects about one-third of patients with obstructive sleep apnea.
- Cognitive behavioral therapy for insomnia concurrent with the treatment of upper airway obstruction improves patient-centered outcomes in comorbid insomnia and obstructive sleep apnea.
- Despite their potential impact, the relationship between obstructive sleep apnea and circadian misalignment (pathogenesis, patient symptoms, and function) is understudied.
- Periodic limb movements of sleep are common in obstructive sleep apnea and are associated with poor sleep quality in those with obstructive sleep apnea that does not improve with positive airway pressure.

INTRODUCTION

Obstructive sleep apnea (OSA) is the most common sleep disordered breathing syndrome, with prevalence ranging from 9% to 38% in the general population.[1] OSA is highly burdensome because it contributes to psychiatric, metabolic, and cardiovascular diseases (CVDs), such as depression, diabetes, hypertension, and stroke,[1–4] and importantly impairs daytime function by potentiating sleep deficiency. The National Institutes of Health defines sleep deficiency as abnormalities in sleep duration, circadian alignment, sleep quality, and sleep-related disorders.[5]

Sleep deficiency in OSA may be a direct consequence of upper airway obstruction, leading to hypoxemia, arousals from sleep, and sympathetic activation. These events result in poor quality sleep and decreased sleep duration, extensively described in prior literature.[6,7]

Sleep deficiency in OSA, however, is also closely linked to comorbid disorders. These disorders may contribute to poor sleep directly or through interactions with OSA. Conditions such as insomnia, circadian misalignment, periodic limb movements of sleep (PLMS) can all impact sleep quantity and quality in patients with OSA hence worsening sleep deficiency. Here, we discuss these relationships as they relate to sleep deficiency in individuals with OSA.

COMORBID INSOMNIA AND OBSTRUCTIVE SLEEP APNEA

Epidemiology

Difficulty initiating, maintaining, or early termination of sleep associated with daytime symptoms (eg, fatigue) or functional impairment are diagnostic characteristics of the insomnia disorder. These are also common in those with OSA. For example, a recent systematic metanalysis by Zhang and colleagues[8] examined the co-occurrence of insomnia symptoms and insomnia disorder in patients with OSA (apnea-hypopnea

[a] Starling Physicians, 533 Cottage Grove Road, Bloomfield, CT 06002, USA; [b] Section of Pulmonary, Critical Care and Sleep Medicine, Department of Internal Medicine, Yale School of Medicine, 300 Cedar Street, The Anlyan Center, 455SE, New Haven, CT 06519, USA
* Corresponding author.
E-mail address: andrey.zinchuk@yale.edu

Clin Chest Med 43 (2022) 353–371
https://doi.org/10.1016/j.ccm.2022.02.013
0272-5231/22/Published by Elsevier Inc.

index [AHI] ≥ 5; n = 28,252). Insomnia was defined based on the insomnia severity index (ISI) score of 15 or higher,[9] *Diagnostic Statistical Manual Mental Disorders*, 5th edition, or the International Classification of Sleep Disorders (ICSD) criteria,[10,11] or physician diagnosis.[12] The prevalence of insomnia was 38% (95% confidence interval, 15%–64%).[8] Difficulty maintaining sleep was the most common presenting symptom (42%). However, other signs such as short sleep duration owing to difficulty falling asleep and early morning awakenings occurred in 18% and 21% of patients with OSA, respectively. In contrast with previous studies,[13] OSA severity did not influence the prevalence of insomnia, suggesting that clinicians should assess for insomnia in all patients with OSA, regardless of the AHI.

Pathophysiology

The co-occurrence of insomnia and OSA may be related to each disorder perpetuating the other (**Fig. 1**).[14] Insomnia may increase susceptibility to apneic episodes. Physiologic arousal is heightened in insomnia patients, as evidenced by elevated cortisol, metabolic rate, electroencephalography (EEG) activity, and prolonged sleep latency.[15–23] This state of hyperarousal increases the propensity for lighter sleep, which in turn increases the vulnerability to apneic episodes.[24] Indeed, a low arousal threshold, or propensity to awaken easily from a respiratory stimulus, is more common in those with comorbid insomnia and OSA (COMISA) versus OSA alone.[25] In those with a low arousal threshold, ventilatory overshoots during arousals lead to greater CO_2 reduction with resultant worsening in upper airway muscle tone and propensity for airway obstruction during sleep.[26] Data suggest that reducing arousability by pharmacotherapy or cognitive behavioral therapy for insomnia (CBT-I) may decrease the AHI.[27,28]

Conversely, OSA contributes to insomnia symptoms. The repetitive arousals and postarousal awakenings may be perceived as recurrent wakefulness during sleep and promote maladaptive cognition about sleep. Repetitive nights of sleep difficulties may activate the sympathetic nervous system and hypothalamic–pituitary–adrenal (HPA) axis.[29] The consistent association of the bedroom environment, the time of night, and the unmet desire to fall asleep along with sympathetic nervous system/HPA axis activation can become conditioned and underlie the development of psychophysiological or conditioned insomnia.[29,30]

How deeply a patient sleeps as measured by the odds ratio product (ORP) may be an intrinsic trait that influences an individual's tendency for arousal when exposed to internal or external stimuli and may be a pathogenic mechanism linking OSA

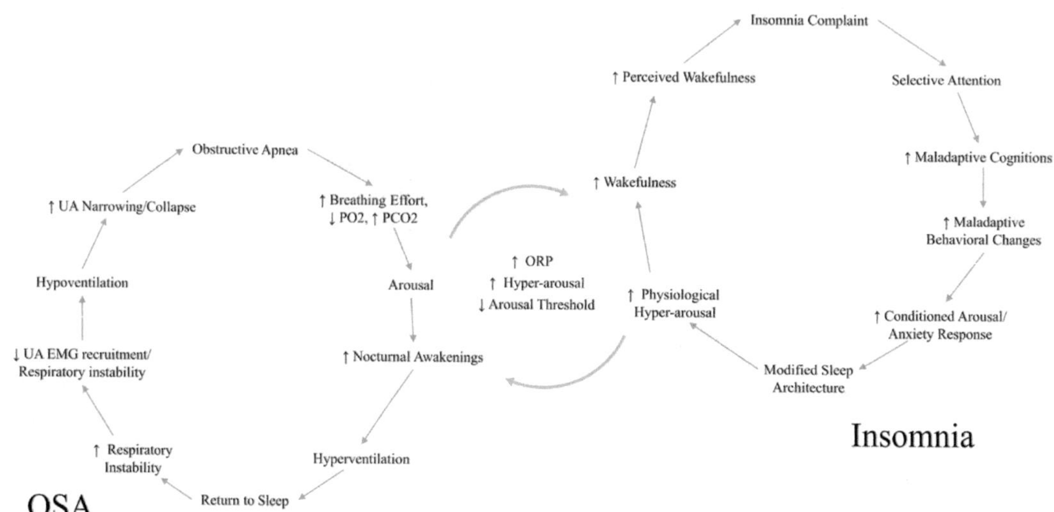

Fig. 1. Potential mechanisms by which OSA and insomnia interact. The physiologic hyperarousal of insomnia may manifest as a low arousal threshold and contribute to respiratory instability in OSA. The frequent arousals and sleep fragmentation from OSA may lead to a conditioned response to arousal and insomnia. The low sleep depth, reflected by the high ORP, may be the intrinsic trait that links OSA and insomnia, with increased susceptibility to arousal, destabilized sleep, and excessive wake time. EMG, electromyographic; P_{O_2}, partial pressure of oxygen; P_{CO_2}, partial pressure of carbon dioxide; UA, upper airway. (*From* Eckert DJ, Sweetman A. Impaired central control of sleep depth propensity as a common mechanism for excessive overnight wake time: implications for sleep apnea, insomnia and beyond. J Clin Sleep Med. 2020 Mar 15;16(3):341 - 343.)

and insomnia. The ORP quantifies the moment-to-moment sleep depth using EEG signal processing from standard polysomnography. An ORP of 2.5 indicates complete alertness/wakefulness, whereas 0 indicates deep sleep/zero likelihood of arousal. Younes and Giannouli[25] investigated the mechanistic origin of excessive wakefulness (defined as a sleep efficiency of <80%) observed in both conditions. They measured the ORP in healthy controls and people referred for polysomnography with and without OSA, PLMS disorder (PLMD), and insomnia symptoms. They found that ORP was higher in those with insomnia symptoms (65% of participants) than those without. Sleep depth in the first 9 seconds after arousal was also lighter, increasing the risk for subsequent arousals.[25] Notably, those with excessive night wake time exhibited a higher ORP than those without, regardless of the comorbid OSA or PLMD. These findings suggest that an individual's sleep propensity is an important determinant of excessive wake time and is not solely owing to disorders characterized by repetitive arousals, such as OSA and PLMD.

Clinical Characteristics and Consequences of Comorbid Insomnia and Obstructive Sleep Apnea

Like all patients suffering from insomnia, those with COMISA have difficulty falling asleep, maintaining sleep owing to frequent awakenings or early morning awakenings, and nonrestorative sleep. Difficulty maintaining sleep is the most common COMISA symptom.[31,32] Individuals with this symptom are older, have a higher body mass index, AHI, and more daytime sleepiness as measured by the Epworth sleepiness score compared with those with other symptoms.[31,33,34] Difficulty initiating sleep, in contrast, is associated with lower OSA severity[34] and is more common in women with COMISA who smoke and manifest poor physical and mental quality of life.[31] Particular attention should be paid to those suffering from mood disorders, chronic pain, and posttraumatic stress disorder, which predict severe insomnia (ISI scores of 23.1 $\pm$ 2.6) and are treatable precipitating and perpetuating factors.[35]

COMISA is associated with adverse consequences, including higher use of sedative and psychotropic medications, greater daytime impairments, and poorer physical and mental quality of life.[31,36,37] Those with COMISA have lower adherence to continuous positive airway pressure (CPAP) therapy (OR, 0.81; $P = .02$) and decreased clinical response to mandibular advancement devices than individuals who have OSA alone.[32,38] CPAP therapy in COMISA improves middle-of-the-night sleep maintenance but may also be associated with the emergence of early morning awakenings.[33]

Both OSA and insomnia are also linked to CVD. The shared mechanistic pathways (**Fig. 2**) suggest the risk from COMISA may be increased compared with each condition alone.[39–46] OSA's negative intrathoracic pressure swings increase transmural pressure of thoracic structures and left ventricular afterload. These changes impede stroke volume, increase myocardial oxygen demand and arrhythmogenesis.[47] Hypoxia leads to pulmonary vasoconstriction, pulmonary hypertension, and right heart dysfunction.[47–49] Insomnia, in contrast, is associated with dysregulation of the hypothalamic–pituitary–adrenal axis. The HPA axis is in turn associated with an increased heart rate, blood pressure, dyslipidemia, and mediators of the CVD pathway, such as impaired glucose metabolism and diabetes.[50–52] Both sleep apnea and insomnia share the pathways of excessive arousals, autonomic dysregulation, increased systemic inflammation, insulin resistance, atherogenesis, and endothelial dysfunction[44,47,48,53–56] Although all these factors are plausible mechanisms for increased risk of CVD in COMISA, further work is needed to determine if this plausibility translates into observed increased CVD risk in COMISA compared with OSA and insomnia alone.

Diagnosis and Treatment

The COMISA-specific diagnostic criteria are yet to be established. Thus, identifying this condition relies on the presence of insomnia and OSA according to current guidelines (*Diagnostic Statistical Manual Mental Disorders*, 5th edition/ICSD and ICSD, respectively).[10,11] A general medical/psychiatric questionnaire, assessment of sleepiness (eg, Epworth sleepiness score), insomnia severity measures (eg, ISI), sleep logs (or actigraphy) in addition to polysomnography or polygraphy are essential to diagnosis and management.[57,58]

Similar to diagnosis, although there are well-established guidelines for treating OSA and insomnia, such guidelines do not exist for COMISA. CPAP therapy is the most common treatment for OSA, with oral appliances, surgery, or upper airway stimulation used in some cases.[59,60] CPAP use, however, is hampered by poor adherence to therapy in those with insomnia symptoms.[61–65] CBT-I is the recommended first-line treatment for insomnia. Recent data suggest that a combination of CBT-I with CPAP therapy may improve outcomes in COMISA.[57,66,67] **Tables 1** and **2** summarize the observational and clinical

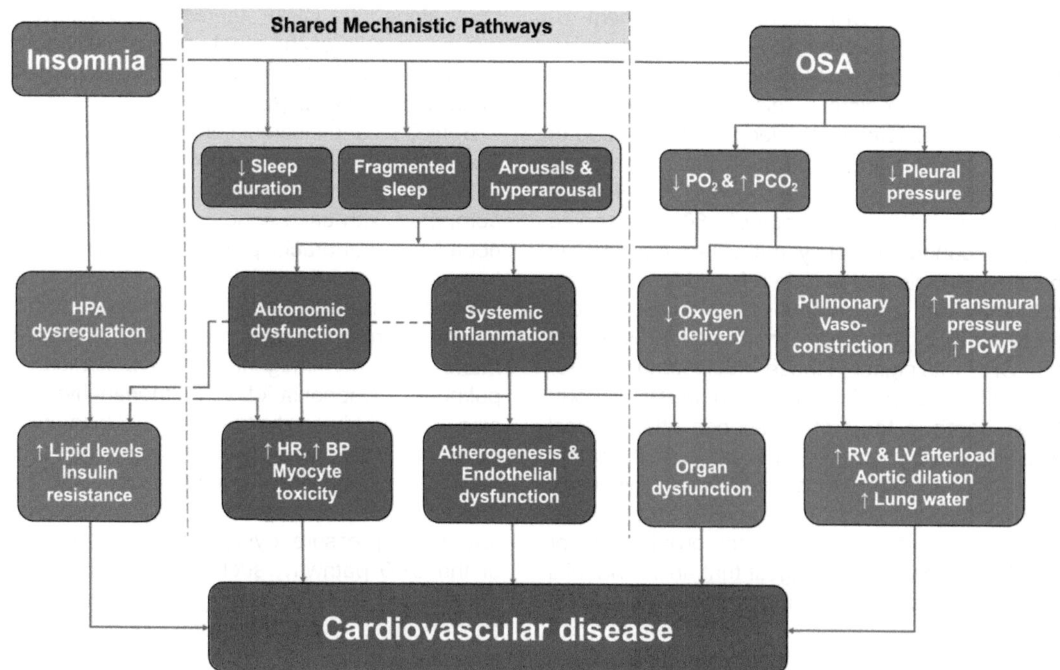

Fig. 2. Potential mechanistic pathways for cardiovascular disease in COMISA. BP, blood pressure; HR, heart rate; LV, left ventricle; PCWP, pulmonary capillary wedge pressure; RV, right ventricle.

trial studies on the treatment of patients with COMISA. Elsewhere in this article, we highlight the findings of the most recent, randomized clinical trials addressing the effect of CBT-I, its delivery method, and when it might be best to administer CBT-I in relation to the initiation of OSA therapy on patient-centered outcomes in COMISA.

Alessi and colleagues[68] compared the effect of concurrent delivery of a 5-session combined CBT-I and behavioral CPAP adherence program administered by trained sleep coaches versus a sleep education control program on insomnia symptoms and CPAP use at 6 months. The CBT-I/adherence intervention was delivered to 125 adult veterans (96% male) with insomnia and an AHI of 15 or more per hour. Compared with sleep education alone, the CBT-I group showed a greater improvement in actigraphy-measured sleep onset latency and efficiency, a clinically significant 6-point decrease in the ISI and 78- and 48-minute greater adherence to CPAP therapy at the 3- and 6-month follow-ups, respectively.[68] Notably, a study by Bjorvatn and colleagues[69] shows that the delivery of CBT-I via a self-help book is not sufficient to derive benefits among patients with COMISA.

To determine if CBT-I administered before OSA therapy can improve outcomes, Sweetman and colleagues compared CBT-I to treatment-as-usual before positive airway pressure (PAP) therapy in 145 patients with COMISA.[70] The CBT-I group demonstrated higher PAP treatment acceptance (99% vs 89%; $P = .034$), nightly adherence to PAP (61 minutes higher; $P = .023$), and greater improvement in insomnia at 6 months (ISI 18.5 vs 9.0; $P = .001$). Notably, the authors identified a 15% increase in sleepiness the week after administering sleep restriction as a part of CBT-I that returned to pretreatment levels in the subsequent weeks.[71] Thus, it may be important to inform patients that a transient worsening in sleepiness may occur, but overall, sleep deficiency will improve.

Finally, Ong and colleagues[72] conducted a 3-arm randomized controlled trial among 121 adults with COMISA comparing the timing of CBT-I and PAP initiation (PAP alone vs CBT-I concurrent with PAP vs CBT-I followed by PAP). Compared with PAP alone, the 2 CBT-I treatment arms reported a significantly greater decrease from baseline in insomnia severity. They had a greater percentage of participants categorized as good sleepers and remitters from insomnia. No significant differences were found between the CBT-I followed by PAP versus concurrent CBT-I/PAP arms on any outcome measure.

In summary, CBT-I, when used with CPAP in patients with COMISA, is more efficacious than CPAP alone.[70,72] Although no data support CBT-I use before versus along with PAP initiation, it is

Table 1
Observational studies examining the impact of insomnia on therapy outcomes in patients with OSA

Study	Design/Setting	Sample Size	Baseline Characteristics (Mean ± SD)	Exposure/Control	Outcome(s)	Findings
Nguyen et al,[124] 2010	Prospective cohort/ sleep clinic (France)	148	Age (years) 54.8 ± 11.8 BMI (kg/m^2) 29.1 ± 6.3 AHI (#/h) 39.0 ± 21.3	High (ISI ≥15) vs low (ISI < 15) insomnia groups	CPAP use at 1 and 6 mo	Insomnia groups did not predict CPAP use or CPAP cessation rates
Wickwire et al,[32] 2010	Retrospective cohort/ sleep clinic (USA)	232	Age 53.6 ± 12.4 BMI 43.4 ± 7.7 AHI 41.8 ± 27.7	Initial (DIS), middle (DMS), and early morning insomnia (EMA) via self-report	CPAP use: average hours/night, and Adherence: ≥4 h/night CPAP use in 70% of the nights in the last 4 wk	Prevalence: DMS (23.7%), EMA (20.6%), DIS (16.6%). DMS associated with a 12 mins/night lower CPAP use and 19% lower adherence (Odds ratio 0.81)
Bjornsdottir et al,[33] 2013	Prospective cohort/ University hospital (Iceland)	705	Age 54.9 ± 10.2 BMI 33.7 ± 5.6 AHI 45.5 ± 20.5	DIS, DMS, EMA insomnia (Basic Nordic Sleep Questionnaire)	Adherence to PAP: 53% APAP 43% CPAP 3% BiPAP 1% ASV Change in Insomnia subtype prevalence in patients using or not using CPAP at 24 mo	Prevalence of DIS, DMS and EMA Insomnia at baseline: 12.9%, 59.4% and 23.3% in PAP users and 20.8%, 59.1% and 36.6% in non-PAP users. DIS insomnia at baseline predicted PAP non adherence at 24 mo. DIS and EMA insomnia at baseline were less likely to adhere to PAP therapy.
Nguyen et al,[125] 2013	Prospective cohort/ sleep clinic (France)	80	Age 54.9 ± 10.6 BMI 30.5 ± 6.0 AHI 45.0 ± 24.6	N/A patients with OSA receiving APAP therapy	Change in ISI score from baseline to 24 mo Responders: ≥ 9-point decline on ISI over 24-mo	Overall ISI decreased from 14 to 8. Of the 39 with Insomnia (ISI ≥ 15), 51% had a decrease in ISI of ≥9 points from baseline to 24-mo

(*continued on next page*)

Table 1
(continued)

Study	Design/Setting	Sample Size	Baseline Characteristics (Mean ± SD)	Exposure/Control	Outcome(s)	Findings
Pieh et al,[126] 2013	Prospective cohort/ sleep center (Germany)	73	Age 55.1 ± 11.5 BMI 30.8 ± 5.0 AHI 39.2 ± 26.7	Insomnia. RIS	Parameters influencing CPAP adherence	Insomnia scores correlate with 6-mo CPAP adherence: Adherence declines by 2.6 h/night per 1 SD of RIS score
Wallace et al,[127] 2013	Retrospective cross-sectional/ Veteran Affairs sleep clinic (USA)	248	Age 59 ± 11 y BMI 33.0 ± 5.0 AHI 40.0 ± 30.0	Factors influencing CPAP adherence	CPAP Adherence	Black race-ethnicity, insomnia symptoms, and self-efficacy associated with mean daily CPAP use. Adherence decreases by 1 h/night per 10-unit ISI increase
Glidewell et al,[128] 2014	Retrospective cohort/sleep center (USA)	68	Age 47.5 ± 12.4 BMI 32.2 ± 7.3 AHI 34.7 ± 32.2	PAP therapy	Change in ISI score	Lower baseline ISI scores, higher baseline RDI and PAP use predict marked reduction of ISI scores (decrease to none/ mild) on PAP therapy; 55% had persistent (moderate or worse) insomnia, exhibited 1.1 h/night lower PAP use

Wohlgemuth et al,[129] 2015	Retrospective cohort/ Veteran Affairs sleep clinic (USA)	207	Age 58.4 ± 11.9 BMI 32.4 ± 5.0 AHI 40.0 ± 29.4	CPAP therapy	CPAP user profiles/ subtypes Predictors of CPAP subgroup membership	Three subgroups were identified and labeled nonadherers, attempters, and adherers. A 1-unit increase in the ISI score increased the likelihood of being an attempter by 9% (OR, 1.09) and a nonadherer by 16% (OR, 1.16).
Eysteinsdottir et al,[130] 2017	Prospective cohort/ sleep clinic (Iceland)	796	Age 54.4 ± 10.6 BMI 33.5 ± 5.7 AHI 44.9 ± 20.7	None	CPAP adherence	Initial and late insomnia predicted CPAP cessation at 1 y only in participants with a BMI of 30 kg/m^2. Higher BMI, AHI and Epworth sleepiness score predicted adherence.
Fung et al,[131] 2016	Prospective cohort/ Veteran Affairs sleep clinic (USA)	134	Age > 60 y BMI AHI < 15/hour	CBT-I (vs sleep education)	Changes in sleep quality (Pittsburgh Sleep Quality Index) Sleep latency, duration	CBT-I improved sleep onset latency and sleep quality regardless of presence of OSA (AHI <5 vs AHI 5 to <15/h)

(*continued on next page*)

Table 1
(continued)

Study	Design/Setting	Sample Size	Baseline Characteristics (Mean ± SD)	Exposure/Control	Outcome(s)	Findings
Krakow B et al,[132] 2017	Retrospective cohort/ sleep clinic (USA)	302	Age 53.4 ± 14.2 BMI 31.6 ± 8.0 AHI 32.0 ± 28.2 Complex insomnia defined as those who failed CPAP owing to intolerance or emergence of treatment-emergent central apneas	Advanced PAP devices (auto BPAP/ASV)	Changes in ISI	Total weekly hours of PAP use correlated inversely with change in ISI scores. In full PAP users (≥20 h/wk, 82% of sample) ISI scores improved by 0.7, 0.9, and 0.7 SDs for DIS, DMS, and EMA subtypes. No difference between ASV and auto-BPAP
Sweetman A et al,[67] 2017	Retrospective cohort/sleep center (Australia)	141	Age 51.7 ± 15.7 BMI 26.3 ± 4.9 AHI 14.3 ± 8.0	CBT-I	Change in insomnia and other patient-centered outcomes at 3 mo	A 10-unit decrease in the ISI score A 58-min increase in the duration of sleep A 19% improvement in sleep efficiency Marked improvement in stress, depressive, and anxiety symptoms

Abbreviations: AHI, apnea- hypopnea index; APAP, auto positive airway pressure; ASV, Adaptive-Servo ventilator; BiPAP, bilevel positive airway pressure; BMI, body mass index; COM-ISA, comorbid insomnia and obstructive sleep apnea; DIS, difficulty initiating sleep; DMS, difficulty maintaining sleep; EMA, early morning awakening; RIS, Regensburg Insomnia Scale.

Nonadherers used CPAP for an average of 37 min nightly, used CPAP 18.2% of nights, and used CPAP for more than 4 h 6.2% of nights. Attempters used CPAP for 156 min on average, used CPAP 68.2% of nights, and used CPAP for more than 4 h 29.3% of nights. Adherers used CPAP for 392 min, used CPAP 95.4% of nights, and used CPAP for more than 4 h 86.2% of nights.

Table 2
Recent randomized controlled trials on CBT-I and PAP therapy in patients with COMISA

Study	Sample	Characteristics	Control	Intervention(s)	Outcome(s)	Findings
Alessi et al,[68] 2021	125	US Veterans Overall Age (years) 63.2 ± 7.1 Male 96%	5 weekly sleep education sessions delivered with CPAP use.	5 weekly CBT-I and CPAP adherence program delivered by a sleep coach.	Primary: CPAP adherence at 3 mo Subjective (D from diary) and objective (A from actigraphy) measures at 3 mo: SOL-D, SE-D, SE-A, WASO-D	CBT-I vs control: 3.2 vs 1.9 h/night CPAP use Greater improvement in SOL-D 16.2 min SE-D 10.5% SE-A 4.4% WASO-D no difference Findings persisted at 6 mo
Bjorvatn et al,[69] 2018	164	Control vs intervention Age (years) 57.0 ± 12.1 vs 55.0 ± 11.6 Male 75% vs 68% BMI 31.9 ± 5.6 vs 32.3 ± 6.0 kg/m^2 AHI 24.9 ± 18.1 vs 25.6 ± 19.9/h	Sleep hygiene advice with CPAP	Delivered self-help CBT-I book with CPAP	Primary: Insomnia severity based on the BIS and ISI. Secondary: CPAP adherence	There was significant improvement in BIS and ISI scores in both groups, no effect of intervention compared with control. No difference in CPAP adherence.
Ong et al,[72] 2020	121	Overall Age (years) 50.0 ± 13.1 Female 53% OSA severity: Mild (51%, 43.2%) Moderate/severe (67%, 56.8%)	CPAP only group	CBT-I before CPAP and CBT-I concurrently with CPAP	Primary: CPAP adherence over 90 d (≥4 h on ≥70% of nights for 30 d) Secondary: ISI and PSQI scores and others	No differences in primary outcome between intervention groups vs control group. Significant decrease in ISI scores and improvement in PSQI scores in intervention vs control groups. No differences between intervention groups.

(*continued on next page*)

Table 2
(*continued*)

Study	Sample	Characteristics	Control	Intervention(s)	Outcome(s)	Findings
Sweetman et al,[70] 2019	145	Control vs intervention Age (years) 59.1 ± 9.9 vs 57.3 ± 9.9) BMI 34.5 ± 6.3 vs 36.2 ± 6.5 kg/m^2 AHI 33.2 ± 19.8 vs 35.8 ± 23.9/h	Treatment as usual	Four session CBT-I before CPAP therapy	Primary: Average CPAP adherence over 6 mo Secondary: CPAP acceptance, insomnia severity, diary sleep metrics, daytime function and others	CBT-I group with 1 h/night greater CPAP adherence 10% greater CPAP acceptance Significant improvement in ISI scores No differences in diary measured sleep metrics No differences in functional outcomes

Abbreviations: BIS, Bergen Insomnia Scale; ; PSQI, Pittsburgh Sleep Quality Index; SE-a, sleep efficiency by 7-day actigraphy; SE-d, sleep efficiency by sleep diary; SOL-d, sleep onset latency by sleep diary; WASO-d, wake after sleep onset by sleep diary

A good sleeper is defined as a PSQI total score of less than 5 at the study end point; insomnia remission is defined as an ISI score of less than 8 at the study end point; insomnia response is defined as a decrease in the ISI score of more than 7 points from baseline to the study end point.

clear that treating insomnia and OSA at least concurrently is needed to improve important patient outcomes.

Owing to the limited availability of qualified CBT-I providers, sedative-hypnotics are often used in patients with COMISA.[73] There are concerns about worsening airway collapsibility in COMISA with hypnotics. Notably, however, the nonbenzodiazepine hypnotics such as eszopiclone or zolpidem do not worsen airway collapsibility among patients with nonsevere OSA.[74,75] In an unselected OSA population, eszopiclone also improved the effectiveness of CPAP titration and initial CPAP adherence (21% more nights and 1.1 more hours per night of CPAP use) at 6 months compared with placebo.[76,77] A notable finding from Sweetman and colleagues' work is that the CBT-I group exhibited a decrease in the AHI that was 7.5 events/h greater than in the control group, suggesting that addressing mechanisms of insomnia and improving sleep quality may also improve OSA control.[28] Targeting patients with OSA and low arousal threshold, which can present as insomnia and responds to nonbenzodiazepine hypnotics, may be an effective way to make therapy for COMISA more precise.[78]

Future Directions

Research is needed to elucidate the relationship between the mechanisms of insomnia and respiratory events. The concept of sleep depth as measured by the ORP is promising. It may be used to investigate the interplay between sleep depth, wakefulness, and upper airway obstruction, especially during treatment with CBT-I, PAP, or both. Insomnia is a disorder of hyperarousal, yet it is unknown whether a low arousal threshold in OSA leads to insomnia or insomnia manifests with a low arousal threshold, or both. The findings of CBT-I reducing OSA severity require validation. When administered with PAP, understanding whether sedative-hypnotics improve OSA severity, sleep quality, and function in those with COMISA is needed. Importantly, whether such use of hypnotics in COMISA is safe in the long term, especially in vulnerable populations, such as the elderly and those on opioid therapy, should be addressed. Finally, data on the efficacy of other treatment combinations such as CBT-I and oral appliance or upper airway stimulation therapy, can help to inform the treatment approaches for those who cannot tolerate PAP.

CIRCADIAN MISALIGNMENT IN OBSTRUCTIVE SLEEP APNEA

Circadian rhythms are patterns of behavior and physiology that follow a 24-hour cycle under the control of a self-sustaining molecular oscillator (ie, circadian clock) that is entrained by external cues such as the solar light–dark cycle and timing of sleep–wake, eating, and exercise.[79] Circadian misalignment includes complex conditions that are characterized by mismatches in timing among solar day–night, the central clock, peripheral clocks, and behaviors such as sleep or feeding.[79] These misalignment phenomena are common in shift workers, individuals who are forced by social and occupational constraints to adhere to a schedule that does not conform to their natural chronotype (social jet lag) and during travel across time zones.

Epidemiology

To our knowledge, no studies have examined the prevalence of circadian misalignment among individuals with OSA. Recent data do suggest that a bidirectional relationship may exist between circadian misalignment and OSA and contribute to sleep deficiency in individuals who suffer from both.

Pathophysiology

Circadian changes in respiratory control and arousability across the 24-hour period may contribute to sleep apnea pathogenesis. Simulations show that circadian changes can augment sleep-induced periodic breathing, a manifestation of high loop gain, in the evening compared with daytime naps.[80] Using a forced desynchrony protocol, Butler and colleagues identified circadian rhythms in the frequency and duration of respiratory events in NREM sleep. At an average clock time of 22:30 (30° from dim light melatonin onset [DLMO]), the AHI was highest, and the duration of apneas and hypopneas was shortest in contrast to the average lowest AHI and longest event duration at an average clock time of 5:30 (135° from DLMO).[81] These changes may be mediated through an increase in arousal threshold, which increases from the onset to the end of a nocturnal sleep period.[82]

OSA, in contrast, may lead to circadian misalignment. For example, circadian variation of oxygen saturation level that helps to synchronize key components of the molecular clock, including the Period and Clock genes,[83] is likely to be disrupted by hypoxia caused by OSA. Hypoxia lengthens the period and dampens the amplitude of circadian rhythmicity of the mammalian molecular clock and can also induce misalignment between peripheral clocks and between peripheral and central clock as observed in mice.[84,85] Such studies provide glimpses of the relationships between circadian rhythms and OSA, and much remains to be elucidated.

Clinical Characteristics and Consequences of Circadian Misalignment in obstructive sleep apnea

Patients with sleep deficiency owing to circadian misalignment in OSA may present with a delay or advance of their major sleep episode with respect to their desired sleep timing. Extreme difficulty with falling asleep at desired bedtimes and waking up at the required or desired times characterize a delayed rhythm. In contrast, the inability to stay awake during evening hours with an undesirably early wake time characterizes an advanced rhythm. Circadian misalignment can worsen excessive daytime sleepiness and depressive symptoms, common features of OSA that confer a great portion of the disability and lost quality of life associated with the disorder.[86,87] Individuals with delayed phase may also present with insomnia symptoms (an inability to fall asleep at conventional evening times) with implications discussed elsewhere in this article. The assessment of circadian timing is, therefore, needed for the success of OSA treatment.

Diagnosis and Treatment

Melatonin-based measurement of the circadian phase is not practical in a clinical setting. Therefore, actigraphy accompanied by a sleep diary as part of the initial assessment of patients with OSA who present with symptoms suggestive of circadian misalignment is important. These data may help to identify individuals who are most likely to benefit from a chronotherapeutic intervention, in addition to CPAP therapy.

Interventions for circadian rhythm disorders include timing of sleep-wake periods, physical activity/exercise, medications, and light therapy (the most effective circadian cue) to phase shift and/or promote sleep or wakefulness. Short amounts (30–60 minutes) of appropriately timed light therapy effectively realigns individuals' circadian rhythm, with associated improvements in sleep duration, self-reported sleep quality, insomnia symptoms, and fatigue.[88] Light therapy is also effective in acutely decreasing sleepiness, fatigue, and increasing alertness.[89–93] Benefits of exercise are multifold in patients with OSA who also have obesity. Buxton and colleagues[94] showed that acute bouts of high-intensity exercise after the DLMO can significantly delay the circadian phase. In contrast, early evening exercise before the DLMO can lead to phase advancement.[94,95] Baehr and colleagues[96] showed that combining bright light therapy and exercise can potentiate their phase-shifting effects.

Future Directions

Much of this discussion is based on research in patients without OSA. This is in part due to the lack of readily applied circadian biomarkers. For example, 24-hour blood, urinary, or salivary melatonin level measurements are impractical in most settings. Developing noninvasive measures can help to define the type of circadian disturbance among patients with OSA and its impact on treatment efficacy and CPAP adherence. Studies assessing the utility of treating circadian misalignment on patient-centered outcomes, such as daytime sleepiness, insomnia, and quality of life are needed.

PERIODIC LIMB MOVEMENTS OF SLEEP IN OBSTRUCTIVE SLEEP APNEA

PLMS are repetitive movements, typically in the lower extremities involving an extension of the toe and flexion of the ankle, knee, and even the hip. PLMS are often associated with a cortical arousal or an awakening.[97] These events can fragment and reduce the duration of sleep already compromised by OSA. Increasing evidence suggests that PLMS are associated with sympathetic activation, inflammation, endothelial dysfunction, and increased cardiovascular risk in those with OSA[98–103] However, the pathophysiology of the relationship between PLMS and OSA and its clinical implications (independent vs synergistic effects) remain understudied, leaving uncertainty about consequences and management. PLMS often coexist with restless leg syndrome (RLS). Because RLS is more readily identified and treated independently of sleep-disordered breathing, we focus the discussion in this section on sleep deficiency associated with PLMS in OSA.

Epidemiology

The reported prevalence of PLMS in OSA ranges widely (8%–59%) and depends on cut-offs of AHI and PLM index (PLMI) used to define OSA and PLMS.[104–106] Similarly, the frequency of PLMS in OSA is different in sleep clinic compared with community populations. In a diverse sleep clinic cohort of 849 patients with OSA (AHI of ≥10/h) randomized to CPAP or sham (Apnea Positive Pressure Long-term Efficacy Study, APPLES), the prevalence of PLMS (PLMI of ≥15/h) was 15%.[107] The prevalence of PLMS increases markedly with age. Among individuals 65 years or older with OSA (AHI of ≥15/h) in community cohorts, PLMS are observed in 52% of women and 60% of men (unpublished data from Study of Osteoporotic Fractures[108] and Outcomes of Sleep

Disorders in Older Men Study[109] cohorts). PLMI is underestimated in those with severe OSA because PLMS are not scored when adjacent to respiratory events. Studies in sleep clinic populations show that, in individuals with OSA and PLMS, a PLMI of 15 or more per hour persists in 65% to 76% after adequate CPAP titration.[106,110] Notably, in 9% to 22% of patients with OSA free of limb movements, PLMS emerge after CPAP use,[106,110] suggesting that monitoring for PLMS as a potential cause of residual symptoms may be warranted. Risk factors include low iron stores; chronic lung, heart, and kidney disease; neurologic disorders (eg, multiple sclerosis, Parkinson's disease); and psychoactive substances (eg, caffeine, antidepressants, antihistamines).

Pathophysiology

The pathophysiology of PLMS is discussed in detail elsewhere.[111] Whether PLMS contribute to the pathogenesis of OSA, are a consequence of respiratory events, or are independent but co-occurring phenomena remains to be understood. Recent studies suggest that a low arousal threshold, a causative trait of OSA, may be a potential mechanism linking PLMS and OSA, whereby the cortical and subcortical arousability observed in PLMS[112] may manifest as a low arousal threshold. In 1 study, 59% of individuals with OSA-PLMS exhibited a low arousal threshold compared with 20% among those with OSA alone, findings also observed in another, independent cohort.[104] In contrast, other work suggests that PLMS may be a consequence of undertreated OSA, with persistent PLMS heralding ongoing airway obstruction (elimination of hypopneas but persistent flow limitation) that improves at higher CPAP pressures.[101] Other studies, including secondary analyses of the APPLES trial, show that PLMI after titration or 6 months of therapy did not differ between sham or in-laboratory titrated CPAP arms (-4.2 ± 25.4 vs -4.8 ± 25.0; $P = .9$).[107] Similar findings in observational studies showing greater rates of PLMS emergence rather than resolution after CPAP titrations suggest that PLMS and OSA may simply co-occur.[106,110]

Clinical Characteristics and Consequences of Periodic Limb Movements of Sleep in Obstructive Sleep Apnea

PLMS may manifest as repeated awakenings, unrefreshing sleep, reports of movements by a bed partner, as well as fatigue, depression, anxiety, and RLS. Without objective testing (eg, PSG on PAP or at-home PLMS monitors), however, one is unlikely to detect PLMS, as demographics, baseline sleep study data, and clinical history only have weak predictive value for PLMI of 15 or more per hour.[113]

Evidence is accumulating that PLMS are associated with adverse consequences in OSA. These include impaired sleep quality (prolonged latency, lower efficiency, and duration) before OSA treatment (independently of AHI) and on CPAP, identified in the APPLES study.[107] These changes did not translate into increased subjective or objective sleepiness, however. Notably, other daytime symptoms such as insomnia and fatigue associated with PLMS in non-OSA samples[114] (and common in OSA) were not reported in this study. Both PLMS and OSA are associated with cyclical alternating pattern. EEG subtypes related to arousals increased sympathetic activation,[111] and heart rate, and blood pressure elevations.[115,116] PLMS may potentiate each of these when associated with respiratory events.[115,116] Small studies also show that inflammation and arterial stiffness are increased in those with PLMS and OSA versus those with OSA or PLMS alone,[99,100] suggesting synergistic effects.

PLMS are associated with increased risk of prevalent hypertension,[117] atrial fibrillation,[118] and incident CVD, and all-cause mortality, independently of the AHI.[119] Few studies, however, have addressed the potential interactive effects of PLMS and OSA. In a cohort of US veterans, a cluster of patients with predominantly mild OSA an elevated PLMI (median of 64/h) was at an increased risk of incident diabetes (adjusted hazard ratio, 2.26; 95% confidence interval, 1.06–4.83)[98] and CVD or death (adjusted hazard ratio, 2.36; 95% confidence interval, 1.61–3.46) compared with a mild cluster.[103] These findings are yet to be replicated, and the impact of therapy for OSA or PLMS on cardiovascular outcomes is unknown.

Diagnosis and Treatment

Objective monitoring is required to diagnose PLMS, and scoring criteria are defined in the American Academy of Sleep Medicine manual.[120] Other approaches to define PLMS and respiratory-related limb movements that may be more relevant in OSA have been proposed.[121–123] The ICSD defines PLMD as a PLMI of more than 15/h and the lack of another explanation for clinical or functional disturbance being observed. Current guidelines suggest the treatment of PLMS in those with OSA should only be considered if they persist after treatment. This approach, however, is challenged by recent findings that in more than 60% of patients with OSA and PLMS, the movements persist after adequate CPAP titration,[106,110] CPAP does not decrease PLMS severity over 6 months, and that movements are associated with impaired sleep quality.[107] These observations raise the question of whether PLMS and OSA should be treated in parallel, or at least monitoring for PLMS be done in those with impaired sleep quality or residual daytime symptoms after OSA therapy.

Approaches to therapy for PLMS are analogous to those for RLS. Addressing modifiable factors (eg, insufficient sleep opportunity, iron storage deficiency, antihistamine, and caffeine use) is important before instituting pharmacotherapy (eg, alpha-2-delta calcium channel ligands, dopamine agonists). Although it is conceptually appealing to use these therapies to improve sleep quality, to our knowledge, no study has assessed whether treatment of PLMS improves sleep or cardiovascular outcomes in OSA.

Future Directions

The key unknowns in those with OSA and PLMS include establishing causal relationships (or lack thereof) between limb movement and respiratory events. This factor is likely to be addressed by signal analysis studies examining the timing and consequences (eg, autonomics, cortical arousability) of both events and randomized interventional trials targeting PLMS in those with OSA. Moreover, although these data suggest potential synergy between PLMS and OSA in risk of intermediate outcomes and CVD, studies aiming to establish whether the risk in OSA is modified by PLMS and in which groups (eg, elderly, without prevalent CVD) are needed. Finally, assessing whether PLMS specific therapies improve patient-centered outcomes in OSA is a domain ripe for exploration.

SUMMARY

Sleep deficiency in patients with OSA can be captured under the domains of short sleep duration, poor quality sleep, circadian misalignment, and influenced by other sleep-related disorders. Conditions including chronic insomnia, circadian misalignment, and PLMS should be considered when evaluating sleep deficiency in patients with OSA.

CLINICS CARE POINTS

- Patients with OSA should be assessed for symptoms of insomnia.
- Co-occurence of OSA and insomnia (COMISA) is associated with greater daytime impairments, poorer physical and mental health outcomes.
- Treating insomnia concurrently with OSA in patietns with COMISA improves patient-centered outcomes (CPAP adherence and daytime function).
- Clinical trials examining concurrent treatment of periodic limb movements or circadian misalignment in patients with OSA do not exist. However, addressing these sources of sleep deficiency, indepedently of OSA, may help ameliorate sleep deficiency in OSA patients.

DISCLOSURES

Dr Odekolu has nothing to disclose. Dr A. Zinchuk is supported by the Parker B. Francis Fellowship Award and by the National Heart, Lung and Blood Institute's K23 Award 1K23HL159259.

REFERENCES

1. Senaratna CV, Perret JL, Lodge CJ, et al. Prevalence of obstructive sleep apnea in the general population: a systematic review. Sleep Med Rev 2017;34:70–81.
2. AlGhanim N, Comondore VR, Fleetham J, et al. The economic impact of obstructive sleep apnea. Lung 2008;186(1):7–12.
3. Hillman DR, Murphy AS, Antic R, et al. The economic cost of sleep disorders. Sleep 2006;29(3): 299–305.
4. Song SO, He K, Narla RR, et al. Metabolic consequences of obstructive sleep apnea especially Pertaining to diabetes Mellitus and insulin sensitivity. Diabetes Metab J 2019;43(2):144–55.
5. National heart LaBI. Sleep Deprivation and deficiency. NHLBI. 2022. Available at: https://www.nhlbi.nih.gov/health-topics/sleep-deprivation-and-deficiency. Accessed July 31, 2022.
6. Strollo PJ, Rogers RM. Obstructive sleep apnea. N Engl J Med 1996;334(2):99–104.
7. Malhotra A, White DP. Obstructive sleep apnoea. Lancet 2002;360(9328):237–45.
8. Zhang Y, Ren R, Lei F, et al. Worldwide and regional prevalence rates of co-occurrence of insomnia and insomnia symptoms with obstructive sleep apnea: a systematic review and meta-analysis. Sleep Med Rev 2019;45:1–17.
9. Cho YW, Kim KT, Moon HJ, et al. Comorbid insomnia with obstructive sleep apnea: clinical characteristics and risk factors. J Clin Sleep Med 2018;14(3):409–17.
10. Diagnostic and statistical manual of mental disorders: DSM-5. 5th edition. Arlington, VA: American Psychiatric Association; 2013.

11. American Academy of Sleep Medicine. International classification of sleep disorders. 3rd edition. Darien, IL: American Academy of Sleep Medicine; 2014.
12. Saaresranta T, Hedner J, Bonsignore MR, et al. Clinical phenotypes and comorbidity in European sleep apnoea patients. PloS one 2016;11(10): e0163439.
13. Bjorvatn B, Lehmann S, Gulati S, et al. Prevalence of excessive sleepiness is higher whereas insomnia is lower with greater severity of obstructive sleep apnea. Sleep Breath 2015;19(4):1387–93.
14. Luyster FS, Buysse DJ, Strollo PJ Jr. Comorbid insomnia and obstructive sleep apnea: challenges for clinical practice and research. J Clin Sleep Med 2010;6(2):196–204.
15. Rodenbeck A, Hajak G. Neuroendocrine dysregulation in primary insomnia. Revue neurologique 2001;157(11 Pt 2):S57–61.
16. Rodenbeck A, Huether G, Rüther E, et al. Interactions between evening and nocturnal cortisol secretion and sleep parameters in patients with severe chronic primary insomnia. Neurosci Lett 2002; 324(2):159–63.
17. Vgontzas AN, Bixler EO, Lin H-M, et al. Chronic insomnia is associated with nyctohemeral activation of the hypothalamic-pituitary-adrenal axis: clinical implications. J Clin Endocrinol Metab 2001; 86(8):3787–94.
18. Campbell SS, Murphy PJ. Relationships between sleep and body temperature in middle-aged and older subjects. J Am Geriatr Soc 1998;46(4):458–62.
19. Bonnet MH, Arand D. 24-Hour metabolic rate in insomniacs and matched normal sleepers. Sleep 1995;18(7):581–8.
20. Bonnet MH, Arand D. Physiological activation in patients with sleep state misperception. Psychosomatic Med 1997;59(5):533–40.
21. Freedman RR. EEG power spectra in sleep-onset insomnia. Electroencephalography Clin Neurophysiol 1986;63(5):408–13.
22. Perlis ML, Smith MT, Andrews PJ, et al. Beta/Gamma EEG activity in patients with primary and secondary insomnia and good sleeper controls. Sleep 2001;24(1):110–7.
23. Lichstein KL, Wilson NM, Noe SL, et al. Daytime sleepiness in insomnia: behavioral, biological and subjective indices. Sleep 1994;17(8):693–702.
24. Ratnavadivel R, Chau N, Stadler D, et al. Marked reduction in obstructive sleep apnea severity in slow wave sleep. J Clin Sleep Med 2009;5(6):519–24.
25. Younes M, Giannouli E. Mechanism of excessive wake time when associated with obstructive sleep apnea or periodic limb movements. J Clin Sleep Med 2020;16(3):389–99.
26. Younes M. Role of arousals in the pathogenesis of obstructive sleep apnea. Am J Respir Crit Care Med 2004;169(5):623–33.
27. Eckert DJ, Owens RL, Kehlmann GB, et al. Eszopiclone increases the respiratory arousal threshold and lowers the apnoea/hypopnoea index in obstructive sleep apnoea patients with a low arousal threshold. Clin Sci (Lond) 2011;120(12):505–14.
28. Sweetman A, Lack L, McEvoy RD, et al. Cognitive behavioural therapy for insomnia reduces sleep apnoea severity: a randomised controlled trial. ERJ Open Res 2020;6(2).
29. Lack L, Sweetman A. Diagnosis and treatment of insomnia comorbid with obstructive sleep apnea. Sleep Med Clin 2016;11(3):379–88.
30. Mercer JD, Bootzin RR, Lack LC. Insomniacs' perception of wake instead of sleep. Sleep 2002; 25(5):559–66.
31. Björnsdóttir E, Janson C, Gíslason T, et al. Insomnia in untreated sleep apnea patients compared to controls. J Sleep Res 2012;21(2):131–8.
32. Wickwire EM, Smith MT, Birnbaum S, et al. Sleep maintenance insomnia complaints predict poor CPAP adherence: a clinical case series. Sleep Med 2010;11(8):772–6.
33. Bjornsdottir E, Janson C, Sigurdsson JF, et al. Symptoms of insomnia among patients with obstructive sleep apnea before and after two years of positive airway pressure treatment. Sleep 2013; 36(12):1901–9.
34. Chung KF. Insomnia subtypes and their relationships to daytime sleepiness in patients with obstructive sleep apnea. Respiration 2005;72(5):460–5.
35. Wallace DM, Wohlgemuth WK. Predictors of insomnia severity index Profiles in United States veterans with obstructive sleep apnea. J Clin Sleep Med 2019;15(12):1827–37.
36. Krakow B, Melendrez D, Ferreira E, et al. Prevalence of insomnia symptoms in patients with sleep-disordered breathing. Chest 2001;120(6): 1923–9.
37. Gupta MA, Knapp K. Cardiovascular and psychiatric Morbidity in obstructive sleep apnea (OSA) with insomnia (sleep apnea Plus) versus obstructive sleep apnea without insomnia: a case-control study from a Nationally Representative US sample. PLOS ONE 2014;9(3):e90021.
38. Machado MA, de Carvalho LB, Juliano ML, et al. Clinical co-morbidities in obstructive sleep apnea syndrome treated with mandibular repositioning appliance. Respir Med 2006;100(6):988–95.
39. Peppard PE, Young T, Palta M, et al. Prospective study of the association between sleep-disordered breathing and hypertension. N Engl J Med 2000;342(19):1378–84.
40. Shahar E, Whitney CW, REdline S, et al. Sleep-disordered breathing and cardiovascular disease: cross-sectional results of the Sleep Heart Health Study. Am J Respir Crit Care Med 2001;163(1): 19–25.

41. Arzt M, Young T, Finn L, et al. Association of sleep-disordered breathing and the occurrence of stroke. Am J Respir Crit Care Med 2005;172(11):1447–51.
42. Phillips B, Mannino DM. Do insomnia complaints cause hypertension or cardiovascular disease? J Clin Sleep Med 2007;3(5):489–94.
43. Lanfranchi PA, Pennestri M-H, Fradette L, et al. Nighttime blood pressure in normotensive subjects with chronic insomnia: implications for cardiovascular risk. Sleep 2009;32(6):760–6.
44. Vgontzas AN, Liao D, Bixler EO, et al. Insomnia with objective short sleep duration is associated with a high risk for hypertension. Sleep 2009; 32(4):491–7.
45. Vgontzas AN, Liao D, Pejovic S, et al. Insomnia with objective short sleep duration is associated with type 2 diabetes: a population-based study. Diabetes care 2009;32(11):1980–5.
46. Schwartz S, Anderson WM, Cole SR, et al. Insomnia and heart disease: a review of epidemiologic studies. J psychosomatic Res 1999;47(4): 313–33.
47. Somers VK, Javaheri S. Cardiovascular effects of sleep-related breathing disorders. Sleep Breathing Disord E-Book. 2016;270.
48. Javaheri S, Barbe F, Campos-Rodriguez F, et al. Sleep apnea: types, mechanisms, and clinical cardiovascular consequences. J Am Coll Cardiol 2017;69(7):841–58.
49. Kholdani C, Fares WH, Mohsenin V. Pulmonary hypertension in obstructive sleep apnea: is it clinically significant? A critical analysis of the association and pathophysiology. Pulm Circ 2015;5(2):220–7.
50. Le-Ha C, Herbison CE, Beilin LJ, et al. Hypothalamic-pituitary-adrenal axis activity under resting conditions and cardiovascular risk factors in adolescents. Psychoneuroendocrinology 2016;66:118–24.
51. Rosmond R, Bjorntorp P. The hypothalamic-pituitary-adrenal axis activity as a predictor of cardiovascular disease, type 2 diabetes and stroke. J Intern Med 2000;247(2):188–97.
52. Javaheri S, Redline S. Insomnia and risk of cardiovascular disease. Chest 2017;152(2):435–44.
53. Parthasarathy S, Vasquez MM, Halonen M, et al. Persistent insomnia is associated with mortality risk. Am J Med 2015;128(3):268–275 e262.
54. Irwin MR. Why sleep is important for health: a psychoneuroimmunology perspective. Annu Rev Psychol 2015;66:143–72.
55. King CR, Knutson KL, Rathouz PJ, et al. Short sleep duration and incident coronary artery calcification. JAMA 2008;300(24):2859–66.
56. Meier-Ewert HK, Ridker PM, Rifai N, et al. Effect of sleep loss on C-reactive protein, an inflammatory marker of cardiovascular risk. J Am Coll Cardiol 2004;43(4):678–83.
57. Schutte-Rodin S, Broch L, Buysse D, et al. Clinical guideline for the evaluation and management of chronic insomnia in adults. J Clin Sleep Med 2008;04(05):487–504.
58. Clinical guideline for the evaluation, management and long-term care of obstructive sleep apnea in adults. J Clin Sleep Med 2009;05(03):263–76.
59. Epstein LJ, Kristo D, Strollo P Jr, et al. Adult Obstructive Sleep Apnea Task Force of the American Academy of Sleep Medicine. Clinical guideline for the evaluation, management and long-term care of obstructive sleep apnea in adults. J Clin Sleep Med 2009;5(3):263–76.
60. Kushida CA, Chediak A, Berry RB, et al. Clinical guidelines for the manual titration of positive airway pressure in patients with obstructive sleep apnea. J Clin Sleep Med 2008;4(2):157–71.
61. Sawyer AM, Gooneratne NS, Marcus CL, et al. A systematic review of CPAP adherence across age groups: clinical and empiric insights for developing CPAP adherence interventions. Sleep Med Rev 2011;15(6):343–56.
62. Rotenberg BW, Murariu D, Pang KP. Trends in CPAP adherence over twenty years of data collection: a flattened curve. J Otolaryngology-Head Neck Surg 2016;45(1):1–9.
63. Barthlen GM, Lange DJ. Unexpectedly severe sleep and respiratory pathology in patients with amyotrophic lateral sclerosis. Eur J Neurol 2000; 7(3):299–302.
64. Smith S, Dunn N, Douglas J, et al. Sleep onset insomnia is associated with reduced adherence to CPAP therapy. Sleep Biol Rhythms 2009;7:A74.
65. Suraiya S, Lavie P. P394 Sleep onset insomnia in sleep apnea patients: influence on acceptance of nCPAP treatment. Sleep Med 2006;(7):S85.
66. Qaseem A, Kansagara D, Forciea MA, et al. Management of chronic insomnia disorder in adults: a clinical practice guideline from the American College of physicians. Ann Intern Med 2016;165(2): 125–33.
67. Sweetman A, Lack L, Lambert S, et al. Does comorbid obstructive sleep apnea impair the effectiveness of cognitive and behavioral therapy for insomnia? Sleep Med 2017;39:38–46.
68. Alessi CA, Fung CH, Dzierzewski JM, et al. Randomized controlled trial of an integrated approach to treating insomnia and improving the use of positive airway pressure therapy in veterans with comorbid insomnia disorder and obstructive sleep apnea. Sleep 2021;44(4).
69. Bjorvatn B, Berge T, Lehmann S, et al. No effect of a self-help book for insomnia in patients with obstructive sleep apnea and comorbid chronic insomnia - a randomized controlled trial. Front Psychol 2018;9:2413.

70. Sweetman A, Lack L, Catcheside PG, et al. Cognitive and behavioral therapy for insomnia increases the use of continuous positive airway pressure therapy in obstructive sleep apnea participants with comorbid insomnia: a randomized clinical trial. Sleep 2019;42(12).
71. Sweetman A, McEvoy R, Smith S, et al. The effect of cognitive and behavioral therapy for insomnia on week-to-week changes in sleepiness and sleep parameters in insomnia patients with comorbid moderate and severe sleep apnea: a randomized controlled trial. Sleep 2020;43(7): zsaa002.
72. Ong JC, Crawford MR, Dawson SC, et al. A randomized controlled trial of CBT-I and PAP for obstructive sleep apnea and comorbid insomnia: main outcomes from the MATRICS study. Sleep 2020;43(9).
73. Krakow B, Ulibarri VA, Romero E. Persistent insomnia in chronic hypnotic users presenting to a sleep medical center: a retrospective chart review of 137 consecutive patients. J nervous Ment Dis 2010;198(10):734–41.
74. Carberry JC, Fisher LP, Grunstein RR, et al. Role of common hypnotics on the phenotypic causes of obstructive sleep apnoea: paradoxical effects of zolpidem. Eur Respir J 2017;50(6).
75. Rosenberg R, Roach JM, Scharf M, et al. A pilot study evaluating acute use of eszopiclone in patients with mild to moderate obstructive sleep apnea syndrome. Sleep Med 2007;8(5):464–70.
76. Lettieri CJ, Quast TN, Eliasson AH, et al. Eszopiclone improves overnight polysomnography and continuous positive airway pressure titration: a prospective, randomized, placebo-controlled trial. Sleep 2008;31(9):1310–6.
77. Lettieri CJ, Shah AA, Holley AB, et al. Effects of a short course of eszopiclone on continuous positive airway pressure adherence: a randomized trial. Ann Intern Med 2009;151(10):696–702.
78. Schmickl CN, Lettieri CJ, Orr JE, et al. The arousal threshold as a Drug Target to improve continuous positive airway pressure adherence: secondary analysis of a randomized trial. Am J Respir Crit Care Med 2020;202(11):1592–5.
79. Baron KG, Reid KJ. Circadian misalignment and health. Int Rev Psychiatry 2014;26(2):139–54.
80. Stephenson R. A theoretical study of the effect of circadian rhythms on sleep-induced periodic breathing and apnoea. Respir Physiol Neurobiol 2004;139(3):303–19.
81. Butler MP, Smales C, Wu H, et al. The circadian system contributes to apnea lengthening across the night in obstructive sleep apnea. Sleep 2015; 38(11):1793–801.
82. Sforza E, Krieger J, Petiau C. Nocturnal evolution of respiratory effort in obstructive sleep apnoea syndrome: influence on arousal threshold. Eur Respir J 1998;12(6):1257–63.
83. Adamovich Y, Ladeuix B, Golik M, et al. Rhythmic oxygen levels reset circadian clocks through HIF1α. Cell Metab 2017;25(1):93–101.
84. Wu Y, Tang D, Liu N, et al. Reciprocal regulation between the circadian clock and hypoxia signaling at the genome level in mammals. Cell Metab 2017; 25(1):73–85.
85. Manella G, Aviram R, Bolshette N, et al. Hypoxia induces a time-and tissue-specific response that elicits intertissue circadian clock misalignment. Proc Natl Acad Sci 2020;117(1):779–86.
86. Smagula SF, Ancoli-Israel S, Blackwell T, et al. Circadian rest–activity rhythms predict future increases in depressive symptoms among community-dwelling older men. Am J Geriatr Psychiatry 2015;23(5):495–505.
87. Maglione JE, Ancoli-Israel S, Peters KW, et al. Depressive symptoms and circadian activity rhythm disturbances in community-dwelling older women. Am J Geriatr Psychiatry 2014;22(4): 349–61.
88. Van Maanen A, Meijer AM, van der Heijden KB, et al. The effects of light therapy on sleep problems: a systematic review and meta-analysis. Sleep Med Rev 2016;29:52–62.
89. Phipps-Nelson J, Redman JR, Dijk D-J, et al. Daytime exposure to bright light, as compared to dim light, decreases sleepiness and improves psychomotor vigilance performance. Sleep 2003;26(6): 695–700.
90. Viola AU, James LM, Schlangen LJ, et al. Blue-enriched white light in the workplace improves self-reported alertness, performance and sleep quality. Scand J work, Environ Health 2008;297–306.
91. Lockley SW, Evans EE, Scheer FA, et al. Short-wavelength sensitivity for the direct effects of light on alertness, vigilance, and the waking electroencephalogram in humans. Sleep 2006;29(2):161–8.
92. Smolders KC, De Kort YA, Cluitmans P. A higher illuminance induces alertness even during office hours: findings on subjective measures, task performance and heart rate measures. Physiol Behav 2012;107(1):7–16.
93. Beaven CM, Ekström J. A comparison of blue light and caffeine effects on cognitive function and alertness in humans. PloS one 2013;8(10):e76707.
94. Buxton OM, Lee CW, L'Hermite-Balériaux M, et al. Exercise elicits phase shifts and acute alterations of melatonin that vary with circadian phase. Am J Physiology-Regulatory, Integr Comp Physiol 2003; 284(3):R714–24.
95. Buxton OM, L'Hermite-Balériaux M, Hirschfeld U, et al. Acute and delayed effects of exercise on human melatonin secretion. J Biol rhythms 1997; 12(6):568–74.

96. Baehr EK, Eastman CI, Revelle W, et al. Circadian phase-shifting effects of nocturnal exercise in older compared with young adults. Am J Physiology-Regulatory, Integr Comp Physiol 2003;284(6): R1542–50.
97. American Academy of Sleep M. International classification of sleep disorders. 3rd edition. Darien, IL: Diagnostic and Coding Manual; 2014.
98. Ding Q, Qin L, Wojeck B, et al. Polysomnographic phenotypes of obstructive sleep apnea and incident type 2 diabetes: results from the DREAM study. Ann Am Thorac Soc 2021;18(12):2067–78.
99. Drakatos P, Higgins S, Pengo MF, et al. Derived arterial stiffness is increased in patients with obstructive sleep apnea and periodic limb movements during sleep. J Clin Sleep Med 2016;12(2): 195–202.
100. Murase K, Hitomi T, Hamada S, et al. The additive impact of periodic limb movements during sleep on inflammation in patients with obstructive sleep apnea. Ann Am Thorac Soc 2014;11(3):375–82.
101. Seo WH, Guilleminault C. Periodic leg movement, nasal CPAP, and expiratory muscles. Chest 2012; 142(1):111–8.
102. Wu MN, Lai CL, Liu CK, et al. Basal sympathetic predominance in periodic limb movements in sleep after continuous positive airway pressure. Sleep Breath 2018;22(4):1005–12.
103. Zinchuk AV, Jeon S, Koo BB, et al. Polysomnographic phenotypes and their cardiovascular implications in obstructive sleep apnoea. Thorax 2018; 73(5):472–80.
104. Wang Q, Li Y, Li J, et al. Low arousal threshold: a potential Bridge between OSA and periodic limb movements of sleep. Nat Sci Sleep 2021;13: 229–38.
105. Lee SA, Kim SJ, Lee SY, et al. Clinical characteristics of periodic limb movements during sleep categorized by continuous positive airway pressure titration polysomnography in patients with obstructive sleep apnea. Sleep Breath 2022;26(1):251–7.
106. Aritake-Okada S, Namba K, Hidano N, et al. Change in frequency of periodic limb movements during sleep with usage of continuous positive airway pressure in obstructive sleep apnea syndrome. J Neurol Sci 2012;317(1–2):13–6.
107. Budhiraja R, Javaheri S, Pavlova MK, et al. Prevalence and correlates of periodic limb movements in OSA and the effect of CPAP therapy. Neurology 2020;94(17):e1820–7.
108. Spira AP, Blackwell T, Stone KL, et al. Sleep-disordered breathing and cognition in older women. J Am Geriatr Soc 2008;56(1):45–50.
109. Zhao YY, Blackwell T, Ensrud KE, et al. Sleep apnea and obstructive airway disease in older men: outcomes of sleep disorders in older men study. Sleep 2016;39(7):1343–51.
110. Ren R, Huang G, Zhang J, et al. Age and severity matched comparison of gender differences in the prevalence of periodic limb movements during sleep in patients with obstructive sleep apnea. Sleep Breath 2016;20(2):821–7.
111. Ferri R, Koo BB, Picchietti DL, et al. Periodic leg movements during sleep: phenotype, neurophysiology, and clinical significance. Sleep Med 2017;31:29–38.
112. Figorilli M, Puligheddu M, Congiu P, et al. The clinical importance of periodic leg movements in sleep. Curr Treat Options Neurol 2017;19(3):10.
113. Moro M, Goparaju B, Castillo J, et al. Periodic limb movements of sleep: empirical and theoretical evidence supporting objective at-home monitoring. Nat Sci Sleep 2016;8:277–89.
114. Hardy De Buisseret FX, Mairesse O, Newell J, et al. While Isolated periodic limb movement disorder significantly impacts sleep depth and efficiency, Co-morbid restless leg syndrome mainly Exacerbates perceived sleep quality. Eur Neurol 2017; 77(5–6):272–80.
115. Yang CK, Jordan AS, White DP, et al. Heart rate response to respiratory events with or without leg movements. Sleep 2006;29(4):553–6.
116. Li X, Covassin N, Zhou J, et al. Interaction effect of obstructive sleep apnea and periodic limb movements during sleep on heart rate variability. J Sleep Res 2019;28(6):e12861.
117. Dean DA, Wang R, Jacobs DR, et al. A systematic assessment of the association of polysomnographic indices with blood pressure: the Multi-Ethnic Study of Atherosclerosis (MESA). Sleep 2015;38(4):587–96.
118. Xie J, Chahal CAA, Covassin N, et al. Periodic limb movements of sleep are associated with an increased prevalence of atrial fibrillation in patients with mild sleep-disordered breathing. Int J Cardiol 2017;241:200–4.
119. Kendzerska T, Kamra M, Murray BJ, et al. Incident cardiovascular events and death in individuals with restless legs syndrome or periodic limb movements in sleep: a systematic review. Sleep 2017; 40(3).
120. Berry RBB R, Gamaldo CE, Harding SM, et al. The AASM manual for the scoring of sleep and associated events: rules terminology and technical pecifications, Version 2.1. Darien, IL: American Academy of Sleep Medicine; 2014. www.aasmnet.org.
121. Ferri R, Fulda S, Allen RP, et al. World Association of Sleep Medicine (WASM) 2016 standards for recording and scoring leg movements in polysomnograms developed by a joint task force from the International and the European Restless Legs Syndrome Study Groups (IRLSSG and EURLSSG). Sleep Med 2016;26:86–95.
122. Aritake S, Blackwell T, Peters KW, et al. Prevalence and associations of respiratory-related leg

movements: the MrOS sleep study. Sleep Med 2015;16(10):1236–44.

123. Manconi M, Zavalko I, Bassetti CL, et al. Respiratory-related leg movements and their relationship with periodic leg movements during sleep. Sleep 2014;37(3):497–504.
124. Nguyen XL, Chaskalovic J, Rakotonanahary D, et al. Insomnia symptoms and CPAP compliance in OSAS patients: a descriptive study using Data Mining methods. Sleep Med 2010;11(8): 777–84.
125. Nguyên XL, Rakotonanahary D, Chaskalovic J, et al. Insomnia related to sleep apnoea: effect of long-term auto-adjusting positive airway pressure treatment. Eur Respir J 2013;41(3):593–600.
126. Pieh C, Bach M, Popp R, et al. Insomnia symptoms influence CPAP compliance. Sleep Breath 2013; 17(1):99–104.
127. Wallace DM, Shafazand S, Aloia MS, et al. The association of age, insomnia, and self-efficacy with continuous positive airway pressure adherence in black, white, and Hispanic U.S. Veterans. J Clin Sleep Med 2013;9(9):885–95.
128. Glidewell RN, Renn BN, Roby E, et al. Predictors and patterns of insomnia symptoms in OSA before and after PAP therapy. Sleep Med 2014;15(8): 899–905.
129. Wohlgemuth WK, Chirinos DA, Domingo S, et al. Attempters, adherers, and non-adherers: latent profile analysis of CPAP use with correlates. Sleep Med 2015;16(3):336–42.
130. Eysteinsdottir B, Gislason T, Pack AI, et al. Insomnia complaints in lean patients with obstructive sleep apnea negatively affect positive airway pressure treatment adherence. J Sleep Res 2017; 26(2):159–65.
131. Fung CH, Martin JL, Josephson K, et al. Efficacy of cognitive behavioral therapy for insomnia in older adults with Occult sleep-disordered breathing. Psychosom Med 2016;78(5):629–39.
132. Krakow B, McIver ND, Ulibarri VA, et al. Retrospective, nonrandomized controlled study on autoadjusting, dual-pressure positive airway pressure therapy for a consecutive series of complex insomnia disorder patients. Nat Sci Sleep 2017;9: 81–95.

9780323897242